RESPIRATORY TECHNOLOGY
PROCEDURE AND
EQUIPMENT MANUAL

RESPIRATORY TECHNOLOGY PROCEDURE AND EQUIPMENT MANUAL

DORIS L. HUNSINGER, R.N., B.S.N.

Graduate Deaconess Hospital School of Nursing
Nursing Care Coordinator, Respiratory Therapy Department, Erie County Medical
  Center, Buffalo, New York
Clinical Instructor of Respiratory Therapy Technology Course at Erie Community
  College
Clinical Instructor, School of Medical Technology, State University of New York at
  Buffalo

KARL J. LISNERSKI, C.R.T.T.

Chief Respiratory Therapist, Millard Fillmore Hospital, Buffalo, New York

JEROME J. MAURIZI, B.S., M.D., F.C.C.P.

Associate Clinical Professor of Medicine, State University of New York at Buffalo
Adjunct Clinical Professor of Respiratory Technology, Erie Community College,
  Williamsville, New York
Director of Respiratory Therapy, Deaconess Hospital, Buffalo, New York

MARY L. PHILLIPS, R.N., B.S.N., C.R.T.T.

Graduate Edward J. Meyer Memorial Hospital School of Nursing
Graduate School of Nursing D'Youville College
Team Leader, Respiratory Therapy Department, Erie County Medical Center, Buffalo,
  New York
Clinical Instructor of Respiratory Therapy Course at Erie Community College

Reston Publishing Company, Inc., Reston, Virginia
A Prentice-Hall Company

Library of Congress Cataloging in Publication Data
Main entry under title:

Respiratory technology procedure and equipment
    manual.

    Bibliography: p. 527
    Includes index.
    1. Inhalation therapy—Handbooks, manuals, etc.
I. Hunsinger, Doris L.   [DNLM: 1. Respiratory
therapy—Methods.   2. Respirators.   WF26 R434]
RM161.R46   615.8′36   80-244
ISBN 0-8359-6670-4

© **1980 by**
Reston Publishing Company, Inc.
A Prentice-Hall Company
Reston, Virginia

10   9   8   7   6   5   4   3   2   1

Printed in the United States of America

CONTENTS

Unit 7   RESPIRATORY THERAPY DEPARTMENT RECORDS   407

Unit 8   INFECTION CONTROL   421

Unit 9   TRACHEOSTOMY AND ENDOTRACHEAL TUBES AND SUCTIONING   441

PREFACE

The authors' intention in preparing this manual has been to make an accurate, up-to-date presentation of those procedures pertinent to a respiratory therapy department.

We wish to thank Diane Lisnerski for her assistance in the preparation of this manual.

We dedicate this manual to the respiratory patient—our goal is the continuing improvement of his care.

Doris L. Hunsinger, R.N., B.S.N.
Karl J. Lisnerski, C.R.T.T.
Jerome J. Maurizi, M.D.
Mary L. Phillips, R.N., B.S.N., C.R.T.T.

RESPIRATORY TECHNOLOGY PROCEDURE AND EQUIPMENT MANUAL

UNIT 1

SCIENCES

This unit is intended as a brief review of those sciences most closely related to respiratory therapy. It is expected that the student will refer to texts which deal exclusively with anatomy, physiology, chemistry, physics, microbiology, and fluid and electrolyte balance.

ANATOMY AND PHYSIOLOGY OF THE RESPIRATORY SYSTEM

Knowledge of the anatomy and physiology of the respiratory system is necessary for the efficient and successful respiratory therapist, to be able to understand and apply scientific principles. You must be able to practice good respiratory care using technical skills. Knowledge and technical skills are not difficult to acquire; however, how you apply them to your patient makes the difference between a mediocre respiratory therapist and an excellent one.

A therapist who can respond intelligently to the patient's questions is fulfilling one of the patient's basic needs—good communication. In addition, it is frequently the respiratory therapist who is the individual responsible for providing patient education. You must make certain that your instructions and comments to the patient are factual, realistic, and current. Encourage the patient to ask questions and be prepared for discussion with him and his family, as well as with the physician and nurses who also participate in his care.

The patient with chronic obstructive pulmonary disease may want to know why you place him in certain positions when performing chest physical therapy. Knowledge of the bronchopulmonary segments aids you in responding to him, as well as improves your care of him. When a patient becomes disoriented and confused, his family becomes upset and anxious. You have the opportunity to talk with the family regarding the carbon dioxide partial pressure in his blood, and this may help them to understand his condition, and perhaps alleviate some of their fears, as this may only be a transient condition.

The patient who is having difficulty raising sputum may benefit from an explanation of the possible loss of the ciliary mechanism. An explanation may help him to understand and result in his following your coughing technique directions more effectively. The respiratory therapist's expertise often aids chronic chest patients during both acute and chronic episodes.

Anatomy of the Respiratory System

The respiratory system is made up of the nose, nasal passages, nasopharynx, larynx, trachea, bronchi and the lungs.

I. The *nose* is a special organ of the sense of smell, and also serves as a passageway for air going to and from the lungs. It filters, warms, and moistens the entering air and also helps in phonation. Under normal conditions breathing should take place through the nose. The nose consists of two parts:

A. The *external nose*, which is composed of a triangular framework of bone and cartilage, covered by skin and lined by mucous membrane. On its under surface are two oval openings, the nostrils (anterior nares), which are the external openings into the nasal cavities. The internal edges of the nose are covered with stiff hairs that stop or inhibit foreign substances from being inhaled.

B. The *nasal cavities* are two irregular, pear-shaped cavities, separated from each other by a partition, or septum. The septum is usually bent more to one side than the other, a condition to be remembered in giving nasal treatment. The nasal cavities communicate with the air in front by the anterior nares, and behind they open into the nasopharynx by the two posterior nares.

II. The *pharynx* is the musculomembranous sac between the mouth and nares and the esophagus. It is continuous below with the esophagus, and above it communicates with the larynx, mouth, nasal passages, and eustachian tubes. The part above the level of the soft palate is the *nasopharynx*, connecting the posterior nares and the eustachian tube. The lower portion consists of two sections, the *oropharynx*, which lies between the soft palate and the upper edge of the epiglottis, and the *hypopharynx*, which lies below the upper edge of the epiglottis and opens into the larynx and esophagus. The pharynx is about 4½ inches long and is considered to be a part of the digestive and respiratory systems.

III.   The *larynx*, or *organ of voice*, is placed in the upper and front part of the neck between the base of the tongue and the trachea. It forms the lower part of the anterior wall of the pharynx, and is covered behind by the mucous lining of that cavity; on either side of it lie the large vessels of the neck. The larynx is broad above, where it presents the form of a triangular box flattened behind and at the sides, and bounded in front by a prominent vertical ridge. Below it is narrow and cylindrical. It is composed of cartilages, which are connected together by ligaments and moved by various muscles. It is lined by mucous membrane continuous above with that of the pharynx and below with that of the trachea.

The *cavity of the larynx* is divided into *two parts* by two folds of mucous membrane stretching from front to back, but not quite meeting in the midline. As such, they produce an elongated fissure called the *glottis*, which is the narrowest section of the air passages. The glottis is protected by a lid of fibrocartilage called the *epiglottis*. The vocal folds, surrounded in mucous membrane at the edges of the slit, are fibrous and elastic ligaments that strengthen the edges of the glottis and give them elasticity. These ligaments, covered with mucous membrane, are firmly attached at both ends to the cartilages of the larynx and are called the *inferior* or *true vocal folds*, because they function in speaking and sound. Above the vocal folds are two ventricular folds, which do not function in the production of the voice. They help keep the true vocal folds moist while holding the breath, and protect the larynx during the swallowing of food.

The *glottis* varies in shape and size according to the action of muscles upon the laryngeal walls. When the larynx is at rest during quiet breathing, the glottis is V-shaped. During a deep inspiration it becomes almost round; during the production of a high note the edges of the folds approximate so closely as to leave scarcely any opening at all.

See Figures 1-1 through 1-4.

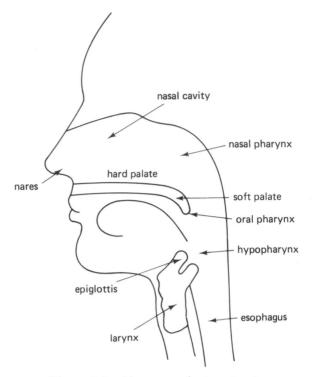

Figure 1-1. Upper respiratory tract.

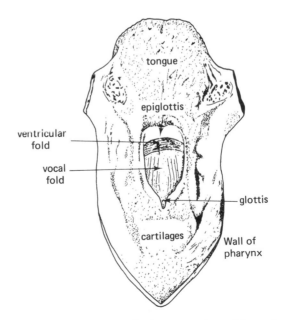

Figure 1-2. Entrance to the larynx, viewed from behind.

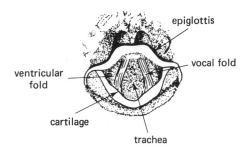

epiglottis

vocal fold

ventricular
fold

cartilage

trachea

Figure 1-3.   Laryngoscopic view of interior of larynx.

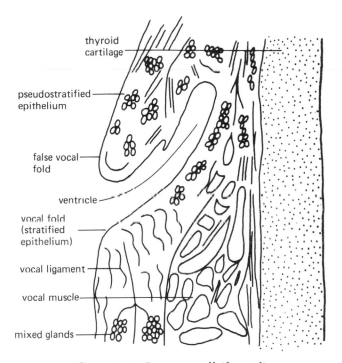

thyroid
cartilage

pseudostratified
epithelium

false vocal
fold

ventricle

vocal fold
(stratified
epithelium)

vocal ligament

vocal muscle

mixed glands

Figure 1-4.   Larynx wall (frontal).

IV.   The *trachea* (windpipe) is a membranous and cartilaginous
tube, almost cylindrical in shape, about 11 centimeters (cm) or
$4\frac{1}{2}$ in. in length and about 2 to 2.5 cm (1 in.) in diameter, always
larger in males than in females. A child's trachea is smaller,
deeper, and moves easier than the adult's. The trachea is anterior to the esophagus and extends from the larynx at the level
of the sixth cervical vertebra to the level of the upper border of
the fifth thoracic vertebra, where it divides into the two

bronchi, one for each lung. The walls of the trachea are made stronger and more rigid by rings of cartilage embedded in the fibrous tissue. There are approximately 16 to 20 cartilages. These rings are C-shaped and incomplete behind, the cartilaginous ring being completed by bands of plain muscular tissue where the trachea is flattened and comes in contact with the esophagus. It is lined with mucous membrane and has a ciliated epithelium upon its inner surface. The mucous membrane, which extends into the bronchial tubes, keeps the inner surface of the air passages free from dust particles and foreign substances. Mucus engulfs particles inhaled, and the continual movement of the cilia sweeps any dust-laden mucus upward into the pharynx. The point at which the trachea bifurcates, forming the right and left main stem bronchi, is known as the *carina*.

V.   The two *bronchi* into which the trachea divides differ slightly, the right bronchus being shorter, wider, and more vertical in direction than the left. They enter the right and left lung, respectively, and then break up into a great number of smaller branches, which are called the *bronchial tubes* and *bronchioles*. The two bronchi are similar to the trachea in structure; but as the bronchial tubes divide and subdivide, their walls become thinner, the plates of cartilage cease, fibrous tissue disappears, and the smallest tubes are made up of only a thin layer of muscular and elastic tissue lined by ciliated epithelium. Each bronchiole terminates in an elongated saccule called the *atrium*. Each atrium has on all parts of its surface small, irregular projections known as *alveoli* or *air cells* or *air sacs*. See Figures 1-5 through 1-9.

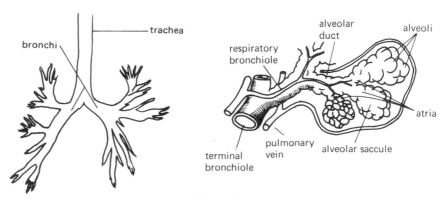

Figure 1-5.

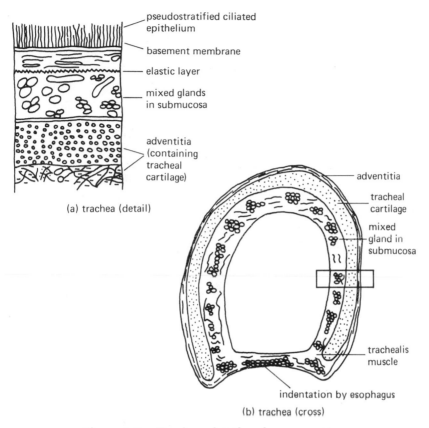

Figure 1-6. Trachea, detail and cross section.

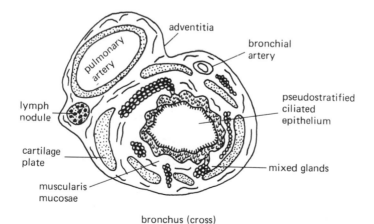

Figure 1-7. Bronchus, cross section.

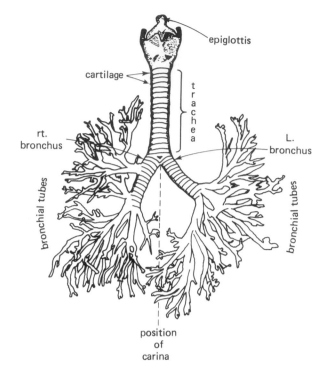

Figure 1-8. Front view of cartilages of trachea and bronchi.

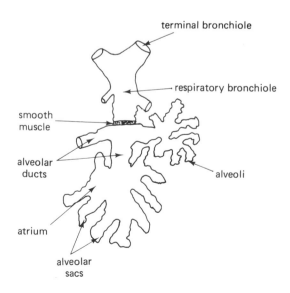

Figure 1-9. Pulmonary, or lung, unit.

VI. The *lungs* are the chief organs of respiration. They are a pair of cone-shaped organs situated one on each side of the chest. The lungs are separated from each other by the heart and great vessels and the other contents of the mediastinum. They consist of a porous, spongy, elastic material that floats in water and crepitates when handled owing to air in the alveoli. The outer surfaces of each lung are rounded outward to accommodate the chest. The bases are somewhat elevated to adjust to the position of the diaphragm. The rounded upper portion of each lung, known as the *apices*, extend upward about 1 to $1\frac{1}{2}$ in. above the level of the sternal end of the first rib. The color of the lungs at birth is pinkish-white. As life progresses the color becomes a dark gray with blotchy patches. These mottled or blotchy patches can become black in later years. The lungs are connected to the heart and trachea via the pulmonary artery, pulmonary vein, bronchial arteries and veins, the bronchus, nerves, lymphatics, and tissue, which are covered by the pleura. These constitute the *roots* of the lungs. The depression on the inner surface of the lung where the bronchus, blood vessels, nerves, etc., enter is called the *hilus*. Below and in front of this area is a deep cavity called the *cardiac impression*, where the heart is situated. It is larger and deeper in the left lung than the right lung, as the heart projects farther to the left side. Both lungs are surrounded by a serous sac, the pleura. One layer of the pleura is closely adhered to the walls of the chest and diaphragm, and is known as the *parietal pleura* (see Figure 1-10). The other layer closely covers the lung and is known as the *visceral* or *pulmonary pleura*. These two layers of the pleural

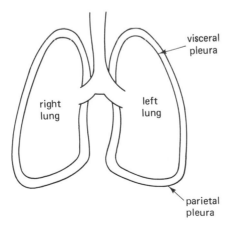

Figure 1-10. Diagram showing parietal and visceral pleura.

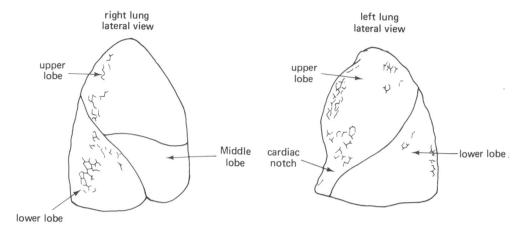

Figure 1-11.   Lobes of the lung.

sacs, moistened by serum, are normally in close contact. Therefore, the pleural cavity is a potential rather than an actual
cavity. The visceral pleura and the parietal pleura move easily
on one another with each respiration.

Characteristics of the Right Lung   (See Figure 1-11.)

Larger and broader than the left lung because the heart projects
farther to the left side.

Usually weighs more than the left lung.

About 1 in. shorter than the left lung because the diaphragm
rises higher on the right side to accommodate the liver.

TABLE 1-1   Bronchopulmonary Segments of the Lung

Right Lung		Left Lung	
Lobes	Segments	Lobes	Segments
Upper	apical posterior anterior	Upper	Superior division — apical posterior anterior
Middle	lateral medial	Inferior (lingular) division	superior inferior
Lower	superior medial basal anterior basal lateral basal posterior basal	Lower	superior anterior-medial basal lateral basal posterior basal

Total capacity is greater than the left lung.

Divided by fissures into three lobes: upper, middle, and lower.

Characteristics of the Left Lung   (See Figure 1-11.)

Smaller than the right lung.

Narrower than the right lung.

Longer than the right lung.

Divided into two lobes: upper and lower.

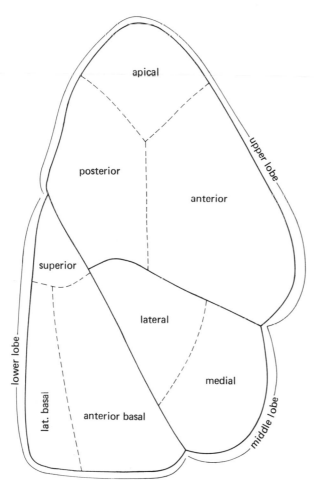

Figure 1-12.   Bronchopulmonary segments: right lung, lateral view.

Each lobe of the lungs is made up of many lobules. A bronchiole enters each lobule and ends in an atrium. The atrium represents a number of air cells/air sacs or alveoli, of which there are about 300 million in the lungs. A network of capillaries surrounds the alveoli, and here the exchange of the important gases, oxygen and carbon dioxide, takes place.

The Bronchopulmonary Segments. These segments represent the portion of a lung that is supplied by a single bronchus. They are bound together by connective tissue, and it is possible to dissect

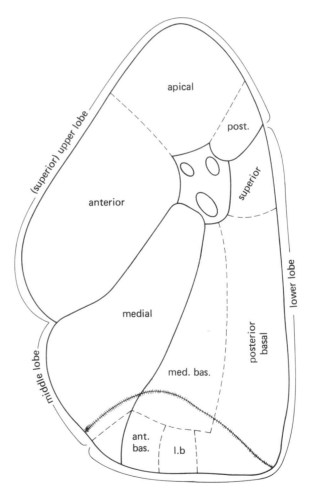

Figure 1-13. Bronchopulmonary segments: right lung, medial and basal view.

them by following along the connective tissue. The right lung has ten bronchopulmonary segments, the left lung, eight, as listed in Table 1-1. See also Figures 1-12 through 1-15.

Cells found in the Respiratory System

1. Squamous
2. Columnar
3. Goblet

See Figure 1-16.

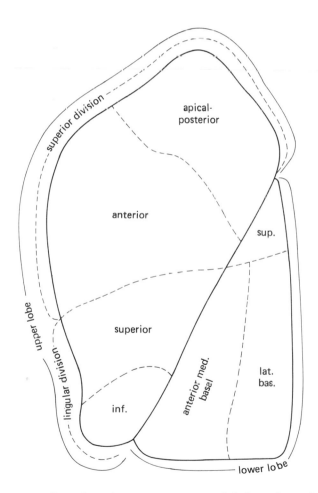

Figure 1-14.   Bronchopulmonary segments: left lung, lateral view.

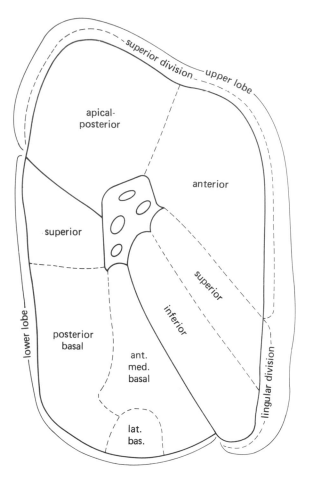

Figure 1-15. Bronchopulmonary segments: left lung, medial and basal view.

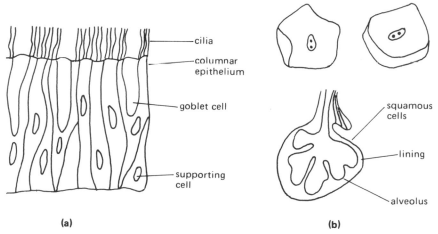

Figure 1-16. Cells found in the respiratory system.

Physiology of Respiration

The primary function of respiration is to supply oxygen to the blood and to remove carbon dioxide. Both the heart and the lungs must work together to transport these gases between atmospheric air and all tissue cells.

Breathing, or *ventilation*, is the movement of air into and out of the lungs. This occurs in the cyclic process of inspiration and expiration. Several muscles of respiration and changes in the shape of the thoracic cage are necessary to accomplish both inspiration and expiration.

The major muscles of inspiration are as follows:

1. Diaphragm
2. External intercostals
3. Scalene and sternomastoids

These inspiratory muscles cause changes in the pleural cavity, the cavity formed by the thoracic cage, which contains the lungs. The pleural cavity enlarges in two ways. The downward movement of the diaphragm pulls this cavity downward, thus lengthening it. The external intercostals and the other muscles of inspiration lift the front of the thoracic cage, thus increasing the thickness and forward movement of the pleural cavity. During inspiration the thoracic cage and the lungs become larger. As we can recall from basic physics, when a volume of gas is enlarged, its pressure will fall. During inspiration, enlargement of the thoracic cage causes a reduction in intrapleural and intrapulmonic pressures, and air will flow in until both of these pressures equal atmospheric pressure. See Figure 1-17.

The major muscles of expiration are as follows:

1. Abdominals
2. Internal intercostals

The abdominal muscles exert a downward pull on the thoracic cage, thus decreasing the thickness of the chest cage. The abdominal contents are forced upward against the diaphragm, decreasing the length of the pleural cavity. The internal intercostals aid expiration by pulling the ribs downward, thus reducing the thickness of the chest. Therefore, during expiration, reducing the size of the thoracic cage around the lungs increases the intrapulmonic pressure, which automatically pushes the air out of the alveoli to the atmosphere.

It is important to remember that to maintain *effective ventilation* requirements such as a patent airway, healthy lungs and tracheo-

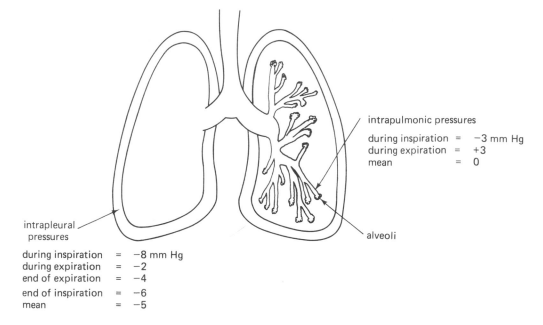

intrapulmonic pressures

during inspiration =   −3 mm Hg
during expiration =   +3
mean   =   0

intrapleural
  pressures

alveoli

during inspiration =   −8 mm Hg
during expiration =   −2
end of expiration =   −4
end of inspiration =   −6
mean   =   −5

Figure 1-17.   Intrapleural and intrapulmonic pressures.

bronchial tree, efficient muscles of the chest wall and related organs, and a normal relation between amount of air inspired each breath and amount of air within the lungs are necessary.

Divisions of the Respiratory Air (see Figure 1-18)

I.   *Volumes*, expressed in cubic centimeters or liters.
    A.   *Tidal volume*—the amount of air moved in or out per breath.
    B.   *Expiratory reserve volume*—the additional amount of air that can be expired at the end of a normal expiration.
    C.   *Inspiratory reserve volume*—the additional amount of air that can be inspired at the end of a normal inspiration.
    D.   *Residual volume*—that amount of air remaining in the lungs at the end of a forced expiration.

II.   *Capacities*, the combination of two or more volumes.
    A.   *Total lung capacity*—sum of all four volumes.
    B.   *Vital capacity*—sum of inspiratory reserve volume, tidal volume, and expiratory reserve volume.
    C.   *Inspiratory capacity*—sum of inspiratory reserve volume and tidal volume.

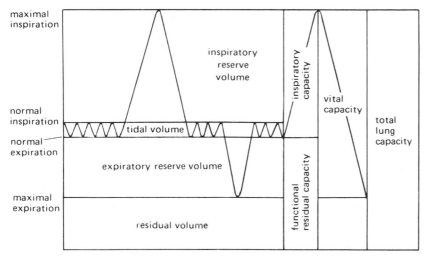

Figure 1-18. Divisions of respiratory air.

D. *Functional residual capacity*—sum of expiratory reserve volume and residual volume.

Regulation of Respiration. Control of respiration takes place principally in the medulla and pons of the brain. The respiratory impulses begin in the respiratory center of these areas and are transmitted to the muscles of ventilation. For instance, the diaphragm receives its stimuli from the phrenic nerve.

1. Inspiratory center
   a. Located in the anterior portion of the medulla.
   b. Causes inspiratory muscles to contract.
2. Expiratory center
   a. Located immediately behind and slightly above the inspiratory center.
   b. Causes expiratory muscles to contract.
3. Apneustic center
   a. Located in lower part of pons.
   b. Causes very prolonged inspiration punctuated by occasional expiratory gasps.
4. Pneumotaxic center
   a. Located in the top of the pons.
   b. Inhibits apneustic type of breathing and accelerates rate of breathing.

The inspiratory center continuously sends impulses to the inspiratory muscles, causing inspiration. At the same time, impulses are sent by way of a delay circuit to the expiratory center, exciting this 2 to 3 seconds later. At the time the expiratory muscles are stimulated, the inspiratory center is inhibited and therefore the inspiratory muscles relax. When the impulses of the expiratory center die out, the inspiratory center becomes active again.

The stimuli from the inspiratory and expiratory centers are relatively weak, but the apneustic and pneumotaxic centers enhance these activities, thus providing deeper respiration and helping to control the ventilation in proportion to the body's need for respiration.

Hering–Breuer Reflex.   Special nerve endings located throughout the lungs are stimulated when the lungs are distended. Impulses go from these endings to the medulla by way of the vagus nerve, causing inhibition of the inspiratory center and stimulation of the expiratory center. This reflex prevents overinflation of the lungs. It also helps maintain the basic rhythm of respiration. This reflex, the Hering–Breuer reflex, inhibits the inspiratory center as the lungs distend, to stop further inspiration. At the same time it excites the expiratory center to begin expiration. Conversely, as the lungs begin to deflate, the Hering–Breuer reflex ceases and the expiratory center is inhibited. See Figure 1-19.

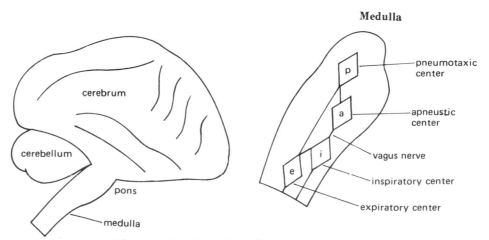

Figure 1-19.   Location of respiratory centers.

Regulation of Alveolar Ventilation.   Carbon dioxide is the most powerful stimulus to the respiratory center. As the carbon dioxide content increases above normal, the center is excited. Thus rate and depth of respiration are increased, perhaps to as much as 15 times normal. The tension of carbon dioxide depends primarily on alveolar ventilation. As alveolar ventilation decreases, alveolar carbon dioxide increases. As alveolar ventilation increases, alveolar carbon dioxide decreases.

One might think that respiration would be governed by the body's need for oxygen. However, at normal ventilatory rates, hemoglobin is almost always completely saturated with oxygen. At times, however, the oxygen concentration in the alveoli becomes too low to adequately supply oxygen to the hemoglobin. This can occur at high altitudes where the oxygen pressure of the air is very low and also in some disease states, such as emphysema, that reduce oxygen in the alveoli. At these times the respiratory system needs to be stimulated by oxygen deficiency. Oxygen deficiency excites the chemoreceptors, which are found in the aortic and carotid bodies. When stimulated, they send impulses along the vagus and glossopharyngeal nerves to the medulla. Here they excite the respiratory center to increase alveolar ventilation. See Figure 1-20.

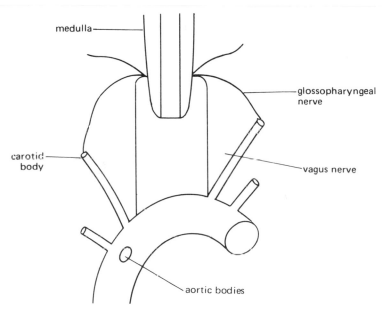

Figure 1-20.   Location of chemoreceptors.

When air is inspired, it is humidified almost immediately by moisture on the linings of the respiratory tract and the alveoli. At normal body temperature of 98.6°F, the partial pressure of water vapor in the lungs is 47 mm Hg. If the body temperature remains stable, this pressure will also remain. When water vapor is mixed with the inspired air, it dilutes the pressure of the other gases slightly.

EXAMPLE	Atmospheric pressure at sea level	= 760 mm Hg.
	Water vapor pressure in the body	= 47 mm Hg.
		713 mm Hg.
	Partial pressure of oxygen	= 0.21 × 713 = 149.73 mm Hg
	Partial pressure of carbon dioxide	= 0.03 × 713 = 0.21 mm Hg
	Partial pressure of nitrogen	= 0.79 × 713 = 563.27 mm Hg

Much of the air we inspire never reaches the alveoli where gas exchange takes place. The respiratory passages not involved with oxygenating the blood are referred to as *dead space.* This volume in the normal adult is about 50 milliliters (ml). With a normal tidal volume of 500 ml, this means that only 350 ml of fresh inspired air actually enters the alveoli.

The Respiratory Gases.   Oxygen and carbon dioxide are the two major gases involved in human functions and functioning. The amounts of these gases in the body fluids are usually measured in terms of their partial pressure. Partial pressure of any gas is referred to as *the pressure that any gas exerts, whether alone or mixed with other gases.* The partial pressure of carbon dioxide (PCO_2) is called the carbon dioxide pressure or carbon dioxide tension. The same rule applies to oxygen. Refer to the following table for the oxygen and carbon dioxide partial pressure/tension (for a normal resting adult breathing quietly).

	Venous Blood	*Arterial Blood*
PCO_2	46 mm Hg	40 mm Hg
PO_2	40 mm Hg	95–100 mm Hg

If the PCO_2 is elevated because of CO_2 retention or owing to CO_2 overproduction, this state is known as *hypercapnia.* When the PCO_2 becomes extremely low owing to hyperventilation, this state is known as *hypocapnia.* If the PO_2 falls to an abnormal state, *hypoxia* results.

CO_2 Transport.   This gas is a deadly acidic substance and must be eliminated by the lungs. It is formed as a by-product of the body's metabolic activities and the oxidation of carbon in foods. There are some changes that occur both in the formation and transportation of this gas. When CO_2 is formed, it is released into the interstitial fluids and from there it passes into the plasma. A certain amount of CO_2 goes to the red blood cells. From the blood plasma it enters the lungs, where it is released.

Changes in CO_2 occur when this gas enters the plasma from the interstitial fluid. They are as follows:

1. A portion of CO_2 remains dissolved in the blood and is measured in terms of the PCO_2. This dissolved CO_2 reacts with water to form carbonic acid: $CO_2 + H_2O \rightleftharpoons H_2CO_3$. This hydration of CO_2 takes place according to this equation.

2. When arterial blood gives up its oxygen to the cells and becomes venous blood again, and with the increase in CO_2, this CO_2 causes carbonic acid to separate into the components of the hydrogen ion and bicarbonate; when carbonic acid is formed, it ionizes according to the equation $H_2CO_3 \longrightarrow H^+ + HCO_3^-$.

3. The hydrogen ions formed are then buffered by the plasma buffers and as a result there is little change in the H^+ concentration.

4. Another reaction is the formation of some carbamino compounds as CO_2 joins the plasma proteins. Therefore, the hydrogen ions so formed are buffered in the plasma.

5. A large portion of CO_2 enters the red blood cells, and here the major buffering of CO_2 occurs.

   a. In the red cells, some CO_2 simply dissolves in the red cell fluid.

   b. Some CO_2 combines with hemoglobin to form carbamino compounds.

   c. A special enzyme, carbonic anhydrase, exists in large amounts in these cells, while there is none in plasma. This enzyme stimulates the reaction of $CO_2 + H_2O \rightleftharpoons H_2CO_3$. H^+ and HCO_3^- do not accumulate in the red blood cells as they do in plasma. The hydrogen ions are buffered by hemoglobin while the bicarbonate ions enter the plasma in exchange for Cl^-. This process is known as the *chloride shift*. Thus the red cell is left with a net positive electric charge, resulting in negatively charged ions entering the cell from the plasma.

   d. The passing of H_2CO_3 into the plasma permits large amounts of CO_2 to be transported to the lungs as bicarbonate ions. When CO_2 reaches the lungs via venous blood, its partial pressure is about 46 mm Hg. The PCO_2 in the alveolar areas of the lungs is about 40 mm Hg. This difference in pressure allows CO_2 to move from venous blood into the alveolar areas.

   e. When CO_2 is entering the alveolar spaces for expiration, a *reverse chloride shift* occurs in the body fluids. Cl^- reenters blood plasma in exchange for HCO_3^-. H_2CO_3 reenters the cell, where it changes into CO_2 and H_2O. CO_2 formed enters the blood plasma. CO_2 formed by these two processes finally is removed from the alveolar spaces into the air.

Although these processes sound lengthy, the actual time of CO_2 transport is very short, a matter of minutes from CO_2 production until it is released from the lungs.

The Transport of Oxygen.   Oxygen is carried in the blood as dissolved oxygen in physical solution in the plasma; this depends on the partial pressure of O_2 in arterial blood.

Oxygen combines very readily with hemoglobin in the red cells of the blood as oxyhemoglobin (HbO_2). This also depends on the partial pressure of O_2 in arterial blood. One gram (g) of hemoglobin (Hb) can combine with 1.34 ml of O_2. Therefore, in the normal person whose Hb content is 15 g/100 ml the blood can carry about 20.10 volumes percent of O_2 as HbO_2. Normally, however, hemoglobin, although capable of combining with this amount of O_2 does not do

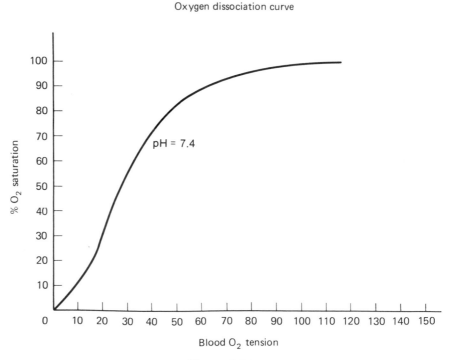

Figure 1-21.

so. A percentage saturation is usually the way in which hemoglobin combining with oxygen is expressed:

$$\% \text{ Saturation} = \frac{\text{oxygen content } (HbO_2)}{\text{oxygen capacity } (HbO_2 + Hb)} \times 100$$

If the O_2 tension is increased, almost all hemoglobin combines with oxygen; however, as in respiratory disease, if O_2 tension is decreased, a very small amount of Hb combines with oxygen. The relationship between the partial pressure of oxygen and the saturation of hemoglobin is known as the oxyhemoglobin dissociation curve, illustrated in Figure 1-21. One can readily see that the amount of O_2 given off to tissues not only depends on the partial pressure of O_2, but is also affected by an increase in CO_2 tension, a decreased pH, or an increased temperature. See Figure 1-22.

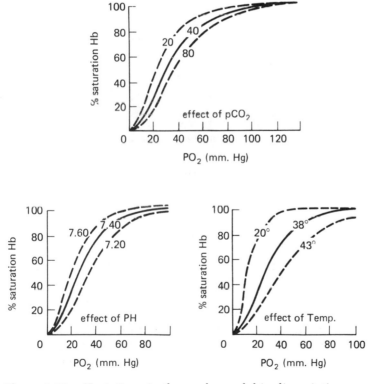

Figure 1-22. Variations in the oxyhemoglobin dissociation curve.

A brief summary of the terms used in the physiology of respiration and the O_2 and CO_2 transport diagram follows:

VENTILATION. The continuous process of moving air in and out of the lungs; usually expressed as volume per unit of time (liters/minute).

DEAD SPACE VENTILATION

1. *Anatomical*—the internal volume of the airway between the mouth, nose, pharynx, larynx, trachea, bronchi and the bronchioles.
2. *Physiological*—includes the volume of the inspired gas that occupies the anatomical dead space and the volume that ventilates alveoli that are not perfused by capillary blood flow.

ALVEOLAR VENTILATION. The amount of air moving in and out of the lungs that is directly involved in gas exchange. For example,

$$\text{Tidal volume} - \text{dead space} = \text{alveolar volume}$$
$$\text{Tidal volume} = 500 \text{ ml}$$
$$\text{Dead space} = -150 \text{ ml}$$
$$\text{Alveolar volume} = 350 \text{ ml}$$
$$\text{Tidal volume} \times \text{rate} = \text{minute ventilation}$$
$$500 \text{ ml} \times 15 = 7500 \text{ ml/min}$$

DISTRIBUTION OF VENTILATION. The allocation of air to the millions of alveoli or gas exchange units.

PERFUSION. The blood flow through the capillary bed of the lungs.

DIFFUSION. The passive process characterized by movement of gases from a place of higher pressure to one of lower pressure.

The air in the alveoli is separated from the blood in the capillaries by the pulmonary membrane, which is made up of endothelium and alveolar lining cells. This membrane has a thickness of 0.24 to 0.4 (microns) μm (micrometers).

One of the principal factors determining the rate of diffusion is the difference between the partial pressures of the gas on the two sides of the membrane. Diffusion depends on the following:

1. The pressure difference of the gases on each side of the membrane.

2. Characteristics of the gas (coefficient of solubility, temperature, and molecular weight)

3. Surface area of the membrane and its thickness.

Transport of Oxygen and Carbon Dioxide

1. Oxygen is carried in the blood attached to hemoglobin; the amount depends on the amount of hemoglobin (1 g of Hb will combine with 1.34 ml of O_2). The amount physically dissolved depends on the partial pressure, temperature, and the coefficient of solubility of the gas.

2. Carbon dioxide is carried physically dissolved attached to hemoglobin and, through the action of carbonic anhydrase, as HCO_3^-.

See Figure 1-23.

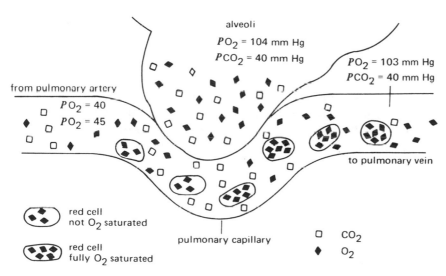

Figure 1-23.   Transport of oxygen and carbon dioxide.

Acid–Base Balance

The normal body fluids are carefully maintained at a slightly alkaline state by a rigid balance between loss and addition of electrolytes, particularly by control of the hydrogen-ion concentration.

This control of hydrogen-ion concentration is achieved by three separate steps:

1. Action of buffers
2. Respiration
3. Renal function

There has been some confusion as to the definition of an acid and a base. A popular classification is to refer to an acid as a proton donor and a base as a proton acceptor. Another definition, which has received some popularity, states that an acid is an electrolyte that dissociates to yield an anion and the hydrogen ion. For example, hydrochloric acid (HCl) in solution would yield an anion, chloride, and a hydrogen ion: $HCl \rightleftharpoons H^+ + Cl^-$. Likewise, a base would be an electrolyte that, when placed in solution, would yield a cation and a hydroxyl, or OH, group: $NaOH \rightleftharpoons Na^+ + OH^-$.

The concentration of the hydrogen ion in blood is extremely small, a very small fraction of a mole per liter of solution (4×10^{-8} mole/liter). A mole of any substance or ion is the number of grams equal to the molecular or ionic weight of the substance. A millimole is one thousandth of a mole or the same number of milligrams instead of grams. To avoid difficulty in handling such numbers, the concept of pH was introduced. This is defined as the negative logarithm of the hydrogen-ion concentration: $pH = -\log (H^+)$. By means of this scheme, the cumbersome number of 4×10^{-8} mole/liter can be expressed as 7.4 on the pH scale. The concentration of hydrogen ion in the arterial blood or the pH can be determined by means of a pH meter with a glass electrode. The normal range of pH of the blood is 7.35 to 7.45. This normal pH range is protected by a number of compounds in blood referred to as buffers.

A buffer can be defined as any substance in solution that resists a change in pH of that solution when an acid or base is added. There are four major buffers in the blood:

1. Hemoglobin
2. Protein
3. Phosphates
4. Bicarbonate system

The clinical evaluation of acid–base problems has been primarily based on the evaluation of the bicarbonate system. This evaluation centers around the determination of the relationship of carbonic acid to bicarbonate. This relationship for bicarbonate can be expressed by means of the Henderson–Hasselbalch equation.

$$pH = pK + \log \frac{(salt)}{(acid)}$$

The pK is that pH at which 50% of the carbonic acid is ionized, and for the bicarbonate system this is equal to 6.1.

$$pH = 6.1 + \log \left[\frac{HCO_3^-}{H_2CO_3} \right]$$

$$pH = 6.1 = \log \left[\frac{24}{1.2} \right]$$

$$pH = 6.1 + \log \left[\frac{20}{1} \right]$$

$$pH = 6.1 + 1.3$$

$$pH = 7.4$$

For clinical purposes, the pH is measured directly by means of the pH meter with the glass electrode. The concentration of carbon dioxide gas (which contributes to the formation of the carbonic acid) is controlled by the degree of alveolar ventilation. Hence, in disease entities causing respiratory insufficiency, there is a retention of carbon dioxide. This increase in the denominator disturbs the 20:1 ratio needed to maintain a pH of 7.4. As the concentration of carbonic acid increases in the denominator, the pH will fall unless the concentration of bicarbonate in the numerator is increased accordingly. In patients experiencing alveolar hypoventilation for significant periods of time, there is a chronic retention of carbon dioxide. In these particular patients, renal compensation comes into play and the kidney retains bicarbonate proportionally so that, despite a PCO_2 of the arterial blood of 60 mm Hg, the bicarbonate will be proportionately elevated, resulting in a pH in the normal range. This is referred to as compensated respiratory acidosis.

In instances of acute respiratory acidosis, such as in an acute asthmatic attack, there is a sudden development of severe hypoventilation with carbon dioxide retention. This occurs rapidly before the kidney has had opportunity to retain bicarbonate. This sudden elevation in carbon dioxide results in a significant lowering of pH. In such an acute problem the rapid administration of bicarbonate may turn out to be lifesaving. In patients who have severe respiratory acidosis resulting from chronic retention, the correction of the pH is a somewhat more complex affair. As a patient is placed on a ventilator and hyperventilated to decrease the P_aCO_2, there is a danger that this may be done too rapidly, and the pH may swing from a very severe respiratory acidosis to an extreme metabolic alkalosis within a relatively short period of time. It is important in the management of patients in respiratory acidosis due to chronic retention of carbon dioxide that particular attention be paid to the pH and not to the PCO_2 alone. The PCO_2 should be decreased at a reasonable rate to allow the kidney to excrete the excess bicarbonate that had been retained. This will avoid a pH swing to a severe alkaline side, which may in itself interfere with body metabolism. This particular set of circumstances has been ignored in many instances, resulting in severe consequences of a metabolic nature. The sudden fluctuations of pH cause interference with enzyme metabolism and with electrolyte movement among the fluid compartments of the body.

Table 1-2 summarizes the preceding discussion.

TABLE 1-2   Quick Reminders and Equations Regarding Acid–Base Balance

P_aCO_2 determines the amount of alveolar ventilation:

P_aCO_2 ↑ = ↓ AV

P_aCO_2 ↓ = ↑ AV

Normally, P_aCO_2 = 35 to 45 mm Hg (40 mm Hg average)

P_aCO_2 ↑ 45 = hypoventilation

P_aCO_2 ↓ 35 = hyperventilation

Acidosis = ↑ H^+ in the blood

Alkalosis = ↓ H^+ in the blood

Normal pH is 7.35 to 7.45 (refers to amount of H^+ in blood)

↓ pH = ↑ H^+ (acidosis)

↑ pH = ↓ H^+ (alkalosis)

Any substance that can give H^+ is an acid

Any substance that can receive H^+ is an alkali

Pure metabolic alkalosis:	HCO_3^- ↑ , PCO_2 ⟶
Pure metabolic acidosis:	HCO_3^- ↓ , PCO_2 ⟶
Pure respiratory acidosis:	HCO_3^- ⟶ , PCO_2 ↑
Pure respiratory alkalosis:	HCO_3^- ⟶ , PCO_2 ↓
Mixed acidosis:	HCO_3^- ↓ , PCO_2 ↑
Mixed alkalosis:	HCO_3^- ↑ , PCO_2 ↓

TABLE 1-2 (continued)

$pH = 7.05$ $PCO_2 = 60$ $HCO_3^- = 16$	Represents mixed acidosis

$pH = 7.18$ $PCO_2 = 25$ $HCO_3^- = 9$	Respiratory alkalosis Metabolic acidosis (predominate—due to pH)

$pH = 7.46$ $PCO_2 = 26$ $HCO_3^- = 18$	Respiratory alkalosis Metabolic acidosis } compensated (see pH)

$pH = 7.51$ $PCO_2 = 35$ $HCO_3^- = 27$	Metabolic alkalosis with slight amount respiratory alkalosis Low normal Metabolic alkalosis

$pH = 7.51$ $PCO_2 = 22$ $HCO_3^- = 17$	Respiratory alkalosis with some metabolic acidosis Respiratory alkalosis—(predominate due to pH) Metabolic acidosis

$pH = 7.40$ $PCO_2 = 38$ $HCO_3^- = 23$	Normal (minimal changes)

$pH = 7.46$ $PCO_2 = 22$ $HCO_3^- = 15$	Normal (minimal alkalosis) Respiratory alkalosis Metabolic acidosis } compensated

$pH = 7.49$ $PCO_2 = 26$ $HCO_3^- = 19$	Respiratory alkalosis with metabolic compensation Respiratory alkalosis—(predominate due to pH) Metabolic acidosis

EXERCISES

1. Oxygen moves across the blood–gas barrier by the process of
   _____.

2. The lungs are divided into segments called _____.

3. The greatest amount of air exhaled after the deepest possible inspiration is called the _____ capacity.

4. What values does the Henderson–Hasselbalch equation give you?

5. The trachea is also called the _____.

6. List the three major muscles of inspiration:

   a. _____

   b. _____

   c. _____

7. In the normal resting adult breathing quietly the arterial PCO_2 is _____ and the arterial PO_2 is _____.

8. What enzyme in the red blood cell aids in buffering CO_2?

9. The normal pH is _____.

10. If P_aCO_2 is elevated, what happens to alveolar ventilation?

11. The blood gases of your patient are as follows. Explain. pH = 7.1; PCO_2 = 60; HCO_3^- = 16.

THE CIRCULATORY SYSTEM

I. The heart is a four-chambered pump which keeps blood flowing through the circulatory system (see Figure 1-24). The unoxygenated blood is returned to the heart from the rest of the body through the superior and inferior vena cavae. The blood first enters the right atrium or upper chamber. From the atrium, blood moves through the tricuspid valve into the right ventricle. The ventricle pumps the blood through the pulmonary valve into the pulmonary artery and then to the lungs.

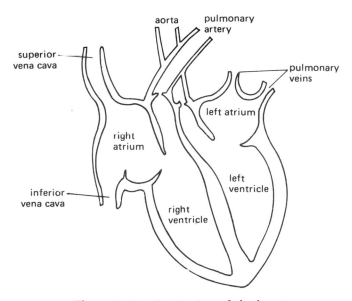

Figure 1-24. Front view of the heart.

In the lungs, the blood gives up carbon dioxide and picks up oxygen. The pulmonary veins return the oxygenated blood to the left atrium of the heart. Again, from the left atrium, blood moves through the bicuspid or mitral valve into the left ventricle. The left ventricle then contracts and forces blood through the aortic valve, into the aorta, and on through the systemic circulation.

II. Arteries, veins, and capillaries
    A. *Arteries*—tubes that carry blood away from the heart to the capillaries.
        1. The aortic and pulmonary arteries have an average diameter of 1.2 in. at their origin within the heart.
        2. Arteries divide and subdivide into smaller branches.
        3. The smallest arteries are called arterioles.
        4. Capillaries begin at the distal end of the arterioles.
    B. *Veins*—carry blood to the heart; they are formed by the joining of capillaries.
        1. Tend to collapse when not filled with blood.
        2. Contain valves to prevent backflow of blood, especially in the extremities.
    C. *Capillaries*—exceedingly minute vessels, with an average diameter of 0.008 mm.
        1. Connect the arterioles and venules (smallest veins).
        2. Capillaries communicate freely with one another to form networks.

GAS LAWS

Boyle's Law.   The volume of a gas varies inversely with the pressure, if the temperature is kept constant (see Figure 1-25).

A mass of oxygen occupies 5 liters under a pressure of 740 mm Hg.   *EXAMPLE*
Determine the volume of the same mass of gas at a standard pressure of (760 mm Hg), when the temperature remains constant.

$$\frac{V_2}{V_1} = \frac{P_1}{P_2}$$

$$V_1 = 5 \text{ liters}$$

$$P_1 = 740 \text{ mm Hg}$$

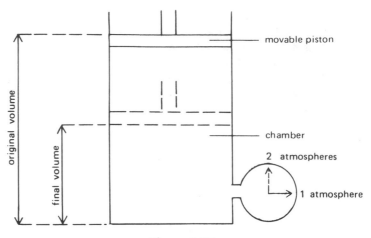

Figure 1-25.

$$P_2 = 760 \text{ mm Hg}$$

$$V_2 = x$$

$$V_2 = \frac{V_1 P_1}{P_2}$$

$$V_2 = \frac{5 \text{ liters} \times 740 \text{ mm Hg}}{760 \text{ mm Hg}}$$

$$V_2 = 4.868 \text{ or } 4.87 \text{ liters}$$

Charles' Law. The volume of a gas is directly proportional to its absolute temperature if the pressure is kept constant. In other words, if the pressure is kept constant, the volume will increase as the temperature increases (see Figure 1-26).

EXAMPLE   A mass of oxygen occupies 200 cc (cubic centimeters) at 100°C. Find its volume at 0°C, when the pressure remains constant.

$$\frac{V_2}{V_1} = \frac{T_2}{T_1}$$

$$V_1 = 200 \text{ cc}$$

$$V_2 = x$$

$$T_1 = 100°C + 273°K = 373°K$$

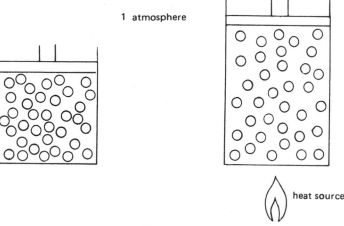

1 atmosphere

heat source

Figure 1-26.

$$T_2 = 0°C + 273°K = 273°K$$

$$V_2 = \frac{V_1 T_2}{T_1}$$

$$V_2 = \frac{200 \text{ cc} \times 273°K}{373°K}$$

$$V_2 = 146.3 \text{ cc}$$

Dalton's Law. The total pressure exerted by a mixture of gases is equal to the sum of the partial pressures of the various gases. The partial pressure of a gas in a mixture is defined as the pressure the gas would exert if it were alone in the container.

Generally, the formula for Dalton's law may be written as

$$\text{Total pressure} = P_1 + P_2 + P_3 + \cdots$$

The atmospheric pressure is 760 mm Hg. Determine the partial pressure of oxygen, nitrogen, and carbon dioxide.   *EXAMPLE*

$$P_1 = \text{partial pressure of oxygen}$$

$$P_1 = 20.96\% \times 760 \text{ mm Hg} = 159.30 \text{ mm Hg}$$

$$P_2 = \text{partial pressure of nitrogen}$$

$$P_2 = 79\% \times 760 \text{ mm Hg} = 600.40 \text{ mm Hg}$$

P_3 = partial pressure of carbon dioxide

P_3 = 0.04% $\times$ 760 mm Hg = 0.30 mm Hg

Henry's Law.   If the temperature is constant, the quantity of a gas that will go into solution is proportional to the partial pressure of that gas. The greater the partial pressure, the more gas will go into solution (see Figure 1-27).

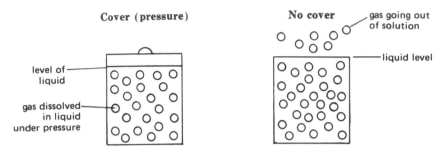

Figure 1-27.

BASIC PHYSICS

Force.   In physics, force is a push or a pull exerted upon an object; it may also be defined as muscular exertion or its equivalent. Forces produce a number of different effects. A force may set an object into motion or it may retard a moving body; or force may produce distortion as, for example, in the compression or the stretching of a spring.

In the metric system the dyne is the absolute unit of force. One dyne acting for 1 second upon 1 gram of mass imparts to it a velocity of 1 centimeter per second. Therefore, the dyne is approximately equal to 1/980 of a gram of force.

Atmospheric Pressure.   This force is due to the weight of the overlying air. The pressure of a column of mercury exactly 76 cm high at 0°C is approximately the average pressure of the atmosphere at sea level, and is called 1 atmosphere or 76 cm of mercury, 760 mm Hg, 29.9 in. Hg, 14.7 lb/in^2., or 1.014×10^{-6} dynes/cm^2.

One of the simplest gauges used to measure this pressure is the open tube manometer. It consists of a U-shaped tube containing a liquid, having one end of the tube at the pressure to be measured, while the other end is open to the atmosphere. Another type of measuring consists of a long glass tube that has been filled with mercury and then inverted into a dish of mercury. Because mercury manometers and barometers are used so frequently in laboratories, it is customary to express atmospheric pressure and other pressure as inches of mercury or centimeters of mercury.

Surface Tension. This force of liquids is the surface energy per unit area of surface, or the force per unit length of surface, and is expressed in dynes per centimeter. See Table 1-3.

TABLE 1-3   Typical Values of Surface Tension

Substance	°C	Surface Tension, dynes/cm
Water	0	75.6
Water	20	72.8
Oxygen	−193	15.7
Helium	−269	0.12
Ethyl alcohol	20	22.3
Glycerine	20	63.1
Soap solution	20	25.0

A piece of glass tubing with an external diameter of 4.0 cm and an internal diameter of 3.5 cm stands vertically with one end immersed in water. What is the downward pull on the tube due to surface tension? Surface tension of water is 74 dynes/cm.   *EXAMPLE*

Force (dynes) = surface tension [dynes/cm × total length of
                surface (cm)]

= 74 dynes/cm × (4.0 + 3.5) π cm

= 74 dynes/cm × 7.5 × $\frac{22}{7}$ = $\frac{165}{7}$

165 ÷ 7 = 23.5

= 74 dynes/cm × 23.5 = 1740 dynes

*PRESSURE DUE TO SURFACE TENSION ONLY IN A
SPHERICAL DROP*

$$P = \frac{2T}{r}$$ where T = surface tension of the liquid
                                  r = radius of the drop

EXAMPLE   Compute the pressure (due to surface tension) within a soap bubble of diameter 4 cm. Surface tension is 30 dynes/cm. The film has two surfaces, inside and outside.

$$P = \frac{2T}{r} + \frac{2T}{r} = \frac{4T}{r} = \frac{4 \times 30/cm}{2\ cm} = 60\ \text{dynes/cm}^2$$

Viscosity.   This force may be described as the internal friction of a fluid. Because of viscosity a force must be exerted to cause one layer of fluid to slide past another or to cause one surface to slide past another. If there is a layer of fluid between the surfaces, both liquids and gases exhibit viscosity, although liquids are much more viscous than gases.

Viscosity is measured in a unit equal to 1 dyne-sec/cm^2 that is called a *poise*. Small viscosities are usually expressed in centipoises or micropoises. Equivalents for calculating viscosity are given in Table 1-4 and typical viscosity values are listed in Table 1-5.

TABLE 1-4   Typical Dyne Calculation

1 dyne	= 1.0197 $\times$ 10^{-6} kg
	2.2481 $\times$ 10^{-6} lb
1 dyne cm	= 1 erg = 9.4805 $\times$ 10^{-11} Btu
	1 erg = 7.3756 $\times$ 10^{-8} ft lb
1 dyne/cm^2	= 9.8692 $\times$ 10^{-7} atm
	0.0010197 g/cm^2
	4.0148 $\times$ 10^{-4} in. H$_2$O
	7.5006 $\times$ 10^{-4} mm Hg
	1.4504 $\times$ 10^{-5} psi
1 poise	= 1 dyne sec/cm^2
	1 g/cm sec
	1 0.067196 lb/ft sec
1 centipoise	= 0.01 poise
	10^{-2} poise (0.01)
1 micropoise	= 10^{-6} poise (0.000001)

TABLE 1-5   Typical Values of Viscosity

$T°C$	Viscosity of Water, centipoise	Viscosity of Air, micropoise
0	1.792	171
20	1.005	181
40	0.656	190

Temperature Scales

1. The *Kelvin scale* was developed by Sir William Thomson, an English physicist whose title was Lord Kelvin. The scale was named after him. The size of each degree is the same as that on the Celsius scale, but the zero point on the Kelvin scale is equal to −273°C. Since 0° Kelvin is considered to be the coldest temperature possible, it is called absolute zero.

Kelvin temperature = Celsius temperature +273

Celsius temperature = Kelvin temperature −273

2. The *Celsius scale* is the most widely used in science today. On this scale the freezing point of water is 0° and the boiling point is 100°. Thus, on the Celsius scale there are 100 degrees between the freezing point and the boiling point of water, as compared with 180 degrees between these two points on the Fahrenheit scale.

3. The *Fahrenheit scale* is most widely used in households and for everyday measurements of temperature. On this scale the freezing point of water is 32° and the boiling point of water is 212°. Often it is desirable to convert a measurement obtained on one scale to another. The formulas below will enable you to make this conversion from Celsius to Fahrenheit and Fahrenheit to Celsius.

$$°C = (°F - 32) \times \tfrac{5}{9}$$

$$°F = (°C \times \tfrac{9}{5}) + 32$$

4. The *Rankine scale* uses the same size of degree as in the Fahrenheit scale but with the zero point shifted to −460°F.

    Figure 1-28 compares readings on the four temperature scales.

Density. The density of a substance is the weight of a unit volume of that substance. In the English system density is expressed as pounds per cubic foot. In the metric system density is usually expressed as grams per cubic centimeter or grams per liter. Usually, the density of liquids and solids is given in grams per cubic centimeter (g/cc), while the density of gases is given as grams per liter (g/liter). The main reason for the use of different units is to obtain numbers of sizes that are convenient for doing calculations.

The density of any substance can be calculated by dividing the weight of a sample of material by its volume. The density of any gas at standard temperature and pressure (STP) is its molecular weight divided by 22.4.

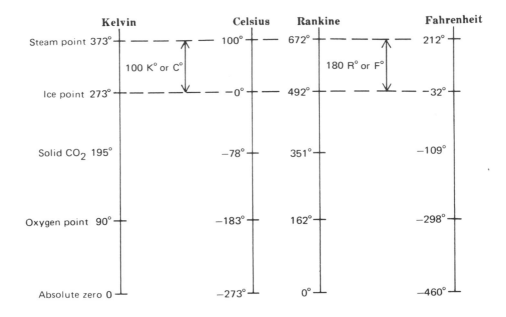

Note: Temperatures have been rounded off to the nearest degree.

Figure 1-28.   Comparison of temperature scales.

EXAMPLE   The density of oxygen is

$$\frac{32}{22.4} \text{ (molecular weight)} = 1.43 \text{ g/liter}$$

$$\text{Density in } \frac{g}{cc} = \frac{\text{weight in g}}{\text{volume in cc}}$$

$$\text{Density in } \frac{g}{\text{liter}} = \frac{\text{weight in g}}{\text{volume in liters}}$$

Density is useful in comparing the relative weights of substances, as shown in Table 1-6.

TABLE 1-6   Densities of Selected Substances

Substance	Density, g/cm³	Gas	Density, g/cm³ at 1 atm, 0°C
Water	1.00	Air	1.2929×10^{-3}
Glycerin	1.26	Carbon dioxide	1.9769×10^{-3}
Ethyl alcohol	0.81	Helium	0.1785×10^{-3}
Steel	7.8	Nitrogen	1.2506×10^{-3}
Ice	0.92	Oxygen	1.4290×10^{-3}

Specific Gravity. The specific gravity of a substance is the number indicating how many times heavier a substance is than the same volume of water. The specific gravity of a substance will tell us, for example, whether a substance will float in water. Any substance with a specific gravity less than that of water (which is 1) will float.

Humidity. Humidity is the measure of water vapor present in the air. Humidity is expressed as absolute or relative humidity. Absolute humidity is the weight of water vapor contained in a unit of volume, and it is usually expressed as percentage of vapor by weight.

When the concentration of water vapor, or the absolute humidity, is such that the partial pressure equals the vapor pressure, the vapor is said to be *saturated*. If the partial pressure is less than the vapor pressure, the vapor is *unsaturated*. The ratio of the partial pressure to the vapor pressure at the same temperature is called the *relative humidity*, and is usually expressed as a percentage.

Percentage relative humidity =

$$100 \times \frac{\text{partial pressure of water vapor}}{\text{vapor pressure at same temperature}}$$

The partial pressure of water vapor in the atmosphere is 10 mm of mercury and the temperature is 20°C. Find the relative humidity. Refer to Table 1-7 (i.e., vapor pressure at 20°C is 17.5 mm Hg).   *EXAMPLE*

$$\text{Relative humidity} = \frac{10}{17.5} \times 100 - 57\%$$

Table 1-7 gives the vapor pressure of water at various temperatures.

TABLE 1-7   Vapor Pressure of Water (absolute)

°C	mm Hg	lb/in.²	°F
0	4.58	0.0886	32
5	6.51	0.1260	41
10	8.94	0.1730	50
15	12.67	0.2450	59
20	17.50	0.3290	68
40	55.10	1.0700	104
60	149.00	2.8900	140
80	355.00	6.8700	176
100	760.00	14.7000	212

TABLE 1-8 Relative Humidity Table (in percent)

Difference Between Wet and Dry Thermometers

Dry Bulb temp F°	0	1	2	3	4	5	6	7	8	9	10	11	12	13	14	15	16	17	18	19	20	21	22	23	24	25
30	100	89	78	67	56	46	36	26	16	6																
32	100	89	79	69	59	49	39	30	20	11	2															
34	100	90	81	71	62	52	43	34	25	16	8															
36	100	91	82	73	64	55	46	38	29	21	13	5														
38	100	91	83	75	66	58	50	42	33	25	17	10	2													
40	100	92	83	75	68	60	52	45	37	29	22	15	8	1												
42	100	92	85	77	69	62	55	47	40	33	26	19	12	5												
44	100	92	85	78	71	65	56	49	43	36	30	23	16	9	2											
46	100	93	86	79	72	65	58	52	45	39	32	26	20	14	8	2										
48	100	93	86	79	73	66	60	54	47	41	35	29	23	17	11	6	1									
50	100	93	87	80	74	67	61	55	49	43	38	32	27	21	16	10	5									
52	100	94	87	81	75	69	63	57	51	46	40	35	30	25	20	15	10	4								
54	100	94	88	82	76	70	64	59	53	48	42	37	32	27	22	17	12	8	5	2						
56	100	94	88	82	76	71	65	60	55	50	44	39	34	29	24	19	16	11	8	6						
58	100	94	89	83	77	72	66	61	56	51	46	41	36	31	26	21	18	14	11	9	1					
60	100	94	89	83	78	73	68	63	58	53	48	43	38	33	29	24	21	17	14	12	5	1				
62	100	94	89	84	79	74	69	64	59	54	50	45	40	36	32	27	24	20	17	15	8	4	1			
64	100	95	90	84	79	74	70	65	60	56	51	47	42	38	34	30	26	22	18	16	11	7	4	0		
66	100	95	90	85	80	75	71	66	61	57	53	48	44	40	36	32	28	25	22	20	14	10	7	3		
68	100	95	90	85	80	76	71	67	62	58	54	50	46	41	37	33	31	27	24	22	16	13	10	6	3	
70	100	95	90	86	81	77	72	68	64	60	55	51	48	44	40	36	33	29	26	24	19	15	12	9	6	3
72	100	95	91	86	82	77	73	69	65	61	57	53	49	45	41	38	34	31	28	26	21	18	15	12	9	6
74	100	95	91	86	82	78	74	70	65	62	58	54	50	47	43	39	36	33	30	28	23	20	17	14	11	8
76	100	96	91	87	83	78	74	71	66	63	59	55	52	48	45	41	38	34	31	30	25	22	19	16	13	11
78	100	96	91	87	83	79	75	71	67	64	60	56	53	49	46	43	39	36	32	31	27	24	21	18	16	13
80	100	96	91	87	83	80	76	72	68	66	61	57	54	50	47	43	41	38	34	32	29	26	23	20	18	15
82	100	96	92	88	84	80	76	72	69	66	61	58	55	51	48	45	42	39	35	33	30	28	25	22	20	17
84	100	96	92	88	84	80	77	73	69	66	62	59	56	52	49	46	43	40	36	35	32	29	26	24	21	19
86	100	96	92	89	85	81	77	73	69	67	63	60	57	53	50	47	46	41	38	36	33	30	28	26	23	21
88	100	96	92	89	85	81	77	74	70	68	64	61	58	54	51	48	47	43	40	37	35	32	30	28	25	22
90	100	96	92	89	85	82	78	74	71	69	65	61	58	55	52	49	47	44	41	39	36	34	31	28	26	24

The temperature at which the water vapor in a given sample of air becomes saturated is called the *dew point*. Measuring the temperature of the dew point is the most accurate method of determining relative humidity.

Also there is a simple, but less accurate, method of determining relative humidity, that of the wet and dry bulb thermometer (Figure 1-29). Another method is the hair hygrometer, which makes use of

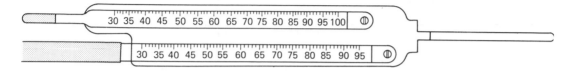

Figure 1-29.   Wet and dry bulb thermometer.

the fact that human hair absorbs or gives up moisture from the air in an amount that varies with relative humidity and changes its length slightly with moisture content. A number of hairs are wrapped around a small pivoted shaft to which is attached a pointer. The hair is kept taut by a light spring, and changes in its length cause the shaft to rotate and move the pointer over a scale.

HOW TO USE THE WET AND DRY HYGROMETER TABLE

1. *Note:* The hygrometer must be swung for 3 full minutes after the wet bulb material is moistened.
2. *Example:* The dry bulb temperature reads 80º; the wet bulb temperature reads 68°. Find the relative humidity. Solution: The difference between the two is *12*. On the humidity table, locate 80° on the dry bulb temperature scale. Follow the line until you reach the vertical wet bulb scale of 12. The relative humidity reading is 54%. See Table 1-8.

BASIC CHEMISTRY

I. Definitions
    A. *Matter*—any substance that occupies space.
    B. *Mass of a body*—the quantity of matter that it contains.
    C. *Weight*—a measure of the gravitational attraction for a body.
    D. *Energy*—the power or ability to do work.

E. *Kinetic energy*—the energy of a moving body.

F. *Potential energy*—stored energy.

G. *Exothermic reactions*—those chemical reactions in which heat is evolved.

H. *Endothermic reactions*—those chemical reactions in which heat is absorbed by the reactants.

II. Laws of the conservation of mass and energy (under ordinary circumstances)

A. *Mass*—can be neither created nor destroyed, but may be transformed from one state to another.

B. *Energy*—can be neither created nor destroyed, but may be transformed from one state to another.

III. Metric conversion factors. See Table 1-9.

IV. Varieties of matter

A. *Elements*—elementary particles of matter that cannot be decomposed by chemical means into simpler substances.

B. *Compounds*—composed of two or more elements and can be decomposed into these elements by chemical means; they are homogeneous, with all the particles of the compound identical in appearance and chemical composition. They have their own characteristic properties, which are different from the properties of their constituent elements; they have a definite and fixed composition.

C. *Mixtures*—are generally heterogeneous and have a variable composition. The various constituents of the mixture can usually be separated by mechanical means.

D. *Solutions*—may be considered as a special type of mixture; arc homogeneous; all particles in the solvent are of molecular dimension.

V. Atoms and molecules

A. *Molecule*—the smallest particle of a compound that still possesses the properties of the compound.

B. *Atoms*—the particles of elements that enter into chemical reaction.

Example: Each *molecule* of oxygen (O_2) contains two *atoms.*

TABLE 1-9   Metric Conversion Factors

| | Approximate *Conversions to Metric Measures* | | | |
Symbol	When You Know	Multiply by	To Find	Symbol
		Length		
in.	inches	*2.5	centimeters	cm
ft	feet	30	centimeters	cm
yd	yards	0.9	meters	m
mi	miles	1.6	kilometers	km
		Area		
in^2	square inches	6.5	square centimeters	cm^2
ft^2	square feet	0.09	square meters	m^2
yd^2	square yards	0.8	square meters	m^2
mi^2	square miles	2.6	square kilometers	km^2
	acres	0.4	hectares	ha
		Mass (weight)		
oz	ounces	28	grams	g
lb	pounds	0.45	kilograms	kg
	short tons (2000 lb)	0.9	tonnes	t
		Volume		
tsp	teaspoons	5	milliliters	ml
Tbsp	tablespoons	15	milliliters	ml
fl oz	fluid ounces	30	milliliters	ml
c.	cups	0.24	liters	l
pt	pints	0.47	liters	l
qt	quarts	0.95	liters	l
gal	gallons	3.8	liters	l
ft^3	cubic feet	0.03	cubic meters	m^3
yd^3	cubic yards	0.76	cubic meters	m^3
		Temperature (exact)		
°F	Fahrenheit temperature	5/9 (after subtracting 32)	Celsius temperature	°C

°F   32   98.6   °F
 −40   0   40   80   120   160   200   212
 −40   −20   0   20   40   60   80   100
 °C   37   °C

*1 in. = 2.54 cm (exactly).

TABLE 1-9 (continued)

Symbol	When You Know	Multiply by	To Find	Symbol
	Approximate *Conversions from Metric Measures*			
mm	millimeters	0.04	inches	in.
cm	centimeters	0.4	inches	in.
m	meters	3.3	feet	ft
m	meters	1.1	yards	yd
km	kilometers	0.6	miles	mi
	Area			
cm^2	square centimeters	0.16	square inches	in^2
m^2	square meters	1.2	square yards	yd^2
km^2	square kilometers	0.4	square miles	mi^2
ha	hectares (10,000 m^2)	2.5	acres	
	Mass (weight)			
g	grams	0.035	ounces	oz
kg	kilograms	2.2	pounds	lb
t	tonnes (1000 kg)	1.1	short tons	
	Volume			
ml	milliliters	0.03	fluid ounces	fl oz
l	liters	2.1	pints	pt
l	liters	1.06	quarts	qt
l	liters	0.26	gallons	gal
m^3	cubic meters	35	cubic feet	ft^3
m^3	cubic meters	1.3	cubic yards	yd^3
	Temperature (exact)			
°C	Celsius temperature	9/5 then add 32)	Fahrenheit temperature	°F

VI. States of matter

    A. *Gases*—have neither a fixed volume nor a fixed shape, spread through and occupy the entire container in which they are placed, and have a high degree of compressibility.

    B. *Liquids*—have a fixed volume but no fixed shape; low degree of compressibility; heat (the latent heat of vaporization) is required to separate the molecules of a liquid and convert it to a gas.

    C. *Solids*—have a fixed size and shape and possess mechanical strength. The latent heat of fusion is the heat required to convert a solid to the liquid state.

VII. *Chemical symbols*—abbreviations, which have various derivations, for the names of the chemical elements.

Examples: O oxygen   He helium
S sulfur   Na sodium
P phosphorus   Hg mercury
H hydrogen   Cl chlorine
N nitrogen   K potassium

VIII. *Formulas*—combinations of symbols of elements that are a simplified method of indicating a compound, as well as the chemical composition of a compound.

> *Examples:* 1. FeS—iron sulfide: 1 atom of iron combined with 1 atom of sulfur
>
> 2. H_2SO_4—sulfuric acid: each molecule contains 2 atoms of hydrogen, 1 atom of sulfur, and 4 atoms of oxygen

HOW THE GAS LAWS ARE APPLIED TO RESPIRATION

Mechanism of Breathing

Boyle's law can be used to explain part of the mechanism of breathing since we consider the temperature of the body to remain constant. During inspiration we have a lowering of the diaphragm and an expansion of the chest wall, allowing the volume of the lungs to increase. This increase in volume (at a constant temperature) causes a decrease in the pressure so that the outside air enters the lungs, because the outside air is at a higher pressure than the air in the lungs, and air flows from an area of higher pressure to an area of lower pressure. During expiration the diaphragm rises, decreasing the volume of the lungs and increasing the pressure, so that the air goes out.

Thus, breathing is due to a difference in pressure between the lungs and the atmosphere. The pressure between the two layers of pleura is below atmospheric pressure (760 mm Hg) at all times in the adult. Intrathoracic pressure varies from −4.5 to −9 mm Hg below atmospheric pressure during inspiration to −3 to −6 mm Hg below atmospheric pressure during expiration.

Mechanism of Respiration

According to Henry's law, the amount of a gas that will dissolve in a liquid is proportional to the partial pressure of that gas. At first, many gas molecules dissolve, but immediately a few escape from solution. As time goes on, the rate changes until as many molecules are escaping as are going into solution. At this time the partial pressure of the dissolved gas would be equal to the partial pressure of the gas above the liquid. Increasing the partial pressure of the gas above the liquid will upset the equilibrium and cause more gas to dissolve, while a decrease in the partial pressure of the gas above the liquid will cause more to escape from solution. Or we can simply say a gas will flow from an area of high pressure to an area of low pressure.

In the Lungs (Figure 1-30)

$$PO_2 \text{ of inspired air} = 159 \text{ mm Hg}$$

$$PO_2 \text{ of alveolar air} = 104 \text{ mm Hg}$$

Therefore, oxygen passes from the inspired air to alveolar air.

$$PCO_2 \text{ of inspired air} = 0.30 \text{ mm Hg}$$

$$PCO_2 \text{ of alveolar air} = 40 \text{ mm Hg}$$

Therefore, carbon dioxide passes from alveolar air to inspired air.

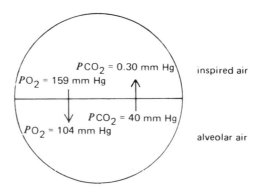

Figure 1-30.

In the Alveoli (Figure 1-31)

$$PO_2 \text{ in alveoli} = 104 \text{ mm Hg}$$

$$PO_2 \text{ in venous blood in capillaries} = 40 \text{ mm Hg}$$

Therefore, oxygen flows from the alveoli into the venous blood.

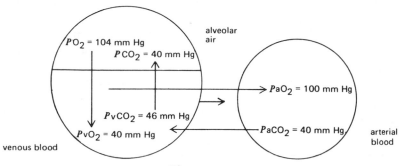

Figure 1-31.

$$PCO_2 \text{ in the alveoli } = 40 \text{ mm Hg}$$

$$PCO_2 \text{ in venous blood } = 46 \text{ mm Hg}$$

Therefore, carbon dioxide passes from venous blood to the alveoli after the venous blood has picked up oxygen from the alveoli and has also lost the carbon dioxide to the alveoli; it becomes arterial blood with a PO_2 equal to 100 mm Hg and a PCO_2 equal to 40 mm Hg.

In the Tissues (Figure 1-32)

$$PO_2 \text{ of the arterial blood } = 100 \text{ mm Hg}$$

$$PO_2 \text{ in the tissues } = 30 \text{ mm Hg}$$

Therefore, oxygen passes from the blood to the tissues through the capillary membranes.

$$PCO_2 \text{ of the arterial blood } = 40 \text{ mm Hg}$$

$$PCO_2 \text{ in the tissues } = 50 \text{ mm Hg}$$

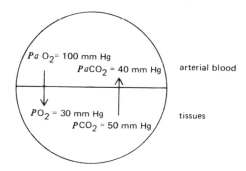

Figure 1-32.

Therefore, CO_2 flows from the tissues into the blood through the capillary membranes.

After the blood has left the tissues and started to return to the heart it becomes venous blood with a PO_2 equal to 40 mm Hg and a PCO_2 equal to 46 mm Hg.

The space surrounding the lungs, the pleural cavity, is at a slightly lower pressure than the lungs themselves. Since the pressure is greater in the lungs, they remain inflated (see Figure 1-33).

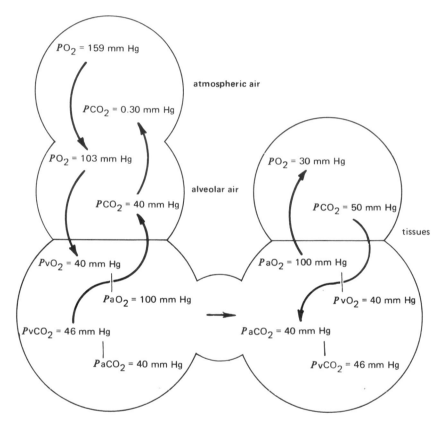

Figure 1-33. Summary diagram of the application of gas laws to respiration.

Mechanics of Respiration

We can use Henry's law to explain how oxygen and carbon dioxide go into solution. By increasing the partial pressure of the gas above a liquid, more gas will dissolve. In a like manner, by decreasing the partial pressure of the gas above a liquid, gas will escape from the liquid. In other words, a gas will flow from an area of high pressure to an area of low pressure. To better understand this, we will trace these flows through the lungs, alveoli, and tissues. See Table 1-10.

When this exchange of oxygen and carbon dioxide has taken place, the venous blood, as a result of losing carbon dioxide, becomes arterial blood. The PO_2 of arterial blood is approximately 100 mm Hg and the PCO_2 approximately 40 mm Hg.

Once the blood leaves the tissues and begins to return to the heart, it again becomes venous blood.

TABLE 1-10   Flow of Oxygen and Carbon Dioxide Through Lungs, Alveoli, and Tissues

Lungs

Inspired air	PO_2 = 159 mm Hg	Oxygen will pass into the
Alveolar air	PO_2 = 104 mm Hg ↓	alveolar air to maintain equilibrium
Inspired air	PCO_2 = 0.3 mm Hg	Carbon dioxide will pass
Alveolar air	PCO_2 = 40 mm Hg ↑	into the inspired air to maintain equilibrium
Alveolar air	PO_2 = 104 mm Hg	Oxygen will pass into the
Venous blood	PO_2 = 40 mm Hg ↓	venous blood in the capillaries to maintain equilibrium
Alveolar air	PCO_2 = 40 mm Hg	Carbon dioxide will pass
Venous blood	PCO_2 = 46 mm Hg ↑	into the alveolar air to maintain equilibrium

Tissues

Arterial blood	PO_2 = 100 mm Hg	Oxygen will pass from
Tissues	PO_2 = 30 mm Hg ↓	the arterial blood into the tissues
Arterial blood	PCO_2 = 40 mm Hg	Carbon dioxide will pass
Tissues	PCO_2 = 50 mm Hg ↑	from the tissues into the arterial blood

Summary

Pulmonary Respiration

Inspired air	PO_2 = 159 mm Hg	PCO_2 = 0.3 mm Hg
Alveolar air	PO_2 = 104 mm Hg ↓	PCO_2 = 40 mm Hg ↑
Venous blood	PO_2 = 40 mm Hg ↓	PCO_2 = 46 mm Hg ↑
Arterial blood	PO_2 = 100 mm Hg	PCO_2 = 40 mm Hg

Tissue Respiration

Arterial blood	PO_2 = 100 mm Hg	PCO_2 = 40 mm Hg
Venous blood	PO_2 = 40 mm Hg ↓	PCO_2 = 46 mm Hg ↑
Tissues	PO_2 = 30 mm Hg	PCO_2 = 50 mm Hg

All values are approximate. Arrows indicate the direction of the flow.

FLUID AND ELECTROLYTE BALANCE: HOMEOSTASIS

This brief study of fluids and electrolytes is important to the respiratory therapist because we are frequently called upon to evaluate humidification devices being used for patient care. In addition, we are involved in the care of patients with tracheostomies and/or endotracheal tubes; these patients have lost approximately 70 to 80% of their ability to humidify their inspired air. It is therefore most important that we understand patient humidification and electrolyte balance. To our patients, fluid and electrolyte balance may mean the difference between a state of well being or a state of discomfort, distress, coma, and even death. All human beings depend on a homeostatic state (a state of balance) of fluid and electrolytes, and the cells of our bodies depend on this proper steady balance to sustain life. It is imperative first that you review the chemical terms and their concepts listed at the end of this chapter.

To provide the therapist with the basic principles of fluid and electrolyte physiology and pathology, in this section we will discuss the major concepts of the following:

1. *Body water*—volume, composition, function, and distribution.
2. *Electrolytes*—distribution and function.
3. *Water and electrolyte exchange* between the fluid compartments.
4. *Mechanisms* that regulate water and electrolyte balance.

Total Body Water (TBW)

Sixty to seventy percent of body weight is composed of water (30 to 40% is composed of solids).

Note: Although the above percentages pertain to the "ideal size and weight of a man," *it must be remembered that body fat is essentially water free.* Therefore, the thinner individual will have more fluid per pound of weight than the fat individual. *Men and women vary in the amount of water their bodies contain.* Women's bodies are composed of a larger amount of fat; therefore, an estimation of a woman's percentage of water is between 50 and 54%, and the solid percentage is estimated at between 46 and 50% solids. *Infants and young adults vary in the percentage of water contained in their bodies.* Until about one year of age, the infant has the highest proportion of body water. Young male adults average about 63% of body weight and about 52% for females. *Age is another factor influencing* total body water. As the aging process takes place, body water gradually diminishes.

Water Balance. This balance depends on the proportion of water intake and output. Gains in water must equal water losses. If water overload occurs, a patient can literally drown in his body fluids. Likewise, if intake is lacking, dehydration can occur. The easiest and most accurate way to monitor water balance is to weigh patients daily. A weight change of 1 kilogram (2.2 pounds) equals a fluid loss or gain of 1 liter. *Body fluid*, that is, water plus electrolytes, is distributed between two fluid compartments.

1. Water within the cells (intracellular fluid compartment, ICF) represents about 70% of total body water, and this fluid gives the cells an internal water medium necessary for chemical function.
2. Water located outside the cells (extracellular fluid compartment, ECF) represents about 30% of total body water, and this fluid serves the body's transportation system as follows (ECF is composed of three different fluids, each having an individual function):
   a. *Interstitial fluid*—occupies the vascular space and the cells; gives the cells an external medium necessary for cell metabolism.
   b. *Plasma*—the liquid portion of blood; with the red blood cells it supports vascular volume (however, the red blood cells do not move out of the vascular compartment, and they do not move from one compartment to another).
   c. *Transcellular fluids*—the body's excretions and secretions (e.g., gastrointestinal juices, urine, saliva, and spinal fluid).

Water Gain and Loss. The greatest gain of water in the body occurs by ingestion—how much water and fluid we drink. In addition, another source is present but somewhat "hidden," that is, the water in solids that are ingested. Lean meats, fruits, and vegetables contain 60 to 90% water. Burning of solids also adds water to our systems; approximately 100 calories of fat, protein, and carbohydrates releases about 14 ml of water.

The greatest loss of water in the body is through the kidneys. The average water loss through this route is about 1500 ml/day. However, the loss of water via the kidneys changes with the amount of food ingested and the level of the antidiuretic hormone (ADH). As the name suggests, this hormone prevents the body from losing fluid under conditions such as surgery, trauma, and/or injury. During these conditions, ADH is released in large amounts and results in increased reabsorption of water. Therapists working in the recovery room or the trauma unit have noted that patients' volume of urine is decreased and is usually more concentrated. Overeating and diabetes mellitus cause the kidneys to excrete enough urine to carry the solids (solutes) to the bladder.

As therapists you should also be aware of some of the conditions and factors that inhibit ADH release and increase diuresis. Increased water load, increased blood volume, alcohol, CO_2 inhalation, diuretics, and diabetes insipidus are some. In the latter, the condition is caused by the lack of ADH production, characterized by extreme thirst and a high fluid intake, resulting in the voiding of large amounts of urine per day.

The other hormone regulator of fluid and electrolyte balance is known as aldosterone. However, aldosterone, instead of being a conserver of water in the body, conserves sodium (Na^+). Since sodium retains fluid in the body, aldosterone, like ADH, becomes a conserver of water in the body.

Water is also lost through the lungs, skin and gastrointestinal tract. The latter water loss is normally very small. Do not confuse water loss from the lungs and skin with sweating (visible water loss). The loss of water from the lungs is eliminated in the vapor of our breath and in the normal moisture that forms on our skin. However, these *insensible water losses* become greatly increased when there is fever or an increase in respiratory rate as in pneumonia. Hot and dry environments will also increase insensible water loss. Respiratory therapists can aid in assessing insensible water loss by keeping accurate patient records regarding rate and depth of respiration, and noting and recording observable water loss such as diaphoresis.

Electrolytes

Whenever a person is ill, the fluid and electrolyte balance is disturbed. Usually the normal daily requirements of electrolytes are increased owing to the stress caused by illness. Therefore, it is necessary for therapists to have some basic knowledge regarding electrolytes, their function, measurement, and concentrations within the body.

The major *cations* of blood serum are sodium (Na^+), potassium (K^+), calcium (Ca^{++}), and magnesium (Mg^{++}).

The major *anions* of blood serum are chloride (Cl^-), bicarbonate (HCO_3^-), phosphate and sulfate (HPO_4^{--}, SO_4^{--}), organic acids, and proteins.

The average total of the concentration of all the cations in blood serum is 150 mEq/liter; the anion concentration must be the same to have a neutral or homeostatic situation within the body.

Electrolytes perform the following physiologic functions in the body:

1. Assist and promote neuromuscular irritability.
2. Help maintain body fluid osmolarity.
3. Regulate H^+ balance.
4. Assist in the distribution of body fluids between the fluid compartments.

The electrolytes in body fluids are expressed in terms of their chemical activity, that is, in milliequivalents per liter (mEq/liter). In the average healthy person the milliequivalents per liter for plasma electrolytes will vary only in a narrow range.

The following are the commonly reported approximate normal values, and basic information regarding each will be discussed.

1. Sodium: 136 to 145 mEq/l.
2. Potassium: 3.8 to 4.5 mEq/l.
3. Calcium: 4.5 to 5.5 mEq/l.
4. Magnesium: 1.5 to 2.5 mEq/l.
5. Chloride: 100 to 106 mEq/l.
6. Bicarbonate: 24 to 31 mEq/l.

Sodium (Na^+). Sodium is found in all fluid compartments; however, most of the sodium is found outside the cells (extracellular). Sodium is the principal cation outside the cell. It regulates fluid volume within the fluid compartments, and, as a result, regulates the size of the compartments. Sodium increases cell membrane permeability, acts as a buffer in conjunction with bicarbonate and phosphate, aids in conduction of nerve impulses, controls body water distribution, and aids in controlling muscle contractility (especially the heart muscle).

The "normal" male of 70 kg (approximately 154 lb) contains 2700 to 3000 mEq of Na^+. A person normally needs 4.5 g of Na^+/day, which is met by a normal diet with salt added to food. Under normal conditions, the sodium level is chiefly regulated through the kidneys.

Potassium (K^+). Potassium is the most important cation inside the cell (intracellular) and is the most abundant cation in the body. It is involved with the conduction of nerve impulses, and is essential for the normal functioning of nerve cells. Potassium is the chief regulator of intracellular or osmolarity and electron neutrality. It also helps to promote proper heart muscle activity.

The body of a normal 154-lb male contains about 3500 mEq of K^+. A normal adult requires 40 mEq of K^+/day. Potassium excretion is predominantly by the kidneys.

Calcium (Ca^{++}). Approximately 99% of the total body calcium is concentrated in the bone. A small fraction of calcium is present in other tissues and in the extracellular fluid. Calcium decreases neuromuscular irritability and decreases capillary membrane permeability. It is necessary for adequate transmission of nerve impulses and is essential to blood clotting time.

Calcium is *not* available in large amounts in our natural foods. *Milk* and *milk products* contribute the greatest amount of calcium, which is needed for building and repairing bones and teeth. Approximate daily calcium requirements vary as follows:

Adults	0.8 to 6 g/day
Children	0.7 to 1.4 g/day
Pregnant and lactating women	1.3 to 1.5 g/day

Calcium is excreted in the urine.

Magnesium (Mg^{++}). The average adult contains 20 g of magnesium; 50% is stored in bone cells, and 49% is distributed in the cells of the liver, heart, and skeletal muscles. Extracellular fluid contains only approximately 1%, and most of this is in the cerebrospinal fluid. Daily requirements vary as follows:

Adults	250 mg
Children	150 mg
Pregnant and lactating women	400 mg

Magnesium is abundant in foods, especially in green plants. It is essential for the functional integrity of the neuromuscular system, on which it has a sedative action. The neuromuscular system is antagonized by calcium. Magnesium activates the enzymes necessary for carbohydrate metabolism.

Most magnesium is excreted in feces; a very small amount is eliminated by the kidneys.

Chloride (Cl⁻).   Chloride is the chief anion of extracellular fluid. Chloride intake occurs when salt (sodium chloride) is added to food, and requirements are approximately the same as for sodium. Chloride has an important role in the osmolarity of respiratory gases in the blood in the occurrence of the chloride shift. Chloride is excreted mainly by the kidneys, chiefly as sodium chloride.

Bicarbonate (HCO$_3^-$).   The diagnosis of metabolic acidosis and metabolic alkalosis is often made from the bicarbonate level in plasma.

$$\text{Normal level } = 24 \text{ to } 31 \text{ mEq/l}$$

Water and Electrolyte Exchange Between the Fluid Compartments

To understand fluid and electrolyte movement, it will be necessary to discuss two subjects, (1) the transportation of fluid and electrolytes between the intracellular and extracellular fluid compartments, and (2) the transportation of fluids between the interstitial fluid compartment and the vascular compartment. *Osmolarity* and *active transport* are two systems involved in the flow of fluid and electrolytes between the ICF and ECF compartments. Osmolarity is the term used to indicate the gram molecular weight of a solute in each liter of solution. Or, to rephrase, osmolarity simply means the number of dissolved particles per liter. When two solutions containing different osmolarities (different concentrations of dissolved particles per liter) are separated by a membrane that is permeable to water, the distribution of water changes, so that the two solutions become equal. In other words, water moves from an area of lesser concentration of particles (solute) to an area of greater concentration of particles in an effort to dilute the greater concentration. As a result, the two solutions will develop equal osmolarities. The physician utilizes the serum Na⁺ level to indirectly measure the osmolarity of the plasma. There is also another mechanism known as the *sodium pump* that allows Na⁺ and other cations to move from the cell to the extracellular fluid. As a result, the body does not have to depend solely on water transport to maintain equilibrium. This process is known as active transport, and avoids the shrinking of some cells and the swelling of other cells, which would otherwise eventually occur if only the water shifted compartments.

Fluid Transport Between the Interstitial Fluid Compartment and the Vascular Compartment.   Plasma proteins (anions) are for the most part found in the intravascular compartment (blood). The capillary membrane is not freely permeable to these large particles, and therefore the normal level of plasma proteins in the blood remains high—in the range of 6 to 8 g percent. Because plasma normally has a greater osmolarity than interstitial fluid, it has a greater ability to attract and hold water. If, for some reason, the plasma osmolarity is reduced, decreased blood volume and edema result.

The maintenance of blood volume depends on three factors:

1. Blood hydrostatic pressure (BHP).
2. Colloid osmotic pressure or oncotic pressure (OP).
3. Filtration pressure (FP).

Blood hydrostatic pressure is the pressure of the blood cells and plasma in the capillaries produced by the pumping action of the heart. Pressure differences within the capillary serve to push and pull fluid. BHP in the arteriolar end of the capillary is 32 mm Hg; therefore, fluid is pushed into the tissue spaces. BHP in the veins (venular end) of the capillary is 12 mm Hg; therefore, fluid is pulled back into the capillary from the tissue space. This pressure is influenced by the level of the arterial blood pressure, the rate of the flow of blood through the capillaries, and the venous pressure. You will recall from physiology that there are factors that can alter the three influencing factors above, such as blood volume, heart rate, blood viscosity, vessel size, respiration, and the condition of the veins.

Another influence on the transportation of fluids between the interstitial and vascular compartments is colloid osmotic pressure, the pressure exerted by the plasma proteins. This pressure works in opposition to the hydrostatic pressure; it tends to hold back water that is escaping from the capillaries. Normal colloid osmotic pressure is 22 mm Hg.

Filtration pressure is another factor in the transportation of fluids between the interstitial and vascular compartments and is equal to the BHP minus the colloid osmotic pressure. In the arteriolar end of the capillary, the filtration pressure is a positive pressure, resulting in fluid being forced out of the capillaries into the tissues. In the venular end of the capillary, filtration pressure is a negative pressure, resulting in fluid being pulled back into the capillary from the tissues. To illustrate, whenever pulmonary edema occurs it indicates that an increase has occurred in the BHP, the colloid osmotic pressure becomes subjected to pressure beyond what it can exert, and thus fluid is pushed into the tissues. When the BHP decreases, the colloid osmotic pressure is able to absorb the fluid back into the blood stream.

Mechanisms That Regulate Water and Electrolyte Balance

The endocrine system plays an important role in controlling fluid and electrolyte balance. We have already discussed two hormones from this system, ADH (the antidiuretic hormone), which prevents the body from losing fluid under certain conditions, and aldosterone, the body's guardian against sodium (Na^+) loss, resulting in water retention. Two other hormones, the thyroid hormone and the diuretic hormone are involved in water and electrolyte balance; however, their role is to increase and promote water loss (diuresis). The gastrointestinal tract assimilates our intake of fluid and electrolytes. This total volume, including glandular and gastrointestinal tract secretions, is estimated to be about 7500 to 10,000 ml/day. However, out of this large volume of fluid, a very small amount of water is lost in feces and a very minute amount of electrolytes. The majority of fluid and electrolytes is reabsorbed by the intestinal mucosa. Osmotic equilibrium is established and maintained between the gastrointestinal tract and extracellular water by rapid bidirectional transfer across the intestinal mucosa. Considering this large volume of fluid and electrolytes, it is not difficult to understand why a very minimum gastrointestinal upset would cause a disturbance of fluid and electrolyte balance.

As respiratory therapists, we are already aware of the lungs' role in homeostasis. The lungs regulate the O_2 and CO_2 levels of the blood. Carbon dioxide is derived from the carbonic acid in the blood; therefore, the lungs serve as an important balance between acids and alkalies in the extracellular fluid. The kidneys, however, are known as the master mechanisms in maintaining homeostasis. It is the *nephron* in the kidneys, of which there are many, that aids in removing waste material from the blood, produces urines, and aids in controlling the acid–base balance in the body. The kidneys literally "sort out" electrolytes as they pass in the blood through the filtering areas of the kidney, eliminating all except those that the body requires and needs. The heart, linked closely to the kidneys, pumps about 1700 to 1800 liters of blood daily to the kidneys for cleansing and purification. Approximately 180 liters of this blood is filtered through the kidneys and only 1.5 liters is excreted as urine, the remainder is reabsorbed. One can readily comprehend the importance of good kidney function, and understand that, if the kidneys malfunction even for a short period of time, fluid and electrolyte balance is impaired. Cardiovascular problems, such as congestive heart failure, and hypertension affect kidney function and result in fluid and electrolyte imbalance.

It will be necessary for us as therapists to read, study, and become more familiar with body fluid and electrolytes. The list of clinical problems in which body fluid disturbance exists is growing: the burn patient, congestive heart failure patients, the patient undergoing surgery, the ventilator patient, and many others. These are the patients we take care of and are involved with every day. The early diagnosis of fluid and electrolyte imbalance depends often upon the close observation of the patient. You, as respiratory therapists, share this responsibility with nurses and physicians; therefore, you are also accountable.

Table 1-11 lists signs and symptoms of electrolyte deficits and excesses as well as their major causes. These may assist you in the assessment of your patients.

Protein Metabolism

Proteins cannot be manufactured within the body. The protein necessary for building muscle and tissues is constantly being used by the body cells to maintain themselves. Therefore, it is essential that each individual consume in his daily diet a certain amount of protein substance so that protein malnutrition does not develop. Protein deficiency may also develop from hemorrhage, draining wounds, and/or decubitus ulcers, severe burns, trauma, and the aftermath of a fracture(s).

Symptoms of Protein Deficiency

Fatigue
Soft, flabby muscles
Pallor
Emotional depression
Gradual loss of weight
Decreased resistance to infection

Therapists can be of help to the physician by carefully noting and evaluating patients' daily dietary intake. You can make your respiratory rounds during mealtimes and ask your patient questions about his diet. Is he satisfied with his diet? Is he eating his entire meal or just his dessert? You can explain to him that his surgical wound will heal more rapidly if his protein intake is satisfactory.

TABLE 1-11 Changes in Composition of Extracellular Fluid

Sodium DEFICIT Symptoms	*Sodium EXCESS Symptoms*
1. Apprehension; sometimes a patient states he feels "impending doom"	1. Dry, sticky mucous membranes
	2. Flushed skin
	3. Intense thirst
2. Abdominal cramps	4. Oliguria
3. Convulsions	5. Anuria
4. Oliguria	6. Increasing temperature
5. Anuria	7. Rough, dry tongue
6. Rapid, thready pulse	
7. Cold, clammy skin; sometimes accompanied with cyanosis	

Causes of Sodium DEFICIT	*Causes of Sodium EXCESS*
1. Decreased intake or increased sodium output	1. Decreased water intake
2. Increased intake or decreased water output	2. Oversalting
3. Heat exhaustion	3. Tracheobronchitis due to increased breathing and increased fever causing increased loss of water via lungs
4. Excessive sweating	4. Watery diarrhea
5. Gastrointestinal suctioning	5. Saltwater near-drowning
6. Diuretics	
7. Freshwater near-drowning	

Potassium DEFICIT Symptoms	*Potassium EXCESS Symptoms*
1. *Early* symptoms may be rather vague; i.e., general malaise or patient may complain of "just not feeling well"	1. *Early:* irritability, nausea, diarrhea
2. *Later* generalized weakness of skeletal muscles	2. *Later:* weakness, paralysis, difficulty in speaking, difficulty in breathing, oliguria progressing to anuria, cardiac arrhythmia resulting in cardiac arrest
3. Decrease or absence of reflexes	
4. Muscles become "flabby"	
5. When condition involves the heart muscle, the patient may have a weak pulse and a decrease in blood pressure	
6. When deficit involves the GI tract, patient may develop vomiting and distention of the intestines	
7. When involving the respiratory muscles, the patient may demonstrate shallow and decreasing respirations	
8. Increased thirst	

TABLE 1-11   (continued)

Causes of Potassium DEFICIT	Causes of Potassium EXCESS
1. Potent diuretics	1. History usually reveals burns or crushing injuries
2. Vomiting, diarrhea	2. Kidney disease
3. Ulcerative colitis	3. Adrenal insufficiency
4. Diabetes acidosis	4. Kidney damage due to mercuric bichloride poisoning
5. Severe burns	

Calcium DEFICIT Symptoms	Calcium EXCESS Symptoms
1. Tingling of the ends of the fingers	1. Hypertonicity of the muscles
2. Tetany	2. Flank pain
3. Muscle cramps	3. Deep bone pain
4. Abdominal cramps	4. Bone cavity pain
5. Convulsions	5. Kidney stones

Causes of Calcium DEFICIT	Causes of Calcium EXCESS
1. Hypoactive parathyroid gland	1. Tumor of the parathyroid gland
2. Massive subcutaneous injections	2. Large doses of vitamin D (example: arthritic treatment)
3. Peritonitis	3. Hyperactivity of the parathyroid glands
4. Removal of the parathyroid gland surgically	4. Multiple myelomas

Magnesium DEFICIT Symptoms	Magnesium EXCESS Symptoms
1. Tremors	1. Warm sensation all through the body
2. Hyperactive deep reflexes	2. Paralysis similar to curare-like medications
3. Positive Chvostek sign	3. Falling blood pressure
4. Convulsions	4. Respiratory embarrassment
5. Confusion, hallucinations	5. Cardiac arrhythmias leading to cardiac arrest
6. Rising blood pressure	
7. Tachycardia	

Causes of Magnesium DEFICIT	Causes of Magnesium EXCESS
1. Chronic and severe malnutrition	1. Renal insufficiency causing magnesium retention
2. Chronic alcoholism with delirium tremens	2. Severe dehydration in which patient develops oliguria and retains magnesium
3. Chronic nephritis	3. Increased usage of antacids that are high in magnesium
4. Prolonged, severe diarrhea	
5. Hypoparathyroidism	
6. Intestinal malabsorption	

This is an area in which you can utilize the holistic approach to patient care. It is not only the job of the hospital dietician and/or nurse to demonstrate interest in the patients' daily intake. This is one aspect of fluid and electrolyte balance in which you play an important role. Whenever the amount of plasma proteins is decreased and is below normal, retention of fluids can occur due to the blood's decreased colloidal osmotic pressure. Fluid from the vascular system flows into the tissues, thus causing edema.

The Hydrogen Ion

Although hydrogen is present in very small quantities in the extracellular fluid, its role is extremely important to health.

If hydrogen increases (pH decreases), the extracellular fluid becomes acid (acidosis).

If hydrogen decreases (pH increases), the extracellular fluid becomes alkaline (alkalosis).

In the extracellular fluid, carbonic acid is formed when CO_2 combines with water.

Cations, such as Na^+, K^+, Ca^{++} and Mg^{++}, combine with the HCO_3^- anion, forming base bicarbonate.

This ratio of carbonic acid to the base bicarbonate of extracellular fluid regulates the concentration of the hydrogen ions; the hydrogen ion concentration is considered normal when there is 1 meq of carbonic acid for each 20 meq of base bicarbonate.

If the carbonic acid increases or base bicarbonate decreases, acidosis results.

If the base bicarbonate increases or carbonic acid decreases, alkalosis results.

Two types of disturbance can result: (1) metabolic (systemic), which affects the base bicarbonate level, and (2) respiratory, which affects the carbonic acid level.

Base Bicarbonate Deficit

1. Known as metabolic acidosis
2. Associated with diabetic ketosis and renal acidosis
3. Caused by decrease in the amount of base bicarbonate as in:
   a. Diabetic acidosis
   b. Renal insufficiency
   c. Systemic infection

4. Symptoms are as follows:
    a. Stupor
    b. Deep rapid breathing (Kussmaul respiration)
    c. Dyspnea on exertion
    d. Weakness
    e. When very severe, unconsciousness may develop

Base Bicarbonate Excess

1. Known as metabolic alkalosis
2. Caused by:
    a. Loss of gastric juices following gastrointestinal suctioning
    b. Vomiting
    c. Chronic ingestion of potent diuretics
3. Symptoms:
    a. Hypertonicity of muscles
    b. Tetany
    c. Decreasing respirations

Carbonic Acid Deficit

1. Known as respiratory alkalosis
2. Caused by:
    a. Lack of oxygen
    b. Fever
    c. Anxiety and emotional states
3. Symptoms:
    a. Tetany
    b. Convulsions
    c. Unconsciousness

Carbonic Acid Excess

1. Known as respiratory acidosis
2. Caused by:
    a. Pneumonia
    b. Emphysema
    c. Asthma
    d. Morphine and barbiturate poisoning
3. Symptoms:
    a. Disorientation
    b. Respiratory embarrassment
    c. Weakness
    d. Coma

Note: Continue with pulmonary physiology to determine if the condition is a result of metabolic acidosis or alkalosis, respiratory acidosis or alkalosis, or kidney or pulmonary compensatory mechanisms.

Terms Related to Fluid and Electrolytes

ADH.   Antidiuretic hormone secreted by the pituitary gland, located in the brain.

Aldosterone.   Hormone that is an inhibitor of renal sodium (Na^+) excretion; is secreted by the adrenal glands.

Anion.   Negatively charged ions; e.g., chloride (Cl^-), bicarbonate (HCO_3^-), phosphate (HPO_4^-), sulfate (SO_4^-).

Atom.   Smallest particle of a chemical element that can exist alone or in combination.

Blood hydrostatic pressure.   Pressure of the blood cells and plasma in the capillaries.

Cation.   Positively charged ions; e.g., sodium (Na^+), calcium (Ca^+), potassium (K^+).

Chloride shift.   Buffering activity in which a chloride ion leaves a red blood cell for each bicarbonate ion entering, or in which a chloride ion enters a red blood cell for each bicarbonate ion leaving it in order to maintain electroneutrality.

Colloid osmotic pressure, oncotic pressure (OP).   Pressure that results from dispersed colloid particles.

Electrolytes.   Substances that dissociate into ions or electrically charged particles when placed in water; electrolytes in body fluid are derived from minerals contained in the foods we eat.

Extracellular fluid.   Water in the spaces between the cells (approximately 30% of total body water).

Filtration pressure (FP).   Transfer of water and dissolved substances through a permeable membrane from a region of high pressure to a region of low pressure.

Hyperkalemia.   Increase in serum potassium.

Hypokalemia.   Decrease in serum potassium.

Hypervolemia.   Increase in body water; ADH release is stopped and aldosterone is not secreted, resulting in an increase of urination and no thirst, resulting in body fluid becoming normal.

Hypovolemia.   Decrease in body water; ADH is released, increasing thirst, resulting in more fluid intake, less urination, and more concentration of urine; aldosterone is released, sodium is conserved water is held in body, resulting in normal water balance.

Interstitial.   Outside of the cells within the tissue spaces.

Intracellular fluid.   Water and electrolytes within the cells; approximately 70% of total body water.

Ion. Electrically charged particle or group of atoms.

Kilogram (kg). Unit of weight in the metric system.

Liter (l). Measure of volume.

Milliequivalent (mEq). Measure of the chemical activity or chemical combining power of an ion.

Milliliter (ml). Cubic centimeter (cc) fluid.

Millimole. 1/1000 of a mole.

mole. Molecular weight of a substance in grams.

Nonelectrolyte. Undissociated substances, such as urea, dextrose, and creatinine.

Osmolarity. Indicates the gram molecular weight of a solute in each liter of solution; used in volume analysis to determine concentration of solutes.

EXERCISES

1. List three ways the body gains water, and discuss those hormones involved in the loss of water from the body.
2. List the major cations and anions of blood serum.
3. What physiologic function do electrolytes perform in the body?
4. Identify those patients assigned to your care today who might develop a fluid and electrolyte imbalance.
5. Discuss homeostasis as related to fluid and electrolyte balance.

MICROBIOLOGY

I. Definition of terms

    A. *Aerobe*—an organism that grows best in the presence of oxygen.

    B. *Anaerobe*—an organism that is able to grow without air or oxygen.

    C. *Antibiosis*—an association between two dissimilar organisms that is harmful to one or both.

    D. *Bacteria*—minute, one-celled miscroscopic organisms; they possess some characteristics of both plants and animals.

    E. *Binary fission*—simple cell division.

    F. *Capsule*—a colorless layer, either mucoid or gelatinous, that surrounds some bacteria.

G. *Commensalism*—the living together of two species; one of the species benefits, while one is neither benefited nor harmed.

H. *Colony*—a group of bacteria on a solid medium, usually the result of multiplication of a single organism; is visible without a microscope.

I. *Flagella*—a whiplike process found on some bacteria; used for motility.

J. *Flora*—the permanent bacterial life of a specific area; for example, in the human body, "the flora of the respiratory tract."

K. *Fungus*—a many-celled plant that lacks chlorophyll; reproduction is primarily by spores.

L. *Hemolysis*—destruction of red blood cells, resulting in the freeing of hemoglobin.

M. *Motility*—the ability to move from one place to another.

N. *Nonpathogen*—a microorganism or material that does not produce a disease.

O. *Nosocomial*—pertaining to a hospital or infirmary; for example, a nosocomial infection would be one acquired in a hospital.

P. *Parasite*—a plant or animal that lives on or in another living organism and benefits from that organism, but does not give anything in return.

Q. *Pathogen*—a disease-producing microorganism or material.

R. *Pyogenic*—pus-forming.

S. *Saprophyte*—an organism that lives on dead organic matter.

T. *Symbiosis*—the living together of two dissimilar organisms, each benefiting from the other.

II. Classification of bacteria

A. Nomenclature—organisms are classified as a means of reference and so that they can be differentiated from others. The general areas of classification are:

1. *Species*—a group in which all members have some characteristics which identify them as members of that particular group and no other

2. *Genus*—a group of similar species

3. *Family*—a group of similar genera

      4. *Order*—a group of similar families

      5. *Class*—a group of similar orders

  B. Common bacterial shapes

      1. *Bacilli*—rod-shaped organisms

      2. *Cocci*—spherical organisms

      3. *Spirilla*—comma-shaped or spiralled; move about

  C. Other means of classification

      1. Chemical composition

      2. Biochemical properties

      3. Physiology

      4. Pathogenic properties

      5. Metabolism

III. Patterns of growth of bacteria

  A. Bacteria increase in number, but not necessarily in size.

  B. *Generation time*—the time it takes an organism to divide in two; varies from 20 minutes to 20 hours depending on the organism.

  C. Growth patterns that may be observed after inoculation of bacteria into a culture medium.

      1. *Lag phase*—a period of adjustment during which little or no multiplication of bacteria occurs

      2. *Logarithmic phase*—period of maximum growth; generation time is constant; reproduction is accomplished by binary fission

      3. *Stationary phase*—death of bacteria occurs at a rate equal to the rate of multiplication

      4. *Death phase*—growth rate steadily declines, while death rate becomes constant

IV. Conditions necessary for bacterial growth

  A. Nutrition—specific to that species.

B. Humidity—necessary for chemical activity, elimination of waste products; composes a large portion of the cell's protoplasm.

C. Temperature—although there are minimum and maximum temperatures at which organisms will grow (usually 0 to 90°C), the optimum temperature is that best suited for growth and varies according to species; the temperature range for most bacterial *survival* is −250° to 160°C.

D. Inorganic salts such as potassium, sodium, phosphorus, chlorine, magnesium, calcium, and sulfur are required to a varying extent by most bacteria.

V. Other growth factors

A. Oxygen—requirements vary from those organisms that require free oxygen for growth (obligate aerobes) to those that cannot grow when any free oxygen is present (obligate anaerobes).

B. Light—most bacteria grow only in the absence of diffused or direct sunlight.

C. Carbon dioxide—some species find this gas necessary for growth.

D. The pH of the medium—while most pathogens grow best at a neutral pH, some bacteria grow best at slightly acid or very acid conditions.

VI. Forms of growth

A. True bacteria divide by binary fission or simple cell division of the cytoplasm and nucleus into two equal parts.

B. *Colony formation*—a group of bacteria, which are all of one kind, having been formed from the reproduction of a single bacterial cell. Colonies are visible to the naked eye. Color, among other properties, may be used for identification purposes.

C. *Spores*—some bacilli are able to form hard, thick-walled granules within the bacterial cell as a method of surviving unfavorable conditions for growth and development. The spores contain the essential portions of the cytoplasm and render it highly resistant to heat, drought, and chemicals.

D. *Bacterial variation*—as with humans, who inherit certain characteristics from their parents, bacteria "inherit" certain characteristics of the species. At some point, however, these distinguishing features may be lost, resulting in a *mutant* or variant. This variation may result in an increased resistance to unfavorable conditions, or increased pathogenicity; the opposite may also be true.

VII. Chemical identification of bacteria—various stains may be used for identification of microorganisms, making it possible to see them under a microscope so that their structure may be studied. The fact that certain bacteria retain a particular stain, while others do not, aids in the identification process.

A. *Gram's differential stain*—probably the most widely used, as well as the most useful. After a slide has been prepared, dried, and fixed, it is flooded with gentian violet. This remains in place for 60 sec, at the end of which time the slide is washed off and flushed with an iodine solution, which remains in place for another 60 sec. The iodine is then washed off. Ninety-five percent alcohol is used for 15 to 30 sec, as a decolorizing agent. The slide may then be counterstained with Bismarck brown or a similar dye.

1. Organisms that take on the color of the counterstain are called gram-negative organisms.

2. Those that are not decolorized by the alcohol are referred to as gram-positive organisms.

B. *Acid-fast (Ziehl–Neelsen) stain*—specifically for the identification of the causative organisms of leprosy and tuberculosis. Carbolfuchsin, a red dye, cannot be removed from the organisms despite an application of a solution of alcohol and 3% hydrochloric acid. For this reason, these organisms are termed acid-fast. The alcohol decolorizes all other organisms.

C. Other stains may be used to identify such characteristics as

1. Capsules

2. Spores

3. Flagella

VIII. Culture media

A. The material in which microorganisms are nourished and, therefore, reproduce is known as the culture medium. The medium used for each species varies according to its nutritional requirements.

B. Classifications

1. According to composition

a. *Nonsynthetic*—made from plant and animal products

b. *Synthetic*—chemical substances with definite components; usually contain nitrogen, carbohydrates, minerals and vitamins

2. According to physical states
   a. *Liquid*—for example, a meat broth to which no agar has been added
   b. *Semiliquid*—a medium to which only a small amount of agar has been added
   c. *Solid*—a medium to which enough agar, gelatin, or albumin has been added to cause it to solidify
   d. *Liquefiable solid*—a medium that upon heating becomes liquefied
   e. *Dehydrated*—a dried, powdered form of medium that is reconstituted by distilled water

3. Other
   a. *Selective media*—those to which agents such as dyes have been added, the purpose of which is to inhibit the growth of some bacteria while not affecting the growth of others; may be used as an identification factor
   b. *Differential media*—those to which, for example, an acid indicator has been added in an attempt to identify those bacteria that produce acids as a by-product.
   c. *Blood agar*—a solid medium containing animal blood and agar

IX. Microorganisms involved in respiratory infections
   A. The following is a partial list of those microorganisms that are considered respiratory tract pathogens:
      1. Gram-negative bacilli—of primary concern; non-spore forming; reproduce rapidly.
         a. *Klebsiella pneumoniae*
         b. *Hemophilus influenzae*
         c. *Pseudomonas* species
         d. *Bordetella pertussis*
      2. Gram-negative cocci
         a. *Neisseria meningitidis*
      3. Gram-positive bacilli
         a. *Corynebacterium diphtheriae*
      4. Gram-positive cocci
         a. *Beta-hemolytic Streptococcus*, group A (especially *Streptococcus pyogenes*)

b. *Diplococcus pneumoniae*
c. *Staphylococcus aureus*
   5. Acid-fast bacilli
      a. *Mycobacterium tuberculosis*
   6. Fungi
      a. *Candida albicans*
      b. *Aspergillus* species
   B. It is important to keep in mind that even those organisms that are generally considered nonpathogenic, given the right set of circumstances (e.g., a debilitated patient, especially with surgical wounds or tracheostomy), could be a source of infection.
   C. Nosocomial (hospital acquired) infections greatly increase the length of a patient's hospital stay. Many of these infections could be avoided if the staff carried out proper technique, especially procedures as basic as handwashing. Many of the organisms responsible for nosocomial infections have developed resistance to the more common drugs used for treatment. As a result, more potent antibiotics, with a much greater potential for adverse reactions, must be employed.

INTRODUCTION TO MEDICAL TERMINOLOGY

Medical terminology is certainly a mystery to those who are uninformed. The purpose of this portion of the text is to remove part of this mystery and provide you with terminology related to respiratory care. However, it is not intended to replace a good medical dictionary. You will continue your education in medical terms each day of your lives on-the-job, while you are pursuing your respiratory career. It is well to remember that all medical personnel communicate vital information to each other constantly, directly through conversations and oral reports and indirectly through written reports. If a physician uses an abbreviation and/or a symbol in his written order for respiratory care to his patient, the therapist must be well acquainted with what the orders mean and be careful to follow them correctly. Other health members communicate via medical terms in order to provide care to patients. Most important, your ability to interpret correctly will also aid rapport with and care of your patient. In addition, words and phrases have been included to aid you to approach your patient with a holistic view. As an example, heart terms are included, as often in the later stages of chronic obstructive disease the heart becomes involved. Terms involving diagnosis have been added, as your chest patient may be having problems with other parts of his body. All these terms will help you in your study and care of the total patient.

Terminology

Abacterial (ay″-back-teer′-ee-ul).   Without bacteria.

Abdominal breathing (ab-dom′-ĭ-nal brēth′-ing).   Alternate relaxation (inspiration) and contraction (expiration) of abdominal muscles, allowing diaphragm to descend fully and the entire lung to expand.

Abduction (ab-duk′-shun).   Movement of a part away from the midline.

ABG.   Arterial blood gases.

Absolute humidity.   The mass of water vapor per unit volume of air.

Absolute pressure.   Pressure in a container that would appear on an ordinary gauge plus the local atmospheric pressure of 15 psi.

Absolute temperature.   Temperature reckoned from the absolute zero, estimated at approximately −273°C or −459°F.

Absolute zero.   A temperature of approximately −273.2°C or −459.8°F; the complete absence of heat.

Acapnia (ah-kap′-ne-ah).   Condition of diminished CO_2 in blood.

Acid–base balance (as′-id bās bal′-ans).   Regulation of hydrogen-ion concentration in the body fluids.

Acidemia (as″-i-de′-me-ah).   Decreased pH of the blood irrespective of changes in blood bicarbonate.

Acid-fast (as′-id fast).   Not readily decolorized by acids or other means when stained; said of bacteria-tubercle bacillus.

Acidosis (as″-ĭ-do′-sis).   Indicates an acidemia or lowered blood bicarbonate with a tendency toward acidemia.

Acidotic (as-i-dot-ik).   Pertaining to or marked by acidosis.

Acute (uh-kute′).   Having a rapid onset, a short course, and pronounced symptoms.

Adduction (ah-duk′shun).   Movement of a part toward the midline.

Aeration (a″-er-a′-shun).   1. Arterialization of the venous blood in the lungs. 2. Changing of a liquid with air or gas.

Aerobic (a-er-o′-bik).   Growing only in the presence of molecular oxygen.

Aerosol (a′-er-o′-sol″).   Suspension of fine solid or liquid particles in air or a gas.

Aerosolization (a″-er-o-sol″-ĭ-za′-shun).   Process of dispensing in a fine mist.

Afebrile (a-feb′-ril).   Without fever.

Air (ār).   The gaseous mixture that makes up the earth's atmosphere.

Airway (ār′-wa).   Passage for a current of air.

Alkalemia (al″-kah-le′-me-ah). Increased pH of blood, irrespective of changes in blood bicarbonate.

Alkalosis (al″-kah-lo′-sis). Indicates an increased blood bicarbonate with a tendency toward alkalemia; can be due to washing out of CO_2 from the blood by overventilation of the lungs.

Altitude alkalosis. Respiratory alkalosis resulting from hyperventilation during accommodation to high altitude.

Altitude sickness. Complex system resulting from the hypoxia and lowered atmospheric pressure at high altitudes. It is of two types: *acute type*— breathlessness, hyperventilation, light headedness, headache, malaise, rarely acute pulmonary edema; *chronic type*—(usually occurs with acclimatization to altitudes above 15,000 feet) polycythemia, vascular occlusions, gastrointestinal ulceration, cardiac failure.

Alveolar capillary block syndrome. Arterial hypoxia due to alteration of the alveolar capillary membrane by various disorders, hindering the diffusion of oxygen from the alveolar gas to the capillary blood.

Alveolar duct (al-ve′-o-lar dukt). Portion of the terminal air passage of the lung from which alveoli arise.

Alveolar ventilation (al-ve′-o-lar ven″-tĭ-la′-shun). Amount of air moving in and out of the lungs that is directly involved in gas exchange.

Alveolus (al-ve′-o-lus). Air sac of the lungs formed by terminal dilatation of a bronchiole (plural: alveoli).

Ambient (am′-bē-ent). Natural atmospheric environment.

Ambulatory (am′-bu-lah-tor″-re). Condition in which the patient walks about; not confined to bed.

Aminophylline (am″-i-no′-fil-in). Mixture of theophylline inducing diuretic action, acting as a myocardial stimulant and relaxing smooth muscle in the airways.

Anaerobic (an″-a-er-o′-bik). Growing only in the absence of molecular oxygen.

Anatomic dead space (an″-ah-tom′-ic ded spās). That internal volume of the airway where no significant exchange of O_2 and CO_2 between gas and blood takes place.

Anemia (ah-ne′-me-ah). Condition in which the blood is deficient either in quantity or in quality.

Anesthesia (an″-es-the′-ze-ah). Partial or complete loss of sensation, with or without loss of consciousness, as a result of disease, injury, or administration of a drug or gas.

Angiogram (an′-je-o-gram). Special type of x-ray that visualizes the blood vessels.

Anoxemia (an-ok′-se′-me-ah). Decrease in the amount of O_2 in arterial blood.

Anoxia (an-ok′-se-ah). Reduction of oxygen in body tissue below physiologic levels.

Anoxic anoxia (an-ok′-sik an-ok′se-ah). Lessened O_2 tension in arterial blood, but with normal O_2 capacity.

Antibiotic (an"-te-bī-ot'-ik).   Chemical substance produced by microorganisms that has the capacity, in dilute solutions, to inhibit the growth of or to destroy bacteria and other microorganisms.

Antiseptic (an"-te-sep'-tik).   Both aseptic and antiseptic; a substance that will inhibit the growth and development of microorganisms without necessarily destroying them.

Antitussive agents (an"-te-tus'-iv 'ā-jent).   Cough medication that inhibits the cough reflex in the cough center.

Antrum (an'-trum).   Cavity or hollow space, especially in a bone, e.g., the maxillary sinus.

Aorta (a-or'-tah).   Main trunk from which the systemic arterial system proceeds.

A–P (anterior–posterior).   X-ray beam directed from front to back.

Apex of lung (a'-peks).   Most superior part of the lung above the clavicle (upper area; most pointed part).

Apnea (ap-ne'-ah).   Transient cessation of the breathing impulse that follows forced breathing.

Apneusis (ap-nu'-sis).   Condition marked by maintained inspiratory activity unrelieved on expiration, each inspiration being long and cramplike; it follows excision of the upper portion of the pons (pneumotaxic center).

ARDS.   Adult respiratory distress syndrome.

ARF.   Acute respiratory failure.

Arrhythmia (a-rith'-mee-uh).   Absence of rhythm; used to designate an alteration or abnormality of normal cardiac rhythm.

Arterial blood.   Blood in the pulmonary vein from the point of origin of the small venules in the lungs to the capillary beds in tissues where oxygen is released and carbon dioxide taken up.

Arteriogram (ar-te"-rē-o-gram').   Artery x-ray.

Arteriole (ar-te-rē-ol).   Minute arterial branch, especially one just proximal to a capillary.

Arteriosclerosis (ahr-teer"-ee-o-skle-ro'-sis).   Any of various proliferative and degenerative changes in arteries, not necessarily related to each other, resulting in thickening of the walls, loss of elasticity, and in some instances calcium deposition.

Artery (ar'-ter-ē).   A vessel through which blood passes on its way *from* the heart to various parts of the body.

Artificial respiration (ar"-te-fish'-al res"-pi-rā'-shun).   Forcing of air in and out of the lungs by artificial means.

Asbestosis.   Diffuse, fibrous pneumoconiosis resulting from the inhalation of asbestos dust.

Asepsis (ah-sep'-sis).   Freedom from infection.

Aseptic (ah-sep'-tik).   Sterile; without sepsis.

ASHD.   Arteriosclerotic heart disease.

Aspergillosis (as"-per-jil-o'sis).   Disease condition caused by species of

Aspergillus and marked by inflammatory granulomatous lesions in the skin, ear, orbit, nasal sinuses, and lungs.

Asphyxia (as-fik'-se-ah). Suffocation.

Aspiration (as"-pı-ra'-shun). 1. The act of breathing or drawing in. 2. Removal of fluids or gases from a cavity by means of an aspirator.

Asthma (az'-mah). Disease marked by recurrent attacks of paroxysmal dyspnea, with wheezing, coughing, and a sense of constriction due to spasmodic contraction of the bronchi and bronchioles.

Asymmetry (ay-sim'-i-tree). Lack of similarity or correspondence of the organs and parts on each side of an organism.

Asystole (ay'-sis'-to-lee). Cessation or weakening of ventricular contraction of the heart.

Atelectasis (at"-e-lek'-tah-sis). 1. Incomplete expansion of the lungs at birth. 2. Collapse or airless condition of the adult lung.

Atmosphere (at'-muh-sfeer). Layer of air surrounding the earth to a height of approximately 200 miles.

Atmospheric pressure (at"-mos-fer'-ik presh'-ur). Pressure exerted by the gases in the atmosphere.

Atrophy (at'-ro-fe). Decrease in size and function; a wasting.

Auscultation (aws"-kul-ta'-shun). Act of listening for sounds within the body, chiefly for determining the condition of the lungs, pleura, abdomen, and other organs.

Autopsy (aw'-top-sē). Postmortem examination of a body.

Bacillus (bah-sil'-us). Genus of Schizomycetes that includes aerobic, grampositive, spore-forming, rod-shaped bacteria; saprophytic forms found in soil and dust.

Bacteria (bak-te'-rē-ah). In general, any microorganisms of the order Eubacteriales, a nonspore-forming, rod-shaped, nonmotile organism.

Bacteriology (bak-te"-rē-ol'-o-jē). Science that studies bacteria.

Bacteriostatic (bak-te"-rē-o-stat'-ik). Inhibiting the growth or multiplication of bacteria.

Barometer (bah-rom'-e-ter). Instrument for determining the atmospheric pressure.

Barrel chest (bar'-el chest). Appearance of the chest, especially in emphysema, due to permanent elevation of the rib cage by increased use of intercostal muscles during breathing.

Base (bās). Substance alkaline in nature.

BCG. A preparation for the prophylactic inoculation of humans against TB. It consists of living cultures of bovine tubercle bacilli. It is administered subcutaneously; its use has declined over the past few years.

Benign (be-nīn'). Not malignant; not recurrent; favorable for recovery.

Bernoulli's principle. When a fluid or gas flows through a tube containing a constriction, the speed of the fluid or gas is greatest in the constricted portion. If the fluid or gas flows in and out of the tube at a constant rate, the amount of fluid or gas flowing per second, in all sections of the pipe, must be the same. Variations in pressure before and after the constriction account for this.

Bicarbonate (bi-kar'-bo-nāt). Any salt having two equivalents of carbonic acid to one of a basic substance; in blood, an index of the alkali reserve.

Bifurcation (bi"-fur-kā'-shun). Division into two branches.

Bilateral (bye-lat'-ur-ul). Pertaining to two sides; pertaining to or affecting both sides of the body.

Biopsy (bi'-op-sē). Removal and examination, usually microscopic, of tissue or other material from the living body for purposes of diagnosis.

Biot's respirations. Type of periodic breathing in which periods of tachypnea, and usually hypopnea, alternate abruptly with apnea. The irregular periods of apnea alternate with periods in which four or five breaths of uniform depth are taken.

Blood (blud). Fluid that circulates through the heart, arteries, capillaries, and veins carrying nutrients and oxygen to the body cells.

Blood gas (blud gas). Refers to the partial pressure of O_2 and CO_2 in the arterial blood; the pressure of each gas is proportional to its percentage in the total mixture.

Blood pressure. Pressure of the blood against the walls of the vessels or of the heart (abbreviated BP).

BMR. Basal metabolic rate.

Bohr's formula. Expired air consists of a mixture of two components, each with a particular composition: a component from the physiologic dead space and an alveolar component that has given up O_2 and received CO_2.

Bolus (bō'-lus). 1. Mass of chewed food or a soft mass that is ready to be swallowed. 2. Quantity of medication that is administered intravenously all at once, as compared to a drip.

Boyle's law (boilz law). If the temperature of a gas remains constant, the volume of the gas will be inversely proportional to the pressure exerted on the gas.

Brachial artery. Artery that originates at the auxillary artery and branches into the radial and ulnar arteries. It distributes blood to the various muscles of the arm, the shaft of the humerus, the elbow joint, the forearm, and the hand. It is a common site for obtaining blood gas samples for analysis.

Bradycardia (brad"-ee-kahr'-dee-uh). Slowness of the heart beat with a heart rate of less than 60 per minute.

Bradypnea (brad"-ee-nee'-ah). Abnormally slow rate of breathing.

Breathing (brēth'-ing). Alternate inspiration and expiration of air into and out of the lungs.

Bronchiectasis (brong"-ke-ek'-tah-sis). Chronic dilatation of the bronchi or bronchioles marked by fetid breath and paroxysmal coughing with the expectoration of mucopurulent matter.

Bronchiole (brong'-ke-ōl). One of the finer subdivisions of the branched bronchial tree.

Bronchiolitis (brong′-kē-ō-lī′-tis).   Infection of the bronchioles.

Bronchiospasm (brong″kē-ō-spasm).   Spasmodic narrowing of the caliber of the bronchial tubes.

Bronchitis (brong-kī′-tis).   Inflammation of the bronchial tubes.

Broncho- (brong″-kō).   Prefix referring to bronchus or bronchiole.

Bronchodilator (brong″-kō-dī-lā′-tor).   Dilating or expanding the lumina of air passages of the lungs.

Bronchogram (brōnk′-ō-gram).   Radiograph of the bronchial tree made after the introduction of a radiopaque substance.

Broncholithiasis (brong″-kō-lĭ-thi′-ah-sis).   Stone in the bronchus.

Bronchopneumonia (brong″-kō-nū-mō′-ne-ah).   Inflammation of the lungs that usually begins in the terminal bronchioles.

Bronchoscopy (brong″-kōs′-kō-pē).   Visual examination of the bronchi.

Bronchospirometry (brong″-kō-spi-rom′-e-trē).   Determination of the vital capacity, O_2 intake, and CO_2 excretion of a single lung.

Bronchostenosis (brong″-kō-ste-nō′-sis).   Narrowing of the bronchus.

Bronchus (brong″-kus).   Either one or two main branches of the trachea.

Brownian movement (brow′-ne-an).   Zigzag motion of colloidal particles caused by the uneven bombardment of the particles by the molecules of the dispersing medium.

BSA.   Body surface area.

Buccal cavity (buk′-al kav-e-tē).   Mouth.

Buffer (buf′-er).   Any substance in a fluid that tends to lessen the change in hydrogen-ion concentration, which otherwise would be produced by adding acids or alkalis.

Bulla (bul′-ah).   Large blister or cutaneous vesicle filled with serous fluid; develops in lungs when several alveoli coalesce because of fragmentation of their interalveolar elastic tissue and subsequent rupture of their attenuated interalveolar septae [plural: bullae (bul′-lae)].

BUN.   Blood urea nitrogen.

Bypass (bī-pas).   Surgical procedure that alters a normal route.

CABG.   Coronary artery bypass graft.

Cachexia (kah-kek′-se-ah).   General ill health and malnutrition.

CAD.   Coronary artery disease.

Calibrations (kal′-ĭ-brā′-shuns).   Graduations.

Calorie (kal′-o-rē).   Unit of heat; the amount of heat required to raise one gram of water one degree centigrade.

Calorimeter (kal″-o-rim′-e-ter).   Instrument for measuring the heat change in any system; in respiration, for measuring the gaseous exchange between a living organism and the atmosphere that surrounds it, and for the simultaneous measurement of the amount of heat produced by that organism.

Capillary (kap′-ĭ-lār″-ē).   Any one of the minute vessels that connects the arterioles and the venules, forming a network in nearly all parts of the body.

Carbogen (kar'-bō-jen).   Mixture of oxygen with 5% carbon dioxide.

Carbohemoglobin (kar"-bō-hē-mō-glō'-bin).   Hemoglobin compounded with carbon dioxide.

Carbon dioxide (kar'-bon dī-ok'-sīd).   Odorless, colorless gas resulting from the oxidation of carbon; formed in the tissues and excreted by the lungs.

Carbon monoxide (kar'-bon mōn-ok'-sīd).   Colorless, poisonous gas formed by burning carbon with a scanty supply of oxygen.

Carboxyhemoglobin (kar-bok"-sē-hē"-mō-glō-bin).   Relatively stable combination of carbon monoxide and hemoglobin that does not take up and give off oxygen or CO_2 during the circulation of the blood and so acts as an asphyxiant.

Cardiac (kar'-dē-ak).   Pertaining to the heart.

Cardiac arrest.   Cessation of cardiac output and effective circulation either because of ventricular asystole or ventricular fibrillation.

Cardiac catheterization (kar'-dē-ak kath"-e-ter-ĭ-zā-shun).   Passage of a small tube through a vein into the heart.

Cardiac failure.   Condition in which the heart is no longer able to pump an adequate supply of blood in relation to the venous return and metabolic needs of the tissues of the body.

Cardiac massage.   Rhythmic compression of the heart, either directly or through the closed chest, in an effort to maintain an effective circulation in cardiac asystole or ventricular fibrillation.

Cardiac tamponade (kar'-dē-ak tam"-pon-ōd).   Acute compression of the heart due to effusion of the fluid into the pericardium or to the collection of blood in the pericardium from rupture of the heart or a coronary vessel.

Cardiogenic shock.   Shock due to impairment of cardiac output, associated with inadequate peripheral circulatory response.

Cardiomegaly (kar"-dē-ō-meg'-ah-lē).   Hypertrophy of the heart.

Cardiopneumatic (kar"-dē-ō-nū-mat'-ik).   Of or pertaining to the heart and respiration.

Cardiopulmonary (kar"-dē-ō-pul'-mō-ner-ē).   Pertaining to the heart and lungs.

Cardioversion (kar"-dē-ō-ver-zhan).   Elective procedure in which electric current is delivered to the heart to terminate dangerous arrhythmias.

Carditis (kar-dey'-tis).   Inflammation of the heart.

Carina, tracheae (kar-ri'-nah, tra'-kē-ae).   Projection of the lowest tracheal cartilage, forming a prominent semilunar ridge running anteroposteriorly between the two orifices of the two bronchi.

Carotid (kar-rot'-id).   1. The carotid artery. 2. A carotid nerve.

Carotid body.   Any one of the several irregular epitheloid masses situated at or near the carotid bifurcation and innervated by the intercarotid or sinus branch of the glossopharyngeal nerve.

Catarrh (kah-tahr').   Inflammation of a mucous membrane, with a free discharge; especially such inflammation of the air passages of the head and throat.

Cavity (kav'-ĭ-tē).   Hollow place or space, especially a space within the body or in one of its organs, such as the pleural cavity.

CBC.   Complete blood count.

CBS.   Chronic brain syndrome.

CC.   Current complaint.

CCU.   Coronary care unit.

Cell (sel).   Any one of the minute protoplasmic masses that make up organized tissue, consisting of a circumscribed mass of protoplasm containing a nucleus.

Centi-.   Prefix meaning: 1. hundredth part, or 2. hundred.

Centimeter (sen'-tĭ-me"-ter).   Unit of linear measure of the metric system; abbreviated cm (2.5 cm = 1 in.).

Centimeter, cubic (sen'-tĭ-me"-ter, kū'-bik).   Unit of mass being that of a cube each side of which measures 1 cm; abbreviated cm^3, cu cm, or cc.

Cerebellum (ser"-e-bel'-um).   That division of the brain behind the cerebrum and above the pons and fourth ventricle; involved in coordination of movements; second largest portion of the brain.

Cerebrum (ser'-e-brum).   Main portion of the brain occupying the upper part of the cranium.

CGA.   Compressed Gas Association.

Charles' law (sharlz).   The volume of a gas is directly proportional to its absolute temperature if the pressure is kept constant. In other words, if the pressure is kept constant, the volume will increase as the temperature increases.

CHD.   Congenital heart disease; coronary heart disease.

Chemoreceptor (ke"-mo-rē-sep'-tor).   Receptor adapted for excitation by chemical substances (or a sense organ, as the carotid body or aortic bodies) that is sensitive to chemical changes in the blood stream, especially reduced oxygen content, and reflexly increases both respiration and blood pressure.

Chemotherapy (ke"-mo-ther'-ah-pē).   Treatment of disease by administering chemicals that affect the causative organisms unfavorably but do not injure the patient.

Chest (chest).   Thorax.

Cheyne–Stokes (chān'-stōks).   Pattern of respirations characterized by rhythmical variations in intensity; occurring in cycles. Each cycle consists of a gradual decrease in intensity of respiratory movements, followed by total cessation of from 5 to 40 seconds, then a gradual increase to maximum, and becomes dyspneic in character.

CHF.   Congestive heart failure.

Chloride (klo'-rid).   A salt of hydrochloric acid; any binary compound of chlorine in which the latter carries a negative charge of electricity (Cl^-).

Chorditis (kor-dī'-tis). Inflammation of the vocal cord.

Chronic (kron'-ick). Long, continued, of long duration.

Cilium (sel'-ē-um). Minute vibratile, hairlike process attached to a free surface of a cell [plural: cilia (sil'-e-ah)].

Circulation (ser"-ku-lā'-shun). Movement in a regular course, as the movement of blood through the heart and blood vessels.

Clinical (klin'-i-kul). 1. Pertaining to the symptoms and course of a disease as observed by the physician, in opposition to the anatomic changes found by the pathologist, or to a theoretical or experimental approach. 2. Pertaining to bedside treatment or to a clinic.

Clot (klot). Semisolidified mass, as of blood or lymph.

Clubbing (of the digits) (klub'-ing). Consists of painless, nontender enlargement of the terminal phalanges of the fingers and toes and is usually a bilateral condition.

CNS. Central nervous system.

CO. Carbon monoxide.

Collateral circulation. That which is carried on through secondary channels after obstruction of the principal vessel supplying the part.

Compliance (of the respiratory system) (kom-pli'-ans). Change in volume that is produced by the application of pressure; defines its elastic resistance to distention.

Congestive heart failure. Failure of the heart to maintain an adequate output, resulting in diminished blood flow to the tissues and congestion in the pulmonary and/or systemic circulation.

Contraindication (kon"-trah-in"-dĭ-kā'-shun). Any condition of disease that renders some particular line of treatment improper or undesirable.

Copious (kō'-pĭ-us). Excessive.

Coronary stenosis. Narrowing of a coronary artery without complete blockage.

Coronary thrombosis. Formation of a thrombus (clot of blood) in a coronary artery of the heart.

Cor pulmonale. Heart disease secondary to disease of the lungs or of their blood vessels; pulmonary heart disease.

Coryza (kŏ-ri'-zah). Cold in the head.

Costal (kos'-tal). Pertaining to a rib or ribs.

Cough (kawf). Sudden noisy expulsion of air from the lungs.

CPAP. Continuous positive airway pressure.

CPPB. Continuous positive pressure breathing; application of positive pressure on both the inspiration phase and the expiration phase of respiration; pressure remains in the lungs at end expiration.

CPPV. Continuous positive pressure ventilation.

Crepitations (krep"-ĭ-tā'-shuns). Rattling or crackling sound (rale).

Cricoid cartilage (kri'-koid kar'-tĭ-lij). Cartilage of the larynx; ring-shaped, lowest part of the larynx.

CRPA. C-reative-protein test.

CS. Central service or supply; an area where hospital supplies are prepared.

CSF. Cerebrospinal fluid.

Culture (kul'-tūr). Propagation of microorganisms of living tissue cells in special media conducive to their growth.

Cutaneous (ku-tā'-nē-us). Pertaining to the skin.

CVA. Cerebrovascular accident; stroke.

CVP. Central venous pressure; pressure exerted by the blood in the major veins.

Cyanosis (sī''-ah-nō'-sis). Any bluish discoloration of the skin; associated with blood oxygen deficiency.

Cystic fibrosis. Inherited disease of exocrine glands, affecting the pancreas, respiratory system, and sweat glands; usually beginning in infancy.

Dalton's law (dawl'-tonz). In a mixture of gases, each part exerts pressure as if it were the only gas present; so the pressure of each gas is proportional to its percentage in the mixture. This pressure is the partial pressure of the gas.

Dead space (ded spās). *Anatomic:* the mouth, nose, pharynx, larynx, trachea, bronchi, and bronchioles. *Mechanical:* space in breathing apparatus outside the patient where the expired air is trapped and then reinhaled. *Physiologic:* includes the volume of the inspired gas that occupies the anatomic dead space and volume that ventilates alveoli that are not perfused by capillary blood flow.

Decompression sickness (dē''-kom-presh'-un). If a man ascends to high altitudes, the PN_2 decreases in inspired air and alveolar gas but is still high in blood and tissues. Dissolved N_2 must then diffuse from tissues to blood and from blood to alveolar gas until tissue, blood, and air tensions of N_2 in tissues are again equal. If the ascent is abrupt, the dissolved N_2 in tissues and blood comes out of solution too rapidly to be carried away by diffusion and gas bubbles form. These bubbles produce pain in the muscles and joints (*bends*), sensory disturbances, weakness or paralysis, shortness of breath, dizziness, deafness, and convulsions. Although O_2 bubbles may form, they can be used locally. N_2 bubbles, however, can be removed only by diffusion.

Decortication (dē''-kor-tĭ-kā'-shun). Removal of portions of the cortical substance of a structure or organ, as the brain, kidney, or lung.

Defibrillation (dē-fib''-rĭ-lā'-shun). Emergency procedure in which an electric current is delivered to the heart to terminate a life-threatening arrhythmia, usually ventricular fibrillation.

Detergent (dē-ter'-jent). Agent that cleanses or purifies; helps to loosen respiratory tract secretions.

Diagnosis (dī''-ag-nō'-sis). Art of distinguishing one disease from another.

Dialysis (dī-al-ĭ-sis). Dialysis or diffusion refers to the passage of particles (ions) from an area of high concentration to an area of low concentration across a semipermeable membrane. There are two types: a. peritoneal, and b. hemodialysis.

Diaphragm (dī'-ah-fram). Musculomembranous partition that separates the abdomen from the thorax.

Diastole (dī-as'-to-le). Period of dilation of the heart, especially of the ventricles.

Diffusion (di-fu'-zhun). Process of becoming diffused or widely spread; dialysis through a membrane, movement of a gas across a membrane due to a greater concentration of blood on one side.

Diffusion capacity. Rate at which oxygen diffuses across the alveolar–capillary membrane; measured in milliliters per minute (mm Hg pressure difference).

DISS. Diameter Index Safety System.

Dissociation curve (dis-sō''-she-ā'-shun). Graph of O_2 content (percentage of saturation) against PO_2; shown as an S-shaped curve.

Diuresis (dī''-u-re'-sis). Increased secretion of urine.

Diuretic (dī''-u-ret'-ik). Increasing the secretion of urine; a medication that promotes the secretion of urine.

DOA. Dead on arrival.

Dorsal (dor'-sul). Pertaining to the back or to the posterior part of an organ.

DOT. Department of Transportation.

Dx. Diagnosis.

Dysphagia (dis-fay'-jee-uh). Difficulty in swallowing, or inability to swallow, whether due to organic or psychic cause.

Dysphonia (dis-fō'-nee-ah). Hoarseness; change in the quality or quantity of the voice due to interference with approximation or tension of the vocal cords.

Dyspnea (disp-ne'-ah). Difficult or labored breathing.

ECG. Electrocardiogram.

Edema (e-dē'-mah). Presence of abnormally large amounts of fluid in the intercellular tissue spaces of the body.

EEG. Electroencephalogram.

EKG. Electrocardiogram.

Electrocardiogram (ē-leck''-trō-kahr'-dee-ō-gram). Graphic record, made by an electrocardiograph, of the electrical forces produced by the contraction of the heart.

Electrocardiogram leads. Electrodes placed on the body surface that record electric potential differences due to contraction of the heart.

Electrolyte (ē-lek'-trō-līt). Any solution that conducts electricity by means of its ions.

Embolism (pulmonary) (em'-bo-lizm). Closure of the pulmonary artery or one of its branches by an embolus (moving clot), resulting in pulmonary edema or hemorrhagic infarction.

Emphysema (em''-fi-sē'-mah). Swelling or inflation due to the presence of air in the interstices of the connective tissues.

Empyema (em''-pi-ē'-mah). Accumulation of pus in a cavity of the body, especially in the chest.

Endotracheal (en″-dō-trā′-kē-al).   Within or through the trachea.

ENT.   Ear, nose, and throat.

Enzyme (en′-zim).   Organic compound, frequently a protein, capable of accelerating or producing by catalytic action some change in its substrate for which it is often specific.

Epiglottis (ep″-ĭ-glot′-is).   Lidlike structure (cartilage) that covers the entrance to the larynx.

EPPB.   Expiratory positive pressure breathing; application of positive pressure on expiration; inspiration occurs at atmospheric pressure.

Erythrocyte (e-rith′-rō-sīt).   Red cell.

Esophagus (e-sof′-ah-gus).   Musculomembranous canal extending from the pharynx to the stomach.

Etiology (ee″-tee-ol′-uh-jee).   Science or study of the *causes* of disease.

Eupnea (ūp-nē′-ah).   Easy or normal respiration.

Exacerbation (ek-as″-er-bā′-shun).   Increase in the severity of any symptoms or disease.

Exhalation (eks″-hah-lā′-shun).   To expel from the lungs by breathing.

Expectorant (eks-peck-to-rant).   Medicine that aids in the expulsion of mucus or exudate from the lungs, bronchi, and trachea.

Expectorate (eks-pek′-to-rat).   To discharge, as phlegm, by coughing and spitting.

Expiration (eks″-pı-rā′-shun).   Act of breathing out or expelling air from the lungs or chest (also means termination or death).

Exsufflation (eck″-suf-lāy′-shun).   Forcible expiration; forcible expulsion of air from the lungs by a mechanical apparatus.

External respiration (eks-ter′-nal res″-pĭ-rā′-shun).   Exchange of gases between the alveoli and the blood.

Extracorporeal circulation.   Circulation of the blood outside the body as through a heart–lung apparatus for carbon dioxide-oxygen exchange.

Extubate (eks-tū′-bat).   To remove a tube that has been inserted for the introduction of air.

Exudate (ĕks′-u-dāt).   Fluid that accumulates as a result of inflammation.

FAA.   Federal Aviation Administration.

Farmer's lung.   Pulmonary disorder resulting from inhaling material in moldy hay and other similar moldy vegetable material. Characterized by dyspnea, fever, cyanosis, and diffuse bronchopneumonia.

FDA.   U.S. Food and Drug Administration.

Febrile (fēb′-ril). Pertaining to fever; feverish.

Femoral artery.   Chief artery of the inferior member or extremity.

Fenestration (fen″-e-stray′-shun).   Creation of an opening or openings; perforation.

FF.   Force fluids, encourage patient to drink.

Fibrosis (pulmonary) (fī-brō′-sis).   Thickening of fibrous tissue of the lung.

Fistula (fis′-tu-lah).   Deep sinous ulcer, often leading to an internal hollow organ.

Flaccid (flak'-sid).   Soft, flabby muscle; lacking tone.

Flail chest.   Results from fractures of multiple ribs or the disruption of several costosternal cartilages; this kind of injury usually causes paradoxical movement of the chest wall at the site of the fractures so that the affected area is drawn in during inspiration and pushed out during expiration.

Fluoroscope (floo-ō'-rō-skōp).   Device used for examining deep structures by means of roentgen rays; it consists of a screen covered with crystals of calcium tungstate.

Fluoroscopy (floo"-or-ōs'-kō-pē).   Examination by means of a fluoroscope; a special x-ray technique that examines the deep parts of the body.

Fomites (fo'-mī-tezs).   Contaminated inanimate objects (desks, chairs).

Fowler's position.   Position in which the head of the patient's bed is raised 18 or 20 inches above the level.

FRA.   Federal Railroad Administration.

Funnel chest (fun'-el).   Chest in which there is a funnel-shaped depression in the middle of the anterior thoracic wall, the deepest part being in the sternum.

FUO.   Fever of undetermined origin.

Fx.   Fracture.

Gag reflex.   Contraction of the constrictor muscles of the pharynx in response to the posterior pharyngeal wall or neighboring structures.

Gas (gas).   Any elastic aeriform fluid in which the molecules are separated from one another and so have free paths.

Gay-Lussac's law (ga"-lū-sahks').   If the volume and mass of a gas remain unchanged, the pressure it exerts will vary proportionately to its absolute temperature.

GI.   Gastrointestinal.

Glossopharyngeal (glos"-ō-fah-rin'-jē-al).   Pertaining to the muscles of the tongue and throat (name of the ninth cranial nerve).

Glottis (glot'-is).   Pharyngeal opening of the larynx.

GU.   Gastrourinary.

Guerney (gur-nĭ).   Stretcher or litter.

Gyne.   Gynecology; care for female reproductive problems.

HAFOE.   High air flow with O_2 enrichment.

Hamman–Rich syndrome (ham'-an).   Spontaneous interstitial fibrosis of the lungs.

Hay fever (hā fē'-ver).   Acute conjunctivitis with nasal catarrh, and often with asthmatic symptoms, regarded as an anaphylactic or allergic condition excited by a specific antigen to which the individual is sensitized.

Heart (hart).   Viscus of cardiac muscle that maintains the circulation of the blood.

Heart block (hart' blok).   Condition in which the muscular interconnection between the auricle and ventricle is interrupted so that the auricle and ventricle beat independently of each other.

Heart failure. Sudden fatal cessation of the heart's action; the clinical condition resulting from inability of the myocardium of the ventricles to maintain an adequate flow of blood to all the tissues of the body.

Heimlach maneuver. An emergency procedure/maneuver designed to dislodge a food bolus (or other foreign body) located in the base of the throat so that it occludes the airway (see CPR procedure).

Hemiplegia. Paralysis on one side of the body.

Hemoglobin (he″-mō-glō′-bin). Oxygen-carrying red pigment of the red blood corpuscles.

Hemolysis (he′-mō′-ly-sis). Rupturing of red blood cells.

Hemoptysis (hee-mop′-ti-sis). Spitting of blood or blood-stained sputum from the lungs, trachea, or bronchi.

Hemothorax (he″-mō-thō′-raks). Presence of blood in the pleural cavity.

Heparin (hep′-ah-rin). Macopoly saccharide acid in various tissues; abundant in the liver. Medication that prolongs the clotting time of blood in man and animals.

Hilus of lung (hi′-lus). Depression in the mediastinal surface of the lung for the entrance of bronchi, blood vessels, nerves, etc.

Histotoxic anoxia (his′-to-tok″-sik). Oxygen deficiency resulting from decreased utilization of O_2 by tissues, as in poisoning of tissue cells.

Homeostasis (ho″-mē-ō-sta′-sis). Constancy.

Humidity (hu-mid′-ĭ-tē). Degree of moisture in the air.

HVD. Hypertensive vascular disease, disease of the blood vessels associated with high blood pressure.

Hyaline membrane disease (hi′-ah-lĭn). Absence or inactivity of the surfactant in the lung, resulting in lung collapse in newborns and atelectasis in patients who die after open-heart surgery in which an artificial heart–lung system was used.

Hydration (hī-drā′-shun). Condition of being combined with water.

Hydrothorax (hī″-drō-thō′-raks). Presence of fluid in the pleural cavity.

Hyperbarism (hī″-per-bār′-izm). Disturbed condition in body, arising from ambient gas pressure or atmospheric pressure exceeding that within body tissues, fluids, and cavities.

Hypercapnia (hī″-per-kap′-nē-ah). Excess of carbon dioxide in the blood.

Hyperthermia. Body temperature elevation to 106°F (41°C) or above.

Hypertonic (hī″-pur-ton′-ick). Having an osmotic pressure greater than that of physiologic salt solution or of any other solution as a standard.

Hypertrophy (hī-pur′-truh-fee). Increase in size of an organ, independent of natural growth.

Hyperventilation (hī″-per-ven″-tĭ-lā′-shun). Abnormally prolonged, rapid, and deep breathing frequently used as a test procedure in epilepsy and tetany; also the condition produced by overbreathing O_2 at high pressures; marked by confusion, dizziness, numbness, and muscular cramping.

Hypervolemia (hī″-per-vo-lē′-mē-ah). Abnormal increase in the volume of circulating fluid (plasma) in the body.

Hypocapnia (hī″-pō-kap′-nee-ah). Subnormal concentration of carbon dioxide in the blood.

Hypostatic pneumonia. Pneumonia in dependent parts of the lungs, seen in patients who remain in one position for long periods of time.

Hypothermia (induced). Controlled reduction of body temperature to a level much below normal (32° to 26°C or 89.6° to 78.8°F) and the maintenance of the temperature at that level.

Hypotonic (hī″-pō-ton′-ick). Refers to a solution whose osmotic pressure is less than that of sodium chloride solution, or any other solution taken as standard.

Hypoventilation (hī″-pō-ven″-tĭ-lā′-shun). Decrease of the air in the lungs below normal amount.

Hypovolemic shock. Shock caused by reduced blood volume, which may be due to loss of blood or plasma as in burns, crush syndrome, perforation of gastrointestinal organs, wounds, or other trauma.

Hypoxemia (hī″-pok-sē′-mē-ah). Deficient oxygenation of the blood.

Hypoxia (hī-pok′-sē-ah). Low oxygen content or tension; deficiency of oxygen in the inspired air.

I&O. Intake and output.

ICU. Intensive care unit.

IMV. Intermittent mandatory ventilation.

Incidence (in′-sĭ-dens). Range of occurrence, as of a disease.

Induration (in″-du-rā′-shun). Abnormally hard spot or place; as the hardening and pigmentation of lung tissue as seen in pneumonia.

Inertia (in-ur′-shuh). Opposition to acceleration, lack of activity; sluggishness.

Infarct (in′-farkt). Area of coagulation necrosis in a tissue due to local anemia resulting from obstruction of circulation to the area.

Infection (in-fek′-shun). Invasion of the body by pathogenic microorganisms and the reaction of the tissues to their presence and to the toxins generated by them.

Infiltration (in″-fil-trā′-shun). Accumulation in a tissue of substances not normal to it.

Inflammation (in″-flah-mā′-shun). Condition into which tissues enter as a reaction to injury.

Inflation (in-flā′-shun). Distention with air, gas, or fluid.

Infradiaphragmatic (in″-frah-dī″-ah-frag-mat′-ik). Below the diaphragm.

Inhale (in-hāl′). To take into the lungs by breathing.

Inhaler (in-hā′-ler). An apparatus for administering vapor or volatilized remedies by inhalation.

Inspiration (in″-spĭ-rā′-shun). Act of drawing air into the lungs.

Inspiratory (in-spi′-rah-to″-rē). Pertaining to or subserving inspiration.

Inspirium (in-spir′-ē-um). An inspiration.

Instillation (in″-stil-lā′-shun). Act or process of dropping a liquid into a cavity.

Insufficiency (in″-su̯-fish′-en-se̅). Condition of being insufficient or inadequate to the performance of the allotted duty.

Insufflation (in″su̯-fla̅′-shun). Act of blowing a powder, vapor, gas, or air into a cavity; as into the lungs.

Interalveolar (in″-ter-al-ve̅′-o̅-lar). Between the alveoli.

Intercostal (in″-ter-kos′-tal). Situated between the ribs.

Interlobar (in″-ter-lo̅′-bar). Situated or occurring between the lobes.

Intermittent (in″-ter-mit′-ent). Having periods of cessation of activity.

Internal respiration (in-ter′-nal res″-pĭ-ra̅-shun). Exchange of gases between the blood and tissue cells.

Interstitial emphysema. Escape of air from the alveoli into the interstices of the lung, commonly due to trauma or a violent cough.

Interstitial pneumonia. Inflammation, particularly of the tissue that makes up the framework of the lungs.

Intracostal (in″-trah-kos′-tal). On the inner surface of the rib.

Intubation (in″-tu-ba̅′-shun). Insertion of a tube for the introduction of air.

IPPB/I. Intermittent positive pressure breathing; active inflation of the lungs during inspiration under positive pressure from a cycling valve.

IPPB/IE. Application of positive pressure on the lungs on both inspiration and expiration; the pressure does not remain at end expiration.

Ischemia (is-kee′-mee-ah). Local diminution in the blood supply due to obstruction or inflow of arterial blood, or to vasoconstriction.

Isotonic (i″-so-ton′-ik). Having the same concentration; said of solutions that have the same concentration as the system with which it is compared.

IV. Intravenous(ly).

kcal. Abbreviation for kilocalorie, or large calorie.

Ketosis (ke″-to̅′-sis). Another name for diabetic coma (acidosis).

kg. Abbreviation for kilogram.

Kilogram (kil′-o-gram). Unit of mass (weight) of the metric system, being 1000 grams, or the equivalent of 2.204622 pounds of avoirdupois and of 2.679228 pounds apothecaries weight; abbreviated kg.

Kinemia (ki-ne′-me-ah). Cardiac output.

Kussmaul–Kien respiration (koos′-mowl-ke̅n). Air hunger; a distressing dyspnea occurring in paroxysms.

Kyphosis (ki-fo̅′-sis). Hunchback or pronounced thorax curve.

Laryngitis (lar″-in-ji̅′-tis). Infection of the larynx.

Laryngo- (lah-ring′-go̅). Prefix meaning or referring to larynx.

Laryngopharyngitis (lah-ring″-go̅-far″-in-ji̅′-tis). Infection of the larynx and pharynx.

Laryngoscope (lah-ring′-go̅-sko̅p). Instrument for examining the larynx.

Laryngospasm (lah-ring′-go̅-spazm). Spasmodic closure of the larynx.

Laryngostomy (lar″-ing-gos′-to-me̅). Creating an opening to the larynx through the neck.

Laryngotomy (lar″-ing-got′-o-mē).   Incision of the larynx.

Laryngotracheitis (lar-ring″-gō-tra″-ke-i′-tis).   Infection of the larynx and trachea.

Laryngotracheobronchitis (lar-ring″-gō-tra″-ke-ō-brong-ki′-tis).   Inflammation or infection of the larynx, trachea, and bronchi.

Larynx (lar′-inks).   Musculocartilaginous structure at the top of the trachea and below the root of the tongue and hyoid bone called the organ of voice; it houses the vocal cords.

Lateral (lat′-ur-ul).   Pertaining to the side part away from the midline.

L & W.   Living and Well.

LBBB.   Left bundle branch block.

LDH.   Lactic dehydrogenase level.

Leukocyte (lu′-kō-sīt).   White cell.

Lipoid pneumonia.   Pneumonia due to aspiration of an oily substance such as mineral oil.

Liter (lē′-ter).   Basic unit of capacity of the metric system; the volume occupied by one kilogram of pure water at its temperature of maximum density and under standard atmospheric pressure; equivalent to 1.0567 quarts liquid measure.

LLL.   Left lower lobe (of the lung).

Lobar (lō′-ber).   Of or pertaining to a lobe.

Lobar pneumonia.   Pneumonia involving one or more lobes of the lung, usually pneumococcal pneumonia.

Lobe (lōb).   More or less well-defined portion of any organ; lobes are demarcated by fissures, sulci, connective tissue, and by their shape.

Lobectomy (lō-bek′-tō-mē).   Excision of a lobe.

Lobotomy (lō-bot′-ō-mē).   Incision into a lobe.

Lobule (lob′-ūl).   Small lobe, or one of the primary divisions of a lobe.

LUL.   Left upper lobe (of the lung).

Lung (lung).   Organ of respiration; either one of a pair of respiratory organs that affect the aeration of the blood.

Lung abscess.   Localized, inflammatory lesion with necrosis of lung and surrounding inflammatory tissue.

Lung scan.   Produces a graphic record of particles in the lung field by administration of a radioisotope. Useful in evaluating pulmonary perfusion when space-occupying disorders or pulmonary infarction are suspected.

Manometer (mah-nom′-e-ter).   Instrument for measuring the pressure or tension of liquids or gases or the blood, etc.

Manual ventilation.   Use of hand-operated bag (e.g., Ambu or Puritan manual resuscitators) to aerate a patient's lungs.

Mask (mask).   Appliance that covers the nose and mouth and can be utilized for administration of a gas, vapor, or aerosol.

Maxillary sinus (mak′-sĕ-ler″-ē sī′-nus).   Cavity in the body of the maxilla that communicates with the middle meatus of the nose.

Medial (mee′-de-ul).   Part close to the midline of the body.

Mediastinal emphysema (mē″-dē-as-ti′-n'l).   Accumulation of air in the tissues of the mediastinum.

Mediastinum (mē″-de-as-ti′-num).   Space between the two pleural sacs from the sternum in front to the thoracic vertebrae behind and from the thoracic inlet above to the diaphragm below; divisions known as inferior and superior, with inferior subdivided into anterior, middle, and posterior.

Membrane (mem′-brān).   Thin layer of tissue that covers a surface or divides a space or organ.

Metabolic acidosis.   Primary fall in blood HCO_3^- concentration; pH and total CO_2 content are reduced.

Metabolic alkalosis.   Primary increase in blood HCO_3^-; pH and CO_2 content are elevated.

MI.   Myocardial infarction.

Milliequivalent (mil″-ē-ē-kwiv′-ah-lent).   Number of grams of a solute contained in one milliliter of a normal solution; abbreviated mEq.

Milligram (mil′-e-gram).   Unit of mass (weight) in the metric system, being 10^{-3} gram; abbreviated mg.

Milliliter (mil′-ē-lē″-ter).   Unit of capacity in the metric system, being 10^{-3} liter; abbreviated ml.

Millimeter (mil′-ē-mē″-ter).   Unit of linear measure of the metric system; 10^{-3} meter or the equivalent of 0.03937 inch; abbreviated mm.

Minimal tuberculosis.   Tuberculosis with lesions of slight to moderate density without cavitation and involving one or both lungs.

MLD.   Minimum lethal dose.

Moderately advanced tuberculosis.   Tuberculosis with scattered lesions of slight to moderate density through one lung or both. Cavitation less than 4 cm in total diameter.

Morbid (mor-bĭd).   Diseased.

Mucopurulent (mu″-ko-pur′-roo-lent).   Containing both mucus and pus.

Mucous membrane (mū′-kus).   Membrane composed of epithelium lining those cavities and canals of the body that communicate with external air.

Naso (na′-zō).   Anterior and posterior orifices into the nasal cavity; the nostrils.

Nasa- (na′-za).   Combining form that refers to nose.

Nasopharyngitis (na″-zō-far″-in-jī′-tis).   Inflammation of nose and throat.

Nasopharynx (na″-zō-far′-inks).   Part of the pharynx just above the soft palate of the mouth opening into the nose.

N.B.   Note well (nota bene).

Nebulization (neb″-u-li-zā′-shun).   Conversion into a spray; treatment by a spray.

Nebulizer (neb′-ū-līz″-er).   Apparatus designed to break a liquid into droplets of microscopic size, which are projected on an air current.

Negative pressure. Subambient pressure; below atmospheric.

Nerve (nerv). Cordlike structure that conveys impulses from one part of the body to another.

Neuro. Neurology; care for patients with nervous system disorders.

NFPA. National Fire Protection Association.

Nitrogen (nī'-trō-jen). Colorless, gaseous element found in the air; symbol, N; specific gravity, 0.9713; atomic number, 7; atomic weight, 14.008; forms about four-fifths of common air.

Nosocomial infection (nos"-ō-kō'-mē-al). Hospital-acquired infection.

Nostril (nos'-tril). Naris.

NPO. Nothing by mouth.

OB. Obstetrics; care of the maternity patient.

OOB. Out of bed; patient may get up.

OR. Operating room.

Oropharynx (ō"-rō-far'-inks). Part of the pharynx between the soft palate and the upper edge of the epiglottis; or the opening between the mouth and the pharynx.

Orthopnea (or"-thop-ne'-ah). Inability to breathe unless in an upright position.

Osmolarity (oz-mol'-lar-ity). Total number of dissolved particles (solute) within a solution, or the number of dissolved particles per liter.

Oxygen (ok'-sĭ-jen). Gaseous element existing free in the air and in combination in most nonelementary solids, liquids, and gases; atomic number, 8; atomic weight, 16; symbol, O_2; constitutes 20% of atmospheric air by weight; the essential agent in the respiration of plants and animals; necessary to support combustion; administered in pulmonary diseases mainly by inhalation.

Oxygenate (ok'-sĭ-je-nāt). To saturate with oxygen.

Oxyhemoglobin (ok"-sē-hē"-mō-glō'-bin). Compound of hemoglobin with two atoms of oxygen; formed in the lungs where hemoglobin combines with oxygen and is carried by arteries to the tissues of the body; in the tissues it gives up its oxygen and is returned by the veins.

Ozone (o'-zōn). Allotropic and more active form of oxygen; symbol, O_3; antiseptic and disinfectant; formed when oxygen is exposed to the silent discharge of electricity.

PAC. Premature atrial contractions.

Pacemaker (pās'-māk-er). Another name for the SA node.

Palpation (pal-pay'-shun). Examination by touch for purposes of diagnosis.

Palpitation (pal"-pi-tay'-shun). Fluttering or throbbing, especially of the heart, often associated with rapid heart rate.

PAP. Primary atypical pneumonia.

Paraplegia. Paralysis of the lower part of the body or of the legs.

Parietal (pah-ri'-ĕ-tal). Surface of the lung or parietal pleura; external layer adherent to inner surface of the chest wall, diaphragm, and mediastinum.

PAT. Paroxysmal atrial tachycardia.

Pathogenesis (path″-ō-jen′-e-sis). Development of diseased conditions or of disease.

Pathology (pah-thol′-ō-jē). That branch of medicine which treats of the essential nature of disease, especially structural and functional changes in the tissue or organs of the body that cause disease or are caused by disease.

Pathophysiology (path″-ō-fiz″-ee-ol′-uh-jee). Study of disordered functions or of functions modified by disease.

PCO_2. Symbol for carbon dioxide pressure (tension).

PE. Pulmonary edema.

Peds. Pediatrics; care for sick children.

PEEP. Positive end expiratory pressure.

Percussion (per-kush′-un). Act of striking a part with short, sharp blows as an aid in diagnosing the condition of the parts beneath by the sound obtained.

Perfusion (per-fu′-zhun). Blood flow.

pH. Symbol commonly used in expressing hydrogen-ion concentration, the measure of alkalinity and acidity; pH 7 is the neutral point: above 7 alkalinity increases, below 7 acidity increases.

Pharynx (far′-inks). Airway between the nasal chambers, mouth, and larynx; also called the throat.

Phlegm (flem). Viscid, stringy mucus, secreted by the mucosa of the air passages.

Phrenic nerve (fren′-ik). Nerve from the cervical spine to the diaphragm.

Physiology (fiz″-ee-ol′-uh-jee). Science that treats functions of living organisms and/or their parts.

Plasma. Liquid portion of the blood; pale yellow fluid.

Plethysmograph (ple-thiz′-mo-graf). Device for ascertaining rapid changes in the volume of an organ or part through an increase in the quantity of the blood therein.

Pleura (ploor′-ah). Serous membrane that invests the lungs and lining of the thoracic cavity and encloses the potential space; the pleural cavity.

Pleural cavity (ploor′-al). Potential space on each side of the chest between the parietal and visceral layers of the lungs.

Pleur-evac. Presterilized disposable plastic apparatus that duplicates in principle the three-bottle chest drainage system.

Pleurisy. Inflammation of the pleura, which may be dry (fibrinous) or serofibrinous accompanied by nonpurulent effusion.

Pleuro- (ploor′-ō). Pertaining to pleura; side or rib.

Pneo- (ne′-ō). Prefix meaning breathe or relating to breath.

Pneumococcal pneumonia. Pneumonia caused by pneumoccoci; because the infection usually involves one or more lobes, it is frequently called *lobar*.

Pneumoconiosis (nū-mō-kō-ne-ō'-sis).   Chronic fibrous reaction in the lungs caused by inhalation of dust, asbestos, or silica.

Pneumonectomy (nū"-mō-nek'-to-me).   Excision of the lung.

Pneumonia (nū"-mō'-ne-ah).   Infection of the lungs.

Pneumothorax (nū"-mō-thō'-raks).   Presence of air in the thoracic cavity; an accumulation of air or gas in the pleural cavity; the air enters either by an external wound, a lung perforation, from burrowing abscesses, or from the rupture of a superficial lung cavity; pneumothorax is attended with sudden and severe pain and rapidly increasing dyspnea.

Polycythemia (pol"-e-si-the'-me-ah).   Excess of red corpuscles in the blood seen in chronic cardiac or pulmonary disease patients due to arterial oxygen unsaturation.

Position (po-zish'-un).   Placement of body members, as a particular position assumed by the patient to achieve comfort in certain conditions, or the particular arrangement of body parts to facilitate the performance of certain diagnostic or therapeutic procedures: dorsal p., the posture of a person lying on his back; prone p., patient lying face down; supine p., dorsal.

Positive pressure.   Pressure above atmospheric pressure.

Posterior (pos-te'-re-or).   Situated behind or toward the rear (back or dorsal).

PPD.   Purified protein derivative of tuberculin.

Pressure (presh'-ur).   Stress or strain, whether by compression, pull, thrust, or shear: intrapulmonic p., the air pressure within the lungs; intrathoracic p., the pressure within the thorax, that is, the pressure in the pleural cavity and mediastinal spaces.

PRN (pro re nata).   As necessary.

Prognosis (prog-nō'-sis).   Prediction as to the probable course and outcome of a disease, injury, or developmental abnormality in a patient based on general knowledge of conditions, including specific information and exercise of clinical judgment on a particular case.

Prone.   Lying with the face downward.

Prophylaxis (pro"-fi-lak'-sis).   Prevention of disease; preventive treatment.

Proximal (prock'-si-mul).   Nearest to the body or the middle line of the body or to some point considered as the center of a septem.

Psych.   Psychiatry; care for the emotionally ill.

Pulmo- (pul'-mō).   Prefix referring to the lung.

Pulmonary (pul'-mo-ner"-e).   Pertaining to the lungs.

Pulmonary circulation.   That carrying the venous blood from the right ventricle to the lungs and returning oxygenated blood to the left atrium of the heart.

Pulmonary edema.   Usually acute condition, however sometimes subacute or chronic, marked by an excess of fluid in the extravascular spaces of the lungs.

Pulmonary embolism.   Lodgement of a clot in a pulmonary artery.

Pulse (puls).   Wave of pressure exerted against walls of arteries in response to ventricular systole.

Pulse pressure (puls presh'ur).   Difference between systolic and diastolic pressure.

Purulent (pu'-roo-lent).   Consisting of or containing pus; associated with the formation of or caused by pus.

Quadraplegia (kwod"-ri-ple'-jē-ah).   Paralysis of all four limbs.

Radiolucent (rā"-dē-ō-lu'-sent).   Allowing for the passage of x-rays.

Radiopaque (rā"-dē-ō-pah'k).   Not permitting the passage of radiant energy (such as x-rays).

Rales (rahlz).   Sound heard in the lungs; may be bubbling, sonorous, or rattling.

RBBB.   Right bundle branch block.

RBC, rbc.   Red blood count.

Rebreathing (ree"-breethe'-ing).   Process of respiring air, or air plus other gases, that has been exhaled.

Rebreathing bag.   Flexible rubber bag into and from which breathing takes place for therapeutic or experimental purposes. A bag used in the administration of gas anesthesia.

Relative humidity.   Amount of water vapor in the air as compared with the total amount the air would hold at a given temperature expressed as a percent.

Remission (rē-mish'-un).   Period of decreased severity of symptoms.

Reserve air (rē-zerv').   Supplemental air.

Residual air (rē-zid'-u-al).   Air remaining in the lungs after forced expiration.

Resonance (rez'-ō-nans).   Prolongation and intensification of sound produced by the transmission of its vibrations to a cavity, especially a sound elicited by percussion.

Respiration (res"-pĭ-rā'-shun).   Act of breathing; the act by which air is drawn in and expelled from the lungs, including inspiration and expiration.

Respiratory acidosis.   Primary increase in PCO_2; pH falls and total CO_2 content is increased.

Respiratory alkalosis.   Primary decrease in PCO_2; blood pH is increased and the total CO_2 content is reduced.

Resuscitation (rē-sus"-ĭ-tā'-shun).   Restoration to life or consciousness of one apparently dead.

RHD.   Rheumatic heart disease; disease of the heart following rheumatic fever.

Rhinitis (ri-ni'-tis).   Infection of the nose.

Rhinolith (ri'-nō-lith).   Calculus or stone in the nose or sinus.

Rhinoplasty (ri'-nō-plas"-tē).   Plastic reconstruction of the nose.

Rhinorrhea (rye"-nō-ree'-uh).   Mucous discharge from the nose.

Rhonchus (rong'-kus).   Whistling or snoring sound heard on auscultation of the chest.

Rib (rib).   Any one of 24 bones each of which extends from a vertebra to or toward the sternum.

RICU.   Respiratory intensive care unit.

R/O.   Rule out.

Roentgen ray.   X-ray.

SA node.   Sinuatrial node acts as the pacemaker for the heart.

Saliva (sah-lī'-vah).   Clear, alkaline, somewhat viscid, secretion from the parotid, submaxillary, sublingual, and smaller mucous glands of the mouth.

Saturated (sat'-u-rāt''-ed).   Having all the chemical affinities satisfied; unable to hold in solution any more of a given substance.

Scintiscanner (sin'-tĭ-skan-r).   Special whole body scanner that picks up gamma radiation from radioactive isotopes.

Secretion (se-krē'-shun).   Process of elaborating a specific product as a result of the activity of a gland.

Segment (seg'-ment).   Piece cut off or marked off, either actually or by an imaginary line.

Semi- (sem'-ē).   Prefix signifying one-half.

Semimembranous (sem''-ē-mem'-brah-nus).   Made up in part of membrane or fascia.

Semivalent (sem-iv'-ah-lent).   Having one-half the power that is normal.

Septicemia (sep''-tĭ-sē'-mē-ah).   Bacteria reproduction in the blood stream.

Septum (sep'-tum).   Dividing wall or partition in the nose that separates it into two nasal cavities; it is called the nasal septum.

Shunt (shunt).   Bypass; a direct communication between the arterial and venous circulation or perfusion of unventilated alveoli or ventilation of alveoli that are not perfused.

Sigh (sī).   Audible and prolonged inspiration followed by a shortened expiration.

Silicosis (sil''-ĭ-kō'-sis).   Pneumoconiosis due to the inhalation of dust of stone, sand, or flint, containing silicon dioxide; grinder's disease.

Singultus.   Involving respirations due to spasms of the diaphragm (hiccough).

Sinus (sī'-nus).   Recess, cavity, or hollow space.

Sinusitis (sī''-nus-ī'-tis).   Infection of the sinuses; may be ethmoid, frontal, maxillary, or sphenoid.

Smear (smeer).   Preparation of secretions or blood for microscopial study, made by spreading them on a glass slide or coverslip.

SOB.   Shortness of breath.

SOB spasm (spaz'-um).   Sudden muscular contraction.

SOP.   Standard operating procedure.

Sphenoid (sfe'-noid). Accessory sinus of the nose, located in the anterior part of the sphenoid bone and opening into the nasal cavity above the superior concha.

Spirogram (spye'-rō-gram). Recorded tracing of the movements and excursion of the chest in respiration.

Spirograph (spye'-rō-graf). Instrument for registering respiration.

Spirometer (spye-rom'-e-tur). Device for measuring and recording the amount of air inhaled and exhaled.

Sputum (spu'-tum). Matter ejected from the mouth; saliva mixed with mucus and other substances from the respiratory tract.

Squeeze (skwēz). Compressed air illness; tussive squeeze; the compression of the lung in coughing that forces fluids out into the bronchi.

Stasis (sta'-sis). Standing still; a stoppage of the flow of body or other fluid in any part.

Stat. Abbreviation for immediately.

Stationary air (stā'-shun-er"-ē). Air that remains in the lungs during normal respiration.

Stenosis (ste-no'-sis). Narrowing or constriction, especially of lumen or orifice.

Sterilization (ster"-ĭ-lī-zā'-shun). Complete destruction of microorganisms by heat (wet steam under pressure at 120°C for 15 minutes or by dry heat at 360° to 380°C for 3 hours) or by bactericidal chemical compounds.

Sternal (ster'-nal). Pertaining to the sternum.

Sterter. Snoring type of respiration.

Stethoscope (steth'-o-skōp). Instrument for auscultation or listening to sounds of the lungs.

Stridor (stri'-dor). Harsh, high-pitched respiratory sound such as the inspiratory sound heard in acute laryngeal obstruction.

Suction (suk'-shun). Act or process of sucking or of aspirating, as in the production of adhesion between two surfaces by exhaustion of the air between them.

Sudden death (cardiac arrest). Occurs when the heart swiftly and without warning stops pumping.

Suffocation (suf"-uh-kay'-shun). Interference with the entrance of air into the lungs with resultant unconsciousness.

Supine (suh-pine'). Lying on the back face upward; or the hand, palm upward.

Supplemental air (sup"-lĕ-men'-tal). Air expelled from the lungs; more than normally breathed out.

Symptom (simp'-tum). Any functional evidence of disease or of a patient's condition; a change in a patient's condition indicative of some bodily or mental state.

Syncope (sing'-kuh-pē). Fainting, temporary suspension of consciousness from cerebral hypoxia.

Syndrome (sin'-drome). Group of signs and symptoms that, when considered together, characterize a disease.

Systemic circulation. General circulation carrying oxygenated blood from the left ventricle to various tissues of the body, and returning the venous blood to the right atrium of the heart.

Systole (sĭs-to-le). Contraction of cardiac muscle.

Tachycardia (tack'-i-kahr'-dee-uh). Excessive rapidity of the heart's action.

Tachypnea (tack"-i-nee'-uh). Abnormally rapid rate of breathing.

TAH. Total abdominal hysterectomy.

TBT. Tracheal bronchial toilet.

TBW. Total body water.

Tenacious (te-nay'-shus). Cohesive.

Terminal (tur'-mi-nul). Pertaining to the end.

Therapy (therr'-uh-pee). Means employed to effect the cure or management of disease or of diseased patients.

Therapeutic (therr"-uh-pew'-tick). 1. Curative. 2. Pertaining to therapy.

Thoracentesis (tho"-ruh-sen-tee'-sis). Aspiration of the chest cavity for the removal of fluid; for example, empyema.

Thoracoplasty (tho"-rah-kō-plas'-tē). Plastic surgery of the chest; operative repair of defects of the chest.

Thoracostomy (tho"-rah-kos'-tom-mē). Operation of forming an opening in the wall of the chest for the purpose of drainage.

Thorax (tho'-raks). Chest; the part of the body between the neck and the abdomen.

THR. Total hip replacement.

Thrombus (throm'bus). Plug or clot in a blood vessel or in one of the cavities of the heart that remains where it was formed.

Tidal volume. Volume of gas inspired or expired per breath.

Tomogram (to'-mo-gram). Special x-ray of a selected layer of tissue.

Torr. On the earth's surface, can be used interchangeably with mm Hg.

TPR. Temperature, pulse, and respiration.

Trachea (tra'-kē-ah). Cartilaginous and membranous tube that extends from the larynx to the bronchi; called the windpipe.

Tracheal rings (trā'-kē-al). Horseshoe-shaped rings of cartilage around the trachea.

Tracheo- (trā'-kē-ō). Prefix that refers to the trachea.

Tracheobronchial tree (trā"-kē-ō-brong'-kē-al). Trachea and bronchial structures, referred to as one structure.

Tracheobronchitis (trā"-kē-ō-brong-kī'-tis). Inflammation of the trachea and bronchus.

Tracheostenosis (trā"-kē-ō-ste-nō'-sis). Narrowing of the trachea.

Tracheostomy (trā"-kē-os'-tō-mē). Creation of an artificial opening into the trachea through the neck.

Tracheotomy (trā"-kē-ot'-ō-mē). Incision of the trachea.

Trendelenburg position. Patient is tilted so head is lower than the trunk.

Tuberculosis or pulmonary tuberculosis (tu-ber″-ku-lō′-sis). Infection of the lungs caused by an organism of Myobacterium tuberculosis.

URI. Upper respiratory infection; involving the nose, throat and trachea, the upper respiratory system.

Uvula (u′-vĭ-lah). Small tab of mucous membrane; covered muscle found between oral cavity and oral pharynx.

Vagus nerve (va′-gus). Nerve from the brain to the chest wall, diaphragm, larynx, heart, bronchi, esophagus, stomach, liver, and abdomen.

Valsalva maneuver (val-sal′-vah). Increase in intrapulmonic pressure by forcible exhalation against the closed glottis.

Vapor (vay′-pur). A gas, especially the gaseous form of a substance that at ordinary temperatures is liquid or solid.

Vaporization (vay′-pur-ĭ-zay′-shun). Conversion of a solid or liquid into a vapor.

Vaporizer (vay′-pur-eye″-zur). Atomizer; a device for converting a substance, usually a liquid, into a vapor.

VA/Q. Refers to ventilation/perfusion ratio; the relationship between the ventilation of the lungs and the pulmonary blood flow.

Varix of trachea (var′-iks). Enlarged and tortuous vein or artery of the trachea (plural: varices).

Vasculature (vas′-ku-lah-tūr″). System of vessels.

Vasoconstrictor (va″-zo-kun-strick′-tur). Nerve or an agent that causes constriction of blood vessels.

Vasodilatation (vay″zo-dil″-uh-tay′-shun). Dilatation of the blood vessels.

Vector (vek′-tor). Animal carrier of microbes.

Venous blood. Blood in the pulmonary arteries from the point of origin of the small venules in tissues to the capillary bed in the lungs where carbon dioxide is released and oxygen taken up.

Ventilate (ven′-ti-lāte). 1. Renew the air in a place. 2. To oxygenate the blood in the capillaries of the lungs.

Ventral (ven′-tral). Front or anterior.

Venturi. Device employed in inhalation therapy equipment designed to draw in a second gas to mix with a main flow gas by blowing a high flow of gas through a restricted area.

Venules (ven′-ūlz). Small veins.

Vestibule (ves′-tĭ-būl). Anterior part of the nostrils.

Visceral pleura (vis′-er-al). Portion of the pleura that invests the lungs and lines their fissures, completely separating the different lobes; also called pulmonary pleura.

Vital capacity (vī′-tal). Measurement of the number of cubic centimeters of air expired forcibly after a full inspiration.

Vital signs. Living signs, such as temperature, pulse, respiration, and blood pressure (v.s.).

Vocal cords (vō′-kal).   Membranous bands in the larynx that produce the sound of the voice; there are superior, or false cords, and inferior, or true cords.

Walking ventilation.   Test of breathing response to mild exercise. The patient walks at a rate of 2 miles per hour on level ground and after 4 minutes the expired air is collected and measured.

WBC.   White blood cell.

WHO.   World Health Organization.

Windpipe (wind′-pīp).   Trachea.

X-rays (eks′-rāz).   Roentgen rays (x-ray picture).

EXERCISES

1. Write the abbreviation for each of the following places or procedures:
   a. Central service _____
   b. Operating room _____
   c. Respiratory intensive care unit _____
   d. Blood pressure _____
   e. ABG _____

2. Define the following terms:
   a. Atelectasis
   b. Dysphonia
   c. Copius
   d. Hyperpnea

3. Complete the following:
   a. O_2 moves across the gas barrier by the process of _____.
   b. The lungs are divided into segments called _____.
   c. The proper name for the condition commonly called hunchback is _____.
   d. The pointed portion of the heart or lungs is called its _____.
   e. The term used to mean vomiting of blood is _____.

4. Cardio- is the prefix to describe the heart; study the following terms and give their meaning:
   a. Cardiogenic _____
   b. Cardiograph _____
   c. Cardiopathy _____
   d. Cardialgia _____
   e. Cardiac arrest _____

5. a. The trachea is also referred to as the _____.
   b. Total lung capacity refers to _____.
   c. Vital capacity is _____.
   d. Fractional concentration of O_2 in inspired gas is abbreviated as _____.
   e. When a patient is lying face downward, he is in the _____ position.

MEDICAL GASES AND SAFETY SYSTEMS

The respiratory therapist employs a variety of medical gases, cylinders, and regulating equipment in his work. It is imperative that he be familiar with the agencies regulating these devices and with the properties of each gas he uses.

REGULATING AGENCIES

I. National Fire Protection Association (NFPA)
   A. A voluntary agency whose purpose is to prevent and detect fires and to promote and improve the methods used for same. It is concerned with hazards created in hospitals by equipment and supplies.
   B. Examples of regulations
      1. Sets standards for installation of nonflammable medical gas supply systems used for respiratory therapy.
      2. Sets standards for cylinder carts and trucks used for transportation of large cylinders that are intended for use in hazardous atmospheres or rooms communicating with same.
      3. Sets standards for storage of cylinders.
      4. Sets standards for grounding of electrical equipment.
      5. Standards also apply to the treatment of ambulatory patients in outpatient clinics, physicians' offices, or similar facilities.

II. United States Department of Transportation (DOT)—regulates cylinder construction, testing, and maintenance; formerly carried out by the Interstate Commerce Commission. In Canada this function is assigned to the Canadian Transport Commission.

III. Compressed Gas Association, Inc. (CGA)
   A. An organization founded by manufacturers of compressed gases and dispensing devices. Its aim is to develop the safest, most efficient methods for handling compressed gases and to standardize equipment used with these gases. Many of the rules compiled by the Compressed Gas Association are intended as guidelines and are the result of the experiences of the industries involved. They by no means supersede regulations set forth by governmental agencies, although the CGA does review and make recommendations.
   B. Examples
      1. Safe handling of compressed gases, including moving and storing cylinders.
      2. Medical vacuum systems in hospitals.
      3. Safety relief devices used on compressed gas cylinders, including design and construction, identification, and maintenance requirements.
      4. Marking of portable compressed gas containers.
      5. Hydrostatic testing of cylinders.
      6. Disposition of unserviceable cylinders.
      7. American–Canadian standard cylinder valve outlet and inlet connections.
      8. Pin-Index Safety System for medical gas flush-type connections.
      9. Diameter-Index Safety System for low-pressure medical gas connections.

IV. Federal Food, Drug, and Cosmetic Act
   A. Regulates shipment of medical gases in interstate commerce.
   B. Provides that medical gases must meet standards established by the Pharmacopeia of the United States (USP) or *National Formulary* regarding quality, purity, potency, and labeling.

V. Federal Occupational Safety and Health Act of 1970—provides for federal inspections of facilities used for storage of flammable gases.

VI. Other agencies on a state and municipal level, including local fire departments, have developed regulations with the intent to safeguard their communities from hazards associated with storage, transportation, and use of compressed gases.

MEDICAL GAS CYLINDERS

Cylinder Manufacture. Cylinders are made either from seamless tubing, which is brazed or welded, or from flat sheets of drawn steel shaped into cylindrical form. The cylinder ends are sealed by spinning in a lathe or by forging.

Commonly Made Cylinder Types. The most commonly made cylinders today are the following:

ICC-3A: seamless steel cylinders used for high pressure, from 150 to 15,000 psig.

ICC-3AA; seamless high-pressure cylinders, but made from heat-treated alloy steel and can withstand higher working pressures than the 3A cylinders.

ICC-3B: a seamless cylinder also, but service pressure is only 150 to 500 psig.

ICC-3E: a seamless cylinder limited to 2 in. maximum diameter and 24 in. maximum length; service pressure, 1800 psig.

ICC-8 or ICC-8AL: a seamless low-pressure cylinder used for acetylene service; service pressure, 250 psig.

Required Cylinder Markings. Cylinders manufactured to DOT (ICC) specifications are to have permanently marked symbols on the shoulder of the cylinder.

First line: ICC 3AA 2015 (ICC 3AA is the ICC specification to which the cylinder was manufactured; 2015 is the service pressure in psig)

Second line: II 396042 (serial number of that cylinder)

Third line: BAP (mark of the cylinder manufacturer)

Fourth Line: 8-70 (month and year of qualification test)

Hydrostatic Testing of Cylinder. The water jacket volumetric expansion method is used on all hydrostatic tests when volumetric expansion determinations are required. The procedure is to enclose a cylinder in a vessel completely filled with water and to measure, by a device connected to the vessel, the amount of water displaced by expansion of the cylinder when under pressure and after pressure is released.

How to Use Test Results. The hydrostatic test results will show the total expansion and the permanent expansion of the cylinder at a given pressure.

The total expansion minus the permanent expansion is the elastic expansion. This elastic expansion at a given pressure is a definite measurement of the average wall thickness of the cylinder.

EXAMPLE Total expansion   180 cc
Permanent expansion   −   6 cc
Elastic expansion   174 cc

EXAMPLE A. Take a permanent expansion reading in cubic centimeters and record.

B. Calculate percentage permanent expansion by dividing permanent expansion by total expansion and record. If over 10%, the cylinder fails under ICC regulations.

$$\text{Total expansion} = 180 \text{ cc}$$

$$\text{Permanent expansion} = 6 \text{ cc}$$

$$\text{Percentage permanent expansion} = \frac{\text{permanent expansion}}{\text{total expansion}}$$

$$= \frac{6}{180}$$

$$= 3.3\%$$

C. Elastic expansion is equal to total expansion minus permanent expansion:

$$180 \text{ cc} - 6 \text{ cc} = 174 \text{ cc}.$$

If elastic expansion indicates that cylinder is thin-walled, it should be scrapped.

D. The test is repeated every ten years.

PIPING SYSTEMS

Basically, a hospital oxygen piping system consists of a centrally located supply of oxygen and pipes or tubing to carry the gas from the central supply to points in the hospital where it is used and station outlets at those points. See Figures 2-1 and 2-2b. Oxygen can be supplied to the system from cylinder manifolds. These can be made to accommodate any practical number of cylinders and are most suitable for small hospitals. See Figure 2-2a.

Bulk storage units are most practical for hospitals having a large oxygen consumption. The unit consists of several permanently fixed high-pressure containers, manifolded together and protected by pressure relief valves. Oxygen is fed to the piping system from the specially designed and insulated containers. The oxygen is stored as a liquid, but is readily converted to a gas as required by the piping system. Each oxygen unit has a reserve cylinder supply.

A piping system must be supplied with a pressure regulating valve that maintains a pressure of not less than 50 psi and not more than 100 psi at the service outlet under normal operating conditions.

The main supply line must be provided with a shutoff valve and an alarm system. In addition, each station must be equipped with a manual or automatic shutoff valve. All personnel should be familiar with the placement and use of these valves in the event of an emergency.

MEDICAL GASES

Definitions and Abbreviations

1. psi, pounds per square inch (English system)—pressure.
2. psig, pounds per square inch gauge (English system)—indicates pressure recorded on calibrated gauges. The zero point on the gauge is equivalent to 1 atmosphere (14.7 psi) of pressure. Any reading above zero, therefore, indicates pressure above atmospheric (positive pressure).
3. psia, pounds per square inch absolute—actual total pressure of a gas, including that exerted by the atmosphere. The psia is always 14.7 psi greater than the psig. For example,

$$14.7 \text{ psig} = 29.4 \text{ psia}$$

$$371.2 \text{ psig} = 385.9 \text{ psia}$$

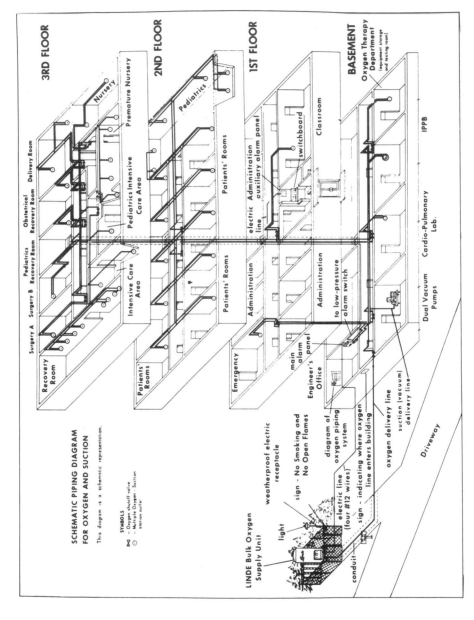

Figure 2-1. (Courtesy of Union Carbide Corp., Linde Division)

104

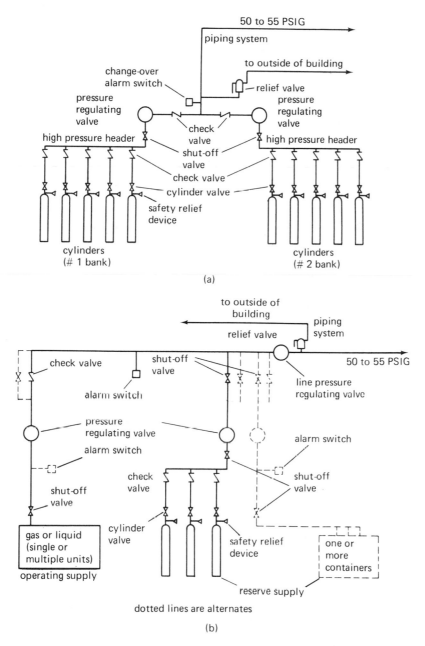

Figure 2-2. (a) Oxygen Cylinder Supply System; (b) Oxygen Bulk Supply System. Reprinted, with permission, from *Nonflammable Medical Gas Systems 1974*, NFPA No. 56F, 1974 Edition. (National Fire Protection Association, Boston, Mass.), pp. 9–11.

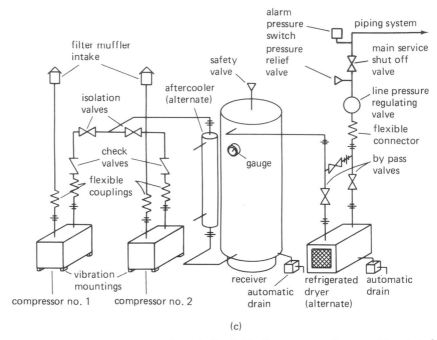

Figure 2-2. (*cont.*)   (c) Duplex Medical Air Compressor System. Reprinted, with permission, from *Nonflammable Medical Gas Systems 1974*, NFPA No. 56F, 1974 Edition. (National Fire Protection Association, Boston, Mass.), pp. 9–11.

Absolute pressure is most commonly used in hyperbaric medicine.

THERAPEUTIC GASES

Air

Air is colorless, odorless, and tasteless. Because of the oxygen content, air does support combustion and is life supporting. Air is nontoxic and nonflammable. For most practical purposes, air composition is taken to be 79% nitrogen and 21% oxygen by volume.

Compressed air has many uses in the health care field. Air is used in conjunction with high-humidity treatments using nebulizers in pediatrics and nurseries as well as in IPPB treatments. Usage of air has been increasing in all respiratory therapy applications where an increase in oxygen content is contraindicated.

Air is produced commercially by mixing of USP oxygen and USP nitrogen, and also by compression and purification of atmospheric air with oil-free-type compressors.

Properties

Molecular weight	28.9752
Color	Colorless
Odor	Odorless
Taste	Tasteless
Physical state in cylinder	Gas
Specific gravity, 70°F	1
Approximate cylinder pressure at 70°F	2200 psig
Critical temperature	−220.3°F
Critical pressure	546.8 psia
Boiling point	−317.8°F
Density of gas at 70°F 1 atm	0.0749 lb/ft^3
Combustion characteristics	Nonflammable

Oxygen

Of the three basic essentials for the maintenance of life—oxygen, water, and food—the deprivation of oxygen leads most rapidly to death. As tissue cells have no reserve, they must be continually supplied with oxygen by means of the circulatory system.

Historical Notes

1794 Oxygen inhalation therapy introduced by Thomas Beddoes in collaboration with James Watt

1868 Oxygen used in anesthesia by Edmund W. Andrews, MD

1885 Oxygen therapy applied to the treatment of pneumonia by George E. Holtzapple, MD

Later developments in the use of oxygen for inhalation therapy coincided with man's increasing knowledge of the function of human blood. As a result, anesthesiologists, biochemists, and chest physicians have discovered innumerable uses for oxygen.

Manufacture of Oxygen. The industrial sources of oxygen are air and water. From air, oxygen is made by liquefaction and fractional distillation. Air, which consists of approximately 21% oxygen, 78% nitrogen, and 1% total of argon, neon, carbon dioxide, and water, is first freed of carbon dioxide and water. It is then compressed, cooled, and expanded until liquefaction results to give liquid air. Since nitrogen has a lower boiling point, it boils away in partial evaporation, leaving the residue rich in oxygen. The cycle is repeated until oxygen is produced that is 99.5% pure.

From water, very pure oxygen can be made by electrolysis as a by-product of hydrogen manufacture. Power compensation makes electrolytic oxygen production more expensive than fractional distillation.

In the laboratory, oxygen is usually manufactured by the terminal decomposition of potassium chlorate (KCl_3). It is catalyzed by the presence of various solids, such as manganese dioxide (MnO_2), ferric oxide (Fe_2O_3), fine sand, or powdered glass. It is thought that the function of the catalyst is to provide a surface on which the evolution of oxygen gas can occur.

Properties

Chemical symbol	O_2
Molecular weight	32.00
Color	Colorless
Odor	Odorless
Taste	Tasteless
Physical state in cylinder	Gas
Specific gravity of gas (air = 1)	1.1052
Approximate cylinder pressure at 70°F	1800 to 2400 psig
Critical temperature	−118.4°C (−181.1°F)
Critical pressure	736.5 psia
Freezing point at 1 atm	−218.4°C (−361.1°F)
Boiling point at 1 atm	−183.0°C (−297.4°F)
Density of gas at 70°F, 1 atm	0.08281 lb/ft.³
Combustion characteristics	Nonflammable; supports combustion

Carbon Dioxide

Carbon dioxide, important in the control of both respiration and circulation, is found in normal air in concentrations of 0.025%. Normally, the tension of carbon dioxide in the body fluids is maintained within narrow limits. During and after anesthesia, carbon dioxide is effective in combating respiratory arrest due to hyperventilation or excessive depression of the respiratory center.

At the conclusion of anesthesia, administration of carbon dioxide increases respiratory minute volume, hastening recovery from anesthesia by speeding up the excretion of anesthesia gases. In some recovery units, carbon dioxide is administered intermittently for a few days to reduce the incidence of postoperative pulmonary complications caused by shallow breathing. It is usually administered in combination with oxygen, and cylinders containing the two gases in varying proportions are available. The value of using carbon dioxide cannot be stated with certainty.

Properties

Chemical symbol	CO_2
Molecular weight	44.01
Color	Colorless
Odor	Odorless
Taste	Slightly acid
Physical state in cylinder	Liquid
Specific gravity of gas (air = 1)	1.5289
Approximate cylinder pressure at 70°F	840 psig
Critical temperature	31.0°C (87.8°F)
Critical pressure	1071.6 psia
Freezing point at 5.2 atm	−56.6°C (−69.9°F)
Sublimation point at 1 atm	−78.5°C (−109.3°F)
Density of gas at 70°F, 1 atm	0.1146 lb/ft³
Combustion characteristics	Nonflammable, does not support combustion

Helium

Helium is one of the chemically inert gases known as the rare gases. It is very light; a mixture of 80% helium and 20% oxygen is only one-third as heavy as air. Helium–oxygen mixtures are used when respiration is embarrassed by obstruction. Helium owes its pharmacologic actions to its physical properties, such as its low coefficient of solubility and high rate of diffusion. Even when breathing occurs under pressure, very little helium is dissolved in body fluids.

Helium is widely used in anesthesia, especially in emergencies when an unexpected obstruction of the respiratory tract occurs or during partial respiratory paralysis. Helium is an expensive gas, but increased usage has made it cheaper and more available. In 1907, it was determined that helium was present in natural gases from certain oil wells in the U.S. Southwest. In 1917, the U.S. Government built plants to obtain helium.

Properties

Chemical symbol	He
Molecular weight	4.003
Color	Colorless
Odor	Odorless
Taste	Tasteless
Physical state in cylinder	Gas
Specific gravity of gas (air = 1)	0.137
Approximate cylinder pressure at 70°F	1800 to 2640 psig
Critical temperature	−267.9°C (−450.2°F)
Critical pressure	33.22 psia
Freezing point at 1 atm	−272.1°C (−457.8°F)
Boiling point at 1 atm	−268.92°C (−452.06°F)
Density of gas at 70°F, 1 atm	0.01034 lb/ft³
Combustion characteristics	Nonflammable, does not support combustion

Nitrous Oxide

Joseph Priestly discovered nitrous oxide in 1776, but it was not until the early 1840s that Colton, a chemist and itinerant lecturer, introduced it to the public as "laughing gas." It continues its long service to anesthesia, with admixture of oxygen and in combination with other agents, through the modern gas machine. To be used safely as an anesthetic, it must be combined with an adequate concentration of oxygen.

Nitrous oxide is the only inorganic gas that is serviceable clinically as an anesthetic agent. It is very soluble in blood, which takes up 45 volumes percent if exposed to the pure gas for a sufficiently long time. However, it does not combine with hemoglobin; it is carried in the blood in physical solution only. Nitrous oxide does not combine chemically with any constituent of the body; it affects only the central nervous system.

Properties

Chemical symbol	N_2O
Molecular weight	44.01
Color	Colorless
Odor	Slightly sweet
Taste	Slightly sweet
Physical state in cylinder	Liquid

Specific gravity of gas (air = 1) at
   15°C   1.530
Approximate cylinder pressure
   at 70°F   745 psig
Critical temperature   36.5°C (97.7°F)
Critical pressure   1054 psia
Freezing point at 1 atm   −90.84°C (−131.5°F)
Boiling point at 1 atm   −89.5°C (−129.1°F)
Density of gas at 20°C, 1 atm   0.1235 lb/ft³
Combustion characteristics   Nonflammable, supports
                                         combustion

Mixtures of Therapeutic Gases

Helium–Oxygen Mixtures. A mixture of 80% helium and 20% oxygen may prove beneficial in the treatment of status asthmaticus. The low density of helium enables the gas to bypass constricted airways. At the same time, the helium carries some oxygen with it, thus preventing atelectasis and relieving hypoxia.

Oxygen–Carbon Dioxide Mixtures. A mixture of 95% oxygen and 5% carbon dioxide may be used to stimulate deep breathing and to relieve cerebral vascular spasm. Close observation of the patient must be maintained during this therapy.

SAFETY SYSTEMS

Diameter-Index Safety Systems

The Diameter-Index Safety System was developed by the Compressed Gas Association, Inc., to provide noninterchangeable threaded connections. DISS applies where make-and-break threaded connections are employed in conjunction with medical-gas-administering equipment at pressures of 200 psig or less, such as medical gas regulator threaded outlets and connections for anesthetic, resuscitation, and therapy apparatus.

    Each connection of DISS consists of a body, nipple, and nut. The system is based on having two concentric and specific bores in the body, *A* and *B*, and two concentric and specific shoulders on the nipple, *C* and *D*. See Figure 2-3. To achieve noninterchangeability between different connections, the two diameters on each part vary in opposite directions so that as one diameter increases, the other decreases. Only properly mated parts fit with each other. Attempts

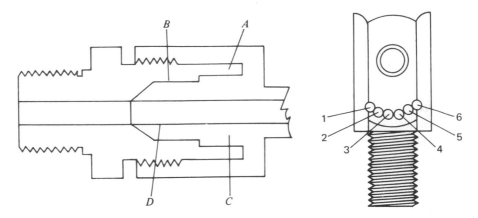

Figure 2-3. Diameter Index Safety System and Pin-Index Safety System.

to connect unintended parts result in interference at either large or small diameter, preventing thread engagement.

Pin-Index Safety System

The use of the Pin-Index Safety System was initiated to prevent the erroneous interchange of medical gas cylinders with flush-type valves. The system consists of two pins installed in the yokes of the apparatus that must match two holes drilled in the body of the cylinder valves. There is only one combination of pins and holes for each gas.

Ten combinations are possible, of which eight are in current use. With this two-pin system, it is impossible for a cylinder of one gas to be unintentionally attached to a yoke pin-indexed for any other gas.

Different Combinations

O_2	2–5
N_2O	3–5
Cyclopropane	3–6
Ethylene	1–3
CO_2–O_2 mixtures (CO_2 not over 7%)	2–6
He–O_2 mixtures (He not over 80%)	2–4
He and He–O_2 mixtures (O_2 less than 20%)	4–6
CO_2 and CO_2–O_2 mixtures (CO_2 over 7%)	1–6

American-Canadian Standard Valve Outlet and Inlet Connections of Compressed Gas Cylinder Valves

I. Thread divisions
   A. Internal
   B. External
   C. Right-handed—nonfuel gases
   D. Left-handed—fuel gases

II. Numbering system identifies
   A. Complete outlet connection — 0
   B. Valve outlet only — 1
   C. Mating assembly — 2
   D. Nipple — 3
   E. Nut — 4
   F. Washers — 5

III. Types of threads
   A. National gas outlet (NGO)—symbol for valve outlet threads
   B. National gas taper threads (NGT)
   C. National pipe threads (NPT)
   D. National straight pipe locking (NSPL)

IV. Inlet threads on valves and cylinder necks have been standardized.

V. Adapters may be required to provide interchangeability of equipment for the same gas, where more than one outlet is provided.

CYLINDER-FILLING DATA

Cylinder Style	Units of Measure	Carbon Dioxide	Oxygen	Helium	Ethylene	Air	Oxygen and Carbon Dioxide
A	Gallons	50.00	20.00	15.00	40.00	19.00	20.00
	Liters	189.00	76.00	57.00	151.00	72.00	76.00
	Cubic feet	6.67	2.67	2.01	5.35	2.56	2.67
B	Gallons	100.00	52.00	40.00	100.00	49.00	40.00
	Liters	378.00	197.00	151.00	378.00	185.00	151.00
	Cubic feet	13.37	6.95	5.35	13.37	6.54	5.35

Cylinder Style	Units of Measure	Carbon Dioxide	Oxygen	Helium	Ethylene	Air	Oxygen and Carbon Dioxide
D	Gallons	250.0	105.0	81.0	200.00	90.0	95.0
	Liters	946.0	397.0	307.0	757.00	374.0	360.0
	Cubic feet	33.4	14.0	10.8	26.74	13.2	12.7
E	Gallons	420.0	175.0	135	330.0	165	165.0
	Liters	1,590.0	662.0	511	1,249.0	623	625.0
	Cubic feet	56.1	23.4	18	44.1	22	22.1
M	Gallons	2,000.0	800	616.0	1,600.0	752.0	800
	Liters	7,570.0	3,028	2,332.0	6,056.0	2,845.0	3,028
	Cubic feet	267.4	107	82.3	213.9	100.5	107
G	Gallons	3,200.0	1,400.0	1,093.0	2,800.0	1,332.0	1,400.0
	Liters	12,112.0	5,300.0	4,137.0	10,598.0	5,043.0	5,299.0
	Cubic feet	427.8	187.2	146.1	374.3	178.1	187.1
H	Gallons		1,850	1,630		1,729	
	Liters		6,909	6,170		6,545	
	Cubic feet		244	218		231	
HH	Gallons		2,244			2,222	
	Liters		8,495			8,410	
	Cubic feet		300			297	

GAS VOLUME CONVERSION FACTORS

Cubic Feet	Liters	Gallons
1.00000	28.300	7.4800
0.03531	1.000	0.2642
0.13370	3.785	1.0000

Duration of Cylinder Flow

$$\frac{\text{Cubic feet of gas in full cylinder} \times \text{conversion factor (cubic feet to liters)}}{\text{Pressure in full cylinder in psig}}$$

= volume of gas leaving the cylinder for every psig drop in pressure

---

EXAMPLE

$$\frac{244 \text{ ft}^3 \times 28.3}{2200 \text{ psig}} = 3.14$$

The volume of gas leaving the cylinder for every psig drop in pressure, 3.14, is a constant, which for simplicity may be rounded off to 3.0.

$$\frac{\text{Gauge pressure in psig} \times \text{volume of gas leaving cylinder}}{\text{Liter flow per minute}}$$

$$= \text{duration of flow in minutes}$$

EXAMPLE

$$\frac{2200 \text{ psig (full cylinder)} \times 3}{10 \text{ liters/min (usual flow for tent)}} = \frac{6600}{10} = 660 \text{ min} \quad \text{or} \quad 11 \text{ h}$$

EXERCISES

1. What would you do in the event the master piping system was shut off or severed?
2. Explain how and why helium may be used in IPPB.
3. Explain why *everyone* should know the location of zone valves.
4. Calculate the length of time an H oxygen cylinder could run if it has a cylinder pressure of 1300 psi and a liter flow of 8 liters/min.
5. Calculate the number of liters and gallons of gas in a 40,000 ft³ reservoir.

OXYGEN THERAPY

This unit will first review some of the basic flow regulation devices; then humidifying devices and nebulization devices will be discussed. Oxygen therapy devices and their procedures will highlight this unit. The unit will end with a review of the Linde Walker Oxygen Reservoir System.

REGULATORS

The purpose of a regulator is to reduce cylinder pressure to a safer level, which is usually about 50 psig, but a higher level may be adjusted. Gas flow from the regulator is adjusted by means of a flowmeter in liters per minute.

Cylinder regulators (see Figure 3-1) may be classified as preset, adjustable, and multiple stage.

1. A preset regulator reduces cylinder pressure to a working pressure of 50 psig by passing the gas through one chamber; it has one safety valve. A Thorpe tube-style flowmeter is attached for regulation of flow.
2. The adjustable regulator reduces cylinder pressure to a working pressure of 50 to 100 psig by passing the gas through one chamber; it has one safety valve. A Bourdon gauge is used to regulate flow or pressure up to 100 psig.
3. The multi-stage regulator reduces cylinder pressure to a working pressure of 50 psig by passing the gas through either two or

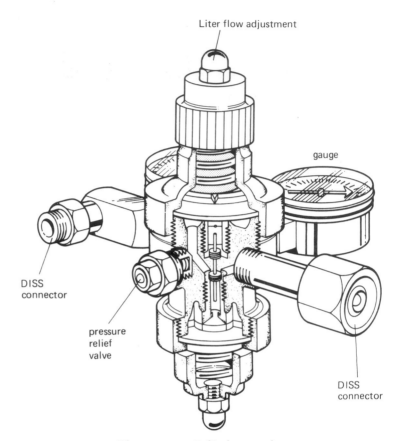

Liter flow adjustment

gauge

DISS connector

pressure relief valve

DISS connector

Figure 3-1.   Cylinder regulator.

three chambers. It has the same number of safety valves as it has chambers.

Attaching Regulator to Cylinder

Thorpe Tube Type (Figure 3-2)

1. Insert regulator inlet in cylinder valve outlet and tighten the inlet nut with a wrench.
2. Close the flow-adjusting valve; this is important and should always be done.
3. Stand to one side of the regulator, not in front or in back of it and open the cylinder valve very slowly until the needle on cylinder contents gauge stops moving; the ball float will rise in the tube

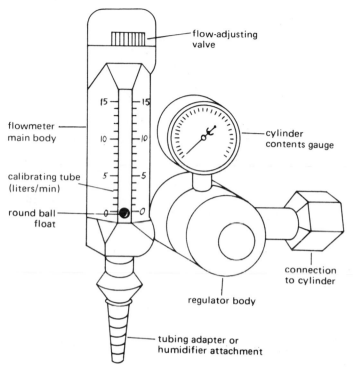

Figure 3-2.   Regulator with flowmeter—Thorpe tube type.

for a moment and then quickly return to zero: this indicates that oxygen has entered the flow indicator tube.

4. Open the flow-adjusting valve; the ball float will rise in the tube; the position of the float indicates the rate of flow in liters per minute.

5. Stop flow by closing the flow-adjusting valve; the float will drop to zero.

Bourdon Type (Figure 3-3)

1. Insert the regulator inlet into the cylinder valve outlet and tighten with a wrench.

2. Loosen regulator flow-adjusting handle.

3. Stand to the side of cylinder and open the cylinder valve slowly until needle on cylinder contents gauge stops moving.

4. Tighten the flow-adjusting handle by turning it to the right until the desired rate of flow in liters per minute is registered on the flow indicator gauge.

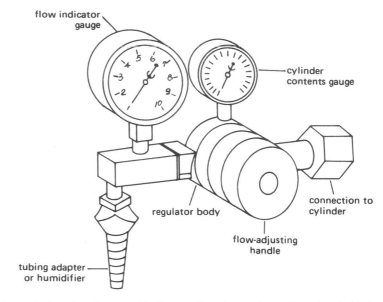

flow indicator
gauge

cylinder
contents gauge

connection to
cylinder

regulator body

flow-adjusting
handle

tubing adapter
or humidifier

Figure 3-3. Regulator with flow-adjusting valve—Bourdon tube type.

5. To disconnect, close the cylinder valve tightly; do not touch the flow-adjusting handle yet.
6. Wait until both the cylinder contents indicator and the flow indicator have returned to zero, then loosen the flow-adjusting handle until it moves freely.
7. Disconnect the regulator by unscrewing the inlet nut.

FLOWMETERS

In hospitals that have oxygen pipeline systems, in order to meter and control the amount of oxygen flow going to the patient, a flow-meter is usually employed. A flowmeter consists of a calibrated tube that indicates oxygen flow in liters per minute and a valve to control rate of flow. The flowmeter must be in an upright position for the reading to be accurate.

When administering equipment is attached to a flowmeter, back pressure is usually created. Items such as humidifiers, fog generators, and nebulizers create back pressure. When any of these devices are employed, the reading on the flowmeter will be incorrect unless the flowmeter is especially designed for use under these conditions. This type of flowmeter is called back-pressure compensated. Pressure compensation in any measuring or regulating device normally means that this device has been so designed that anticipated changes in pressure will not affect its calibration or setting. Medical oxygen flowmeters are commonly used in conjunction with nebulizers, humidifiers, and similar types of equipment. These develop flow restrictions and create a pressure at the outlet of the flowmeter, which varies with the type of equipment used and the rate of flow. Figures 3-4 through 3-6 show why only pressure-compensated flowmeters indicate actual oxygen flow to the patient regardless of the equipment being used with the flowmeter.

Thorpe Flowmeter (Uncompensated)

In this unit, shown in Figure 3-4, pressure is applied to the flowmeter inlet and controlled by the needle valve. The more the valve is opened, the greater the flow and the higher the flow indicator goes. Its position is read in liters per minute on the calibrated flow scale. Units of this type are calibrated to atmosphere (no restriction). When, due to restriction from equipment attached to the outlet of the flowmeter, the pressure at the outlet increases, the oxygen within the flow tube becomes compressed (more dense), causing the ball to drop. However,

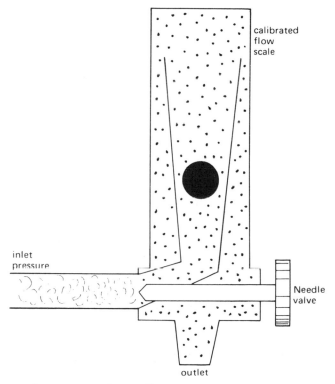

Figure 3-4. Thorpe flowmeter (uncompensated).

as the gas passes the restriction, it expands. The indicated flow under these conditions is incorrect in that the patient will receive higher flows than that indicated.

Bourdon Flow Gauge

This unit is actually a pressure gauge, calibrated in liters per minute, which operates against a fixed-sized orifice (see Figure 3-5). As the needle valve is opened, more pressure is applied to the gauge (giving a high liter-flow reading) and consequently more gas passes the fixed orifice. The Bourdon flow gauge is normally calibrated on the assumption that the gas passes through the orifice to the atmosphere.

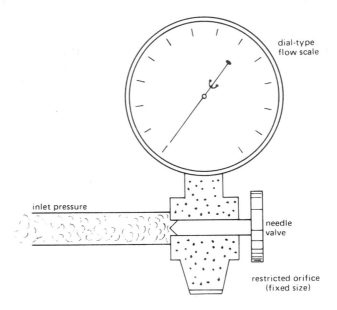

Figure 3-5.   Bourdon flow gauge.

If the free flow of gas is restricted, less oxygen passes, but more flow is indicated on the dial, since it is activated by pressure rather than flow. A unit of this type will indicate maximum flow even when the outlet is closed off completely, since pressure will still be against the gauge. The patient will receive a flow less than that indicated on the dial.

Pressure-Compensated Flowmeter (Figure 3-6)

Inlet pressure is applied to this unit through a calibrated flow scale to a needle valve control at a constant 50 psi. As the needle control

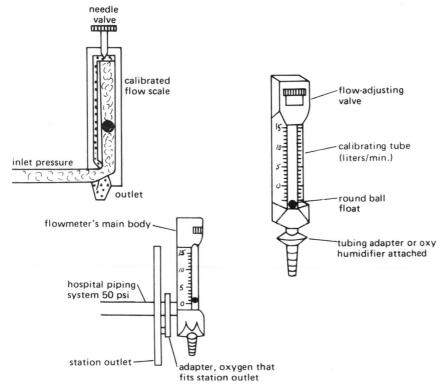

Figure 3-6. Pressure-compensated flowmeter.

valve is opened and gas is allowed to flow, the ball is lifted in the gas stream. The more the valve is opened, the more gas will flow. Back pressure will cause the ball to drop since the flow of oxygen passing the restricting orifice is lower; since the amount of back pressure can never be greater than the pressure within the tube, the flowmeter will accurately indicate the flow. With this design the accuracy of flow is never affected by back pressure. The patient receives the amount indicated on the scale.

To Attach a Flowmeter to Outlet

1. Close the flow-adjusting valve on the flowmeter.
2. Insert the inlet of the flowmeter into the opening of the outlet and press until a firm connection is made.
3. Slowly open the flow-adjusting valve of the flowmeter; as oxygen flows into the flowmeter, the float will rise.
4. To disconnect the flowmeter, close the flow-adjusting valve; when the float has dropped to zero, gently push the flowmeter into the outlet; the flowmeter will then come out.

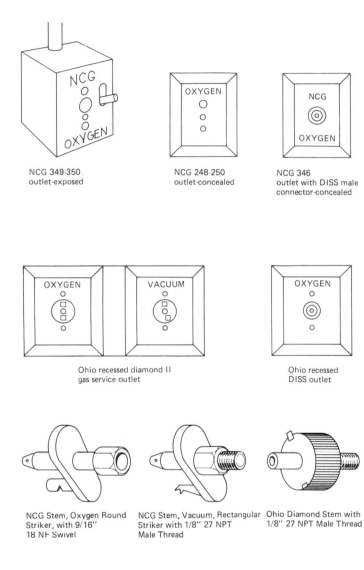

NCG 349-350
outlet-exposed

NCG 248-250
outlet-concealed

NCG 346
outlet with DISS male
connector-concealed

Ohio recessed diamond II
gas service outlet

Ohio recessed
DISS outlet

NCG Stem, Oxygen Round
Striker, with 9/16"
18 NF Swivel

NCG Stem, Vacuum, Rectangular
Striker with 1/8" 27 NPT
Male Thread

Ohio Diamond Stem with
1/8" 27 NPT Male Thread

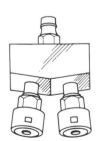

Duplex Adapter with Puritan Inlet
Stem and Two Puritan Quick-Connect
Valve Outlets

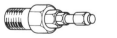

Schrader Quick Connect-System
Oxygen, Non Swivel with 1/4"
Male Thread

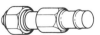

Puritan Quick-Connect Stem
with 9/16" 18 Swivel Nut

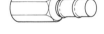

Puritan Quick-Connect
Stem with 1/8" 27 NPT
Female Thread

Figure 3-7.   Wall outlets and adapters.

WALL OUTLETS AND ADAPTERS

A station outlet is located at each point in a "piped" hospital where oxygen is to be withdrawn. Outlets are usually of two types—either threaded or of the quick-connect variety. See Figure 3-7.

I. Quick-connect Outlets
    A. To Attach the Flowmeter
        1. Close the flow-adjusting valve on the flowmeter.
        2. Insert the gas inlet of the flowmeter into the opening of the wall outlet; press until a firm connection is made. Pull back slightly on the flowmeter to check.
        3. Slowly open the flow-adjusting valve of the flowmeter until the desired flow is obtained.
    B. To Disconnect the Flowmeter
        1. Close the flow-adjusting valve.
        2. When the float has dropped to zero, gently push forward on the flowmeter and then pull back from the station outlet valve.
        3. Some outlets have release levers that must be disengaged before the flowmeter is withdrawn.

II. Threaded Outlets
    A. To Attach the Flowmeter
        1. Close the flow-adjusting valve on the flowmeter.
        2. Seat the gas inlet of the flowmeter into the station outlet valve. The Diameter Index Safety System prevents connection of the wrong regulating equipment to a station outlet.
        3. Tighten the knurled inlet nut, securing the flowmeter to the outlet. This assures a gas seal.
        4. Adjust the oxygen flow by turning the flow-adjusting control.
    B. To Disconnect the Flowmeter
        1. Close the flow-adjusting valve.
        2. When the indicator float returns to zero, unscrew the knurled inlet nut on the flowmeter.

HUMIDIFIERS

Medical gases that are administered through a cylinder or master pipeline system are dry. We know that if a dry gas is administered to the patient dehydration usually occurs. To protect the patient from dehydration, humidifiers are used for most administration devices. A humidifier uses a simple means of passing the medical gas through sterile water, so that water vapor is picked up. One of the most popular types of humidifiers uses a porous stone to create tiny bubbles, since the greater the number of bubbles, the more water vapor is produced. Three examples of this are the Ohio Jet Humidifier (Figure 3-8), the Puritan-Bennett Bubble-Jet Humidifier (Figures 3-9 and 3-10), and the Bennett Cascade Humidifier (Figures 3-11 and 3-12).

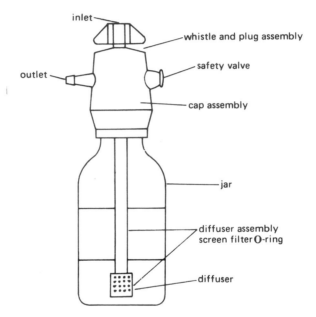

Figure 3-8. Ohio Jet Humidifier.

Bennett Cascade Humidifier

The Bennett Cascade Humidifier is designed primarily for use with Puritan-Bennett IPPB equipment and Puritan-Bennett respiration units. Its function is to humidify the gas delivered to the patient. (The cascade humidifier unit is referred to as "the cascade" in the following instructions.)

Installation

1. Remove the mainstream humidifier and the bracket from the respirator pedestal.

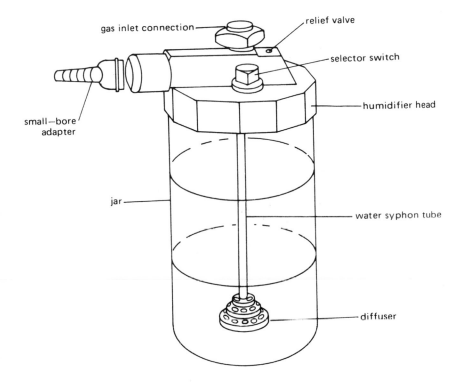

Figure 3-9. Puritan-Bennett Bubble-Jet Humidifier.

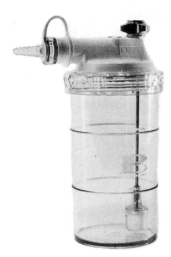

Figure 3-10. Puritan-Bennett Bubble-Jet Humidifier. (*Courtesy of Puritan-Bennett Corp., Kansas City, Mo.*)

127

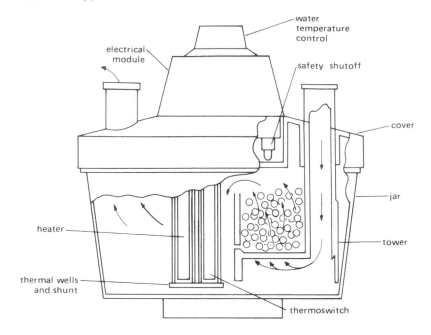

Figure 3-11.   Cascade Humidifier diagram.

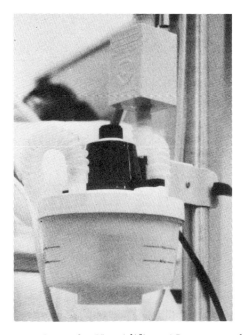

Figure 3-12.   Bennett Cascade Humidifier. (*Courtesy of Puritan-Bennett Corp., Kansas City, Mo.*)

2. Remove the respirator head from the column.

3. Slip the cascade over the column and replace the respirator head.

4. Connect the flex tube (long) or extension tubing to the Bennett valve outlet and to the cascade inlet and adjust the bracket as needed.

5. Connect the exhalation valve tube and nebulizer tubes, and connect the main air hose to the cascade outlet.

6. Slip the thermometer manifold into the exhalation manifold and connect the main tube to the thermometer manifold.

7. Fill the plastic container with sterile water.

8. Plug in the unit.

9. Set the temperature control knob at the desired setting.

Solutions Used

1. Sterile water should be used in the cascade; do not let water go below the refill line.

2. Medications are to be added to the small nebulizer assembly in the usual manner.

Temperature Settings

1. The cascade must be plugged into a suitable electrical outlet.

2. The blue numbers on the cascade represent temperatures below body temperature; the unit must be set at least to number 3 for adequate humidity.

3. The white numbers represent body temperature.

4. The red numbers represent temperatures above body temperature (up to 120°F).

5. The temperature should be checked frequently by means of the thermometer.

Cleaning and Sterilization

1. Disconnect the electrical cord; then allow a few minutes for the heater assembly to cool.

2. Remove the flex tube from the Bennett valve outlet and the main tube from the cascade outlet.

3. Hold the bottom of the jar and turn the two blue knobs on the cascade cover, and lower the cover and jar from the electrical unit.

4. Unscrew the jar from the cover, and empty the water from the jar.

5. Loosen the white thumb nut, and remove the tower from the cover.

6. Wash the jar, cover, tower, thumb nut, and flex tube in warm, soapy water; rinse carefully and put to soak in Cidex for 10 minutes; rinse, dry, and reassemble; the unit may also be gas sterilized.

7. The electrical unit is not in the patient circuit; it should periodically be wiped clean conventionally.

8. The thermometer manifold is cleaned in the usual manner; the thermometer, however, cannot be cleaned other than by wiping it off.

Cascade II Servocontrolled Heated Humidifier for MA-I Volume Ventilator

The Cascade II (Figure 3-13) is a solid-state unit that maintains and displays preselected temperatures of delivered gas. One hundred

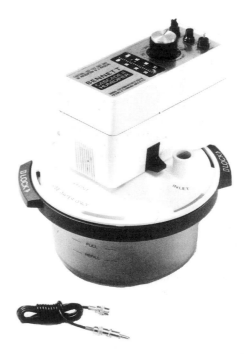

Figure 3-13.   Bennett Cascade II Humidifier. (*Courtesy of Puritan-Bennett Corp., Kansas City, Mo.*)

percent relative humidity at body temperature at the patient wye can be approached, equaled, or exceeded by relating temperature of delivered gas to body temperature.

Installation Procedure for Model MA-1

1. Attach the servocontroller to the mounting plate using the screws provided (longer screws go into the top holes).
2. Attach the protector bar to the mounting plate.
3. Remove the mounting plate screws from their holes in the side of the unit. Attach the plate, with the protector bar and the controller.
4. Assemble the jar and cover to the controller. Align the front of the cover (marked FRONT) with the front of the controller (the side with the grill). Engage the latches in the slots in either side of the controller housing; push upward until the latches snap into place.
5. Fit the angled connectors to the main-flow bacteria filter outlet and to the humidifier outlet.

Operation

Note: These instructions refer to the operation of the Cascade II humidifier only; there is no change in the operation of the Model MA-1 Ventilator.

1. Grasp the jar locking ring handles; turn clockwise. The jar and locking ring will separate easily from the cover.
2. Remove and fill the jar with sterile distilled water only to the Full level. If prescribed medications are ordered by the physician, they should be administered via the nebulizer.
3. Mate the jar to the cover; turn the locking ring counterclockwise until snug. Be certain that the sections of the locking ring mate properly to the cover.
4. Install the sensor probe in the patient tubing and connect it to the controller module.
5. Set the temperature control to the desired gas temperature to be delivered at the location of the probe.
6. Adjust the Alarm Set level to a temperature approximately 3 degrees above the selected temperature. Do not exceed temperature limits, which could be harmful to the patient.
7. Turn on power. Begin cycling the ventilator; allow warm-up time, observing the temperature display on the controller. Under

normal conditions, the water will reach temperature in 15 to 20 min. Monitor the temperature display and adjust the control as required to secure the desired setting.

8. For extended treatment, drape the main tube so that condensate drains back into the humidifier jar. Frequently drain condensate from the main tube. If condensate is allowed to collect in the tube, it may finally block the tube and prevent flow, or may allow condensate to reach the patient.

9. Replace water as necessary. *Do not allow the water level to go below the lower line.*

Disassembly

1. Be sure that the humidifier has had sufficient time to *cool*.
2. Turn the jar locking ring clockwise; remove the jar. Empty the water from the jar; remove the ring seal.
3. Loosen the stud, and remove the tower.
4. Grasp the cover; turn knurled ring counterclockwise to loosen, and remove the heater from beneath the cover.

Cleaning and Sterilization

1. Wash all parts in warm detergent solution. Use care not to damage the ring seal of the cover. If there is a deposit on the heater, remove with scouring powder or fine steel wool.
2. All parts may be cold sterilized or gas sterilized.
3. The control module and the sensor cord are not in the patient circuit. They may be periodically wiped with 70% isopropyl alcohol and dried well. Do *not* autoclave or immerse in a solution.
4. The removable sensor may be cold sterilized, gas sterilized, or autoclaved. Disconnect the sensor from the cord with a push twist motion.

Disposable Humidifiers and Nebulizers

Today in the field of respiratory therapy, a great quantity of disposable items is being used. One of the newer areas of disposable equipment is that of the plastic disposable humidifier–nebulizer, which is manufactured by a number of firms. See Figure 3-14 for examples.

Most humidifier–nebulizers are packed for single-patient use only. They have the standard $\frac{9}{16}$-in. nut for connection to a standard flowmeter or other optional equipment. The newest feature in the disposable humidifier–nebulizer is that of air entrainment for variable concentration and adaptation to ventilators.

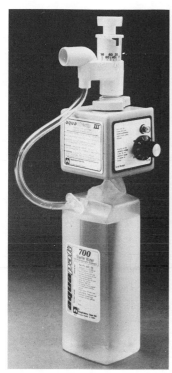
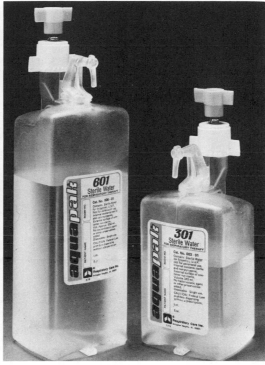

Figure 3-14. Disposable humidifiers and nebulizers. *(Courtesy of Respiratory Care, Inc., Arlington Heights, Ill.)*

Disposable prefilled units are also available in a variety of sizes. As humidifiers, they may be used for up to 5 days continuously for a single patient with their sterility intact. The nebulizer may last for approximately 24 to 48 hours, depending on flow rate; it may also be used with adjustable heaters to provide a wide degree of humidification.

The units are also available for use with ultrasonic nebulizers. Most units have a scale on the bottle so that a record of consumption may be kept. The use of disposable prefilled units in the administration of oxygen and aerosol therapy has helped to decrease the danger of cross-infection.

AEROSOL THERAPY APPARATUS

An aerosol is a suspension of fine particles or droplets in a gas. It is created by means of the Bernoulli principle, which is a law of hydrodynamics that relates the velocity, pressure, and density of a fluid

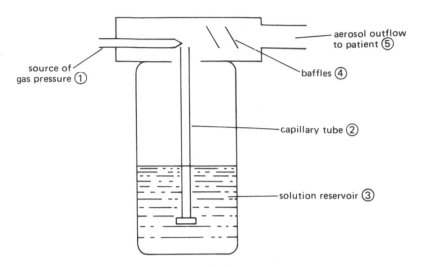

Figure 3-15. Aerosol therapy apparatus.

(gas or liquid) in motion. According to the Bernoulli principle, the greater the velocity of the fluid, the lower its pressure.

Refer to Figure 3-15. A source gas pressure is supplied to the inlet of the nebulizer (1). This causes a fine jet stream of gas across the capillary tube (2), which is immersed in solution (3); this causes a differential in pressure to occur, and the solution comes up the capillary tube. As it reaches the top, the solution is forced against the gas flow and against a baffle (4), which breaks the solution into fine particles. The gas then flows through the outlet of the nebulizer (5) and then to the patient. One of the most popular nebulizers used is the Puritan All-Purpose Nebulizer.

Puritan All-Purpose Nebulizer (Figures 3-16 and 3-17)

Inlet Connection.   The inlet connection is a threaded nut for oxygen. After connecting the nebulizer to a regulated source of oxygen, the unit may be swiveled around the inlet connection for convenience.

Dilution Control.   The dilution control can be set to mix oxygen and air for concentrations of 40%, 70%, or 100%. To set percentage, lift control knob from recess and set concentration to the desired position opposite the percentage-of-oxygen arrow. (Make sure control knob reseats in recess.) The 40% or 70% oxygen concentrations should be used only with an unrestricted ¾-in. large-bore breathing tube no longer than 5 ft, or when nebulizing directly from the large-bore outlet. The dilution control will not function when set at 40% or 70% if used with a catheter, cannula, or other restricting attach-

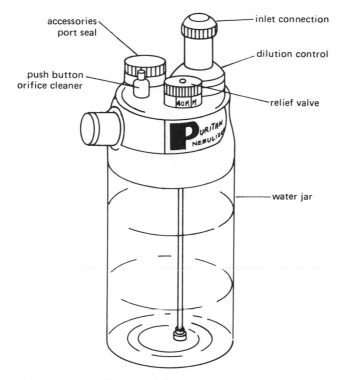

accessories
port seal

inlet connection

dilution control

push button
orifice cleaner

relief valve

water jar

Figure 3-16.   Puritan All-Purpose Nebulizer diagram.

ments. When used with an IPPB unit, always set control to "IPPB 100%" position.

Small-bore Outlet Adapter.   The small-bore outlet adapter snaps into the large-bore nebulizer outlet and permits the use of $\frac{3}{16}$- to $\frac{5}{16}$-in. inside diameter supply tubing. When using this adapter, make sure dilution control is set for 100% oxygen concentration.

Water Jar.   Fill jar with sterile water or prescribed solution to top line on jar. When liquid reaches lower line, refill to top line.

Push-button Orifice Cleaner.   This button permits cleaning of the small jet orifice without interrupting operation. If, when the unit is in operation, water droplets do not fall from the baffle tube within the nebulizer head, this indicates the orifice needs cleaning. Depress push-button orifice cleaner two or three times to clean orifice.

Accessories Port Seal.   The accessories port seal permits interchange of the relief valve or accessories. Never operate nebulizer with ports open.

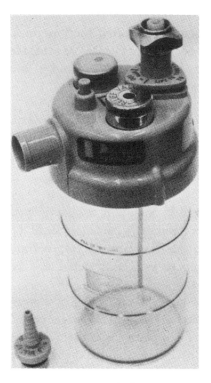

Figure 3-17. Puritan All-Purpose Nebulizer. (*Courtesy of Puritan-Bennett Corp., Kansas City, Mo.*)

Relief Valves. Puritan nebulizers are equipped with one of two relief valves. For patient protection when using catheters, it is recommended that the 40 mm Hg relief valve be installed. The 2-psi relief valve can be used for mask, tents, etc., or other open systems. The relief valves require only a 90° twist to install and seal or remove.

Important: When releasing internal pressure of 40 mm Hg or 2 psi, the relief valves are both audible and visible. However, when the dilution control is set to 40% or 70% oxygen, excessive pressure within the nebulizer or outlet connective system will vent through the dilution control and bypass the relief valves. Pressure buildup is thus avoided, but no audible or visible indication will be evident.

Medication. The Puritan nebulizer is designed to be used with sterile water or solutions. To prevent the possibility of cross-infection, the nebulizer should be cleaned after use on each patient.

Puritan Immersion Heater. This heater is interchangeable with the accessory port seal so that the unit may be used either hot or cold. (A relief valve should always be used with this unit.)

Note: If heater interferes with oxygen-regulating equipment, the relief valve and heater position may be interchanged.

The purpose of heated nebulization is to increase the moisture or medicant content of the inspired oxygen or air–oxygen mixture. In normal usage the Puritan nebulizer with the immersion heater will deliver the moist gas at body temperature or slightly above.

Due to the higher operating temperatures and the higher moisture output in heated nebulization, a considerable quantity of moisture may collect on the walls of the outlet tubing between the nebulizer and the patient. In the event water or medicants collect in the patient delivery tube, drain the solution.

It is recommended that, if possible, the nebulizer be placed below the level of the patient and the supply tube so arranged that moisture occurring in the tube will automatically drain back into the nebulizer jar. Periodic inspection of the tube to determine the amount of condensate is very important.

The thermostat control in the heater is factory set to hold the temperature of water or solution to approximately 135° to 145°F. The issuant temperature of the moist gas stream will be approximately 100° to 110°F, depending on the type of administering equipment used.

Caution: 1. *Do not operate unit dry when immersion heater is heating; the result will be the issuance of extremely dry warm gas to the patient, contributing to patient dehydration and drying of the respiratory tissues.*

2. The heater is equipped with a three-prong grounding plug for use with 110 to 120 volts, 25-, 50-, or 60-cycle alternating current only. If three-hole grounding outlets are not available, the grounding adapter should be connected to a suitable ground, such as a cold-water pipe. Always unplug heater from electrical outlet when not in use. Do not touch the barrel of the heater with bare hand until electrical cord has been disconnected for 5 min.

3. The immersion heater has been factory sealed to preclude moisture. *It should not be disassembled under any circumstances.*

Hudson Cloud Chamber

The Hudson Cloud Chamber synchronizes the continuous flow of the nebulizer with the intermittent flow of the patient's breathing. When driven by an oxygen or compressed-air source, the nebulizer generates aerosol particles, which are accumulated in the aerosol chamber until inhalation. When the patient inhales, the particles are drawn through the mouthpiece and into the lungs. A fluidic valve with no moving parts creates a wall-hugging effect, which forces exhaled gases to exit through the chamber. As the patient exhales, the nebulizer refills the aerosol chamber for the next inhalation.

Operation of Unit (refer to Figure 3-18)

1. Pull nebulizer from aerosol chamber. Pull graduated reservoir from nebulizer housing. Fill reservoir with desired medication

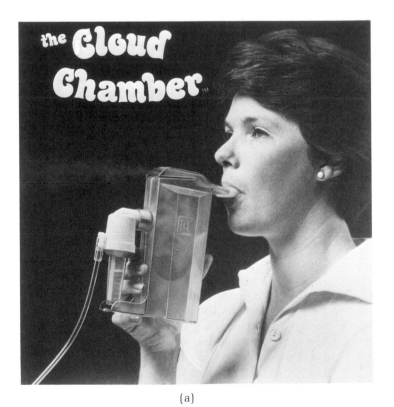

(a)

Figure 3-18. Hudson Cloud Chamber. (*Courtesy of Hudson Oxygen Therapy Sales Company, Temecula, Calif.*)

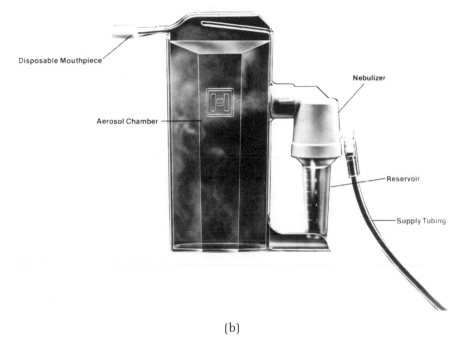

(b)

Figure 3-18.   (*cont.*)

(reservoir will hold a maximum of 10 ml). Reinsert reservoir into nebulizer housing until it snaps into place.

2. Firmly insert nebulizer into aerosol chamber.
3. Attach short connector of supply tubing to inlet fitting on nebulizer housing. Attach long connector end of tubing to regulated compressed-air or medical-oxygen source.
4. Install mouthpiece into chamber.
5. Have patient hold unit around body of chamber and breathe normally through mouthpiece as directed by physician.

Note: Do not block outlet opposite mouthpiece or opening at bottom of unit.

Cleaning and Sterilization

1. Wash all components in warm water and detergent. Rinse in warm water.
2. Sterilize components in a chemical sterilent (Cidex). Immerse parts in the solution for 10 min, remove, and immerse in sterile

water for 10 additional minutes. Remove parts from sterile water
and thoroughly dry.

3. Unit also may be sterilized with ethylene oxide.

Note: Aeration time must be sufficient to remove all traces of sterilizing agent.

Concha Pak Humidifier

The Concha Pak system (see Figure 3-19) is designed to provide continuous heated, humidified gas for volume ventilators for 24 hours
without changing the reservoir. It will humidify continuous-flow gas
systems, as well as oxygen diluter systems. The Concha Pak may be
converted into a heated nebulizer with a nebulizer adapter.

Unit Assembly

1. Mount heater at appropriate location, using a Concha universal
   clamp, or on an MA-1 ventilator, using a Concha permanent
   MA-1 bracket or universal MA-1 bracket.
2. Plug unit into 100-V service outlet.
3. Remove Concha column from packaging and insert, from top to

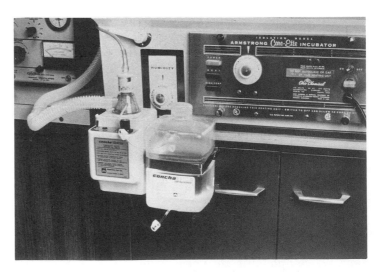

(a)

Figure 3-19. Concha Pak Humidifier. (*Courtesy of Respiratory Care, Inc.,*
Arlington Heights, Ill.)

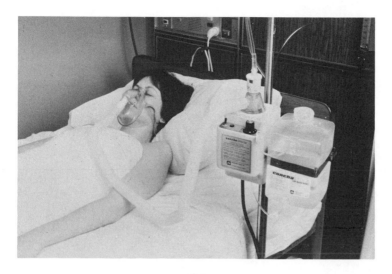

(b)

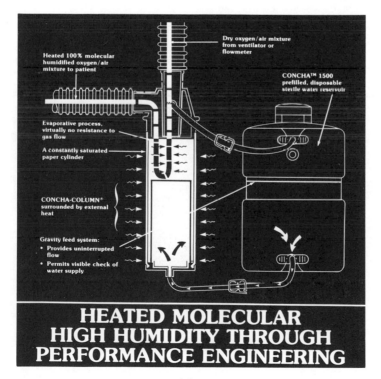

HEATED MOLECULAR
HIGH HUMIDITY THROUGH
PERFORMANCE ENGINEERING

(c)

Figure 3-19. (*cont.*)

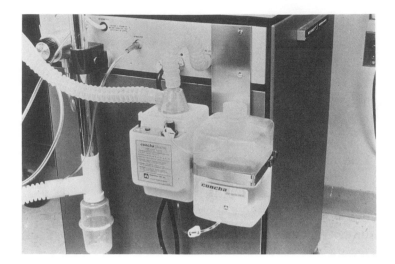

(d)

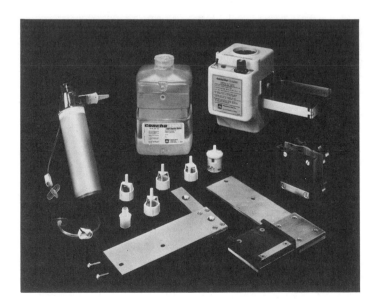

(e)

Figure 3-19.   (*cont.*)

bottom, with bottom puncture pin and tubing passing through heater chamber first.

4. Remove Concha 1500 reservoir from package. Place it in the reservoir bracket on the heater and close the bracket latch. The label on the reservoir bottle should be right side up.

5. Remove sheath from bottom pin on tubing and press pin through the puncture site at the bottom of the reservoir.

6. Remove sheath from pin on tubing at the top of the Concha column and press pin through the puncture site directly above the yellow cap on the Concha reservoir.

7. Be certain both clamps on tubes from Concha column are open. Water should flow into Concha column cylinder.

8. Connect hose from gas source or ventilator to top port of Concha column and patient hose to side port. When input gas is supplied by narrow-bore tubing, the adapter is mounted into the top port.

9. Switch heater and ventilator on (or turn gas flow on), and adjust thermostat dial to desired setting. Warm-up time for the column is approximately 15 min. The dial setting may be set anywhere above no. 1 for the warm-up procedure.

10. The Concha 1500 reservoir bottle will last over 24 hours when the volume ventilator has been set at normal settings of 12 liters/min, volume setting of 1000 cc, and cycle time of 12 to 14 times/min.

11. When the thermostat setting is at no. 6, the temperature of the gas at the patient wye connection will be slightly above body temperature.

12. For heated and humidified oxygen dilution therapy, simply place one of the four fixed or adjustable Concha oxygen dilutors onto the top part of the Concha column. Connect corrugated hose to the outlet part of the column.

13. For heated aerosol therapy, use the Concha nebulizer adapter. Insert the tube from the bottom of the adapter into the top of the column; press adapter securely onto the column. Adjust to desired oxygen concentration.

ULTRASONIC THERAPY

DeVilbiss Ultrasonic Nebulizer

General Remarks.   The DeVilbiss Ultrasonic Nebulizer was developed so that a very fine aerosol with more uniform particles could be delivered to the patient. Such an aerosol has the capacity to penetrate deeper into the bronchial tree, reaching airways that could not be reached before by normal aerosol devices.

The beneficial aerosol is produced through the atomizing of a given medication by means of high-frequency sound waves (1.35 megacycles). High-frequency sound is the number of complete waves there are in a given time period. When ultrasonic energy is used to produce an aerosol, the frequency of the signal generated will determine the particle size of the aerosol produced. The higher the frequency, the smaller the particle, and the lower the frequency, the larger the particles.

The DeVilbiss unit may be used alone or may be used with various ventilators to give ultrasonic treatments to patients who require long-term ventilation.

The basic technique of attaching the two units (ultrasonic nebulizer and ventilator) is relatively simple. All it requires is to introduce the ultrasonic unit into the main stream of the ventilator. This can be accomplished by means of a tubing connection from the ventilator outlet, to the nebulizer inlet, and then continuing on from the outlet on the nebulizer to the patient setup.

Assembly (refer to Figures 3-20 and 3-21)

1. Mounting of modules (5) and (2)
   a. Mount nebulizer module (2) on lower bracket and secure unit by tightening two knurled nuts mounted on unit.
   b. Mount the air supply module (5) on the upper bracket and secure unit by tightening two knurled nuts.
2. Insert elbow (8) to side of air supply module; point elbow outlet downward; insert the two remaining elbows (9) to the nebulizer chamber (4); point elbows so that they are in an upward direction.
3. Remove front cover from the couplant compartment (3).
4. Place nebulizer flange under each cover of couplant compartment.
5. Fill couplant compartment with distilled water until the water level is about $\frac{1}{4}$ in. above the nebulizer's base.
6. Observe the level of water in compartment during operation of unit.
7. Replace front cover of compartment, check indication button (10); if there is adequate water supply it will appear black; if not it will appear light.
8. Attach small- and large-bore tubing from top of liquid reservoir bottle (6) to the side of the nebulizer chamber.

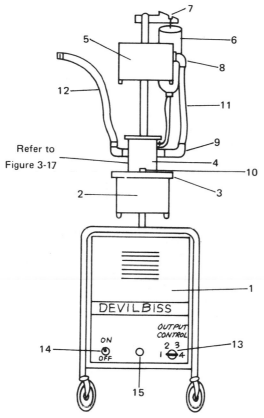

Figure 3-20. DeVilbiss Ultrasonic Nebulizer.

9. Connect air supply tubing (11) to the elbow on the air module (5) and the other end to the elbow (9) on the nebulizer chamber (4).

10. Connect the main aerosol tubing (12) to the nebulizer chamber elbow, and attach mask or various other apparatus for patient use.

11. Fill liquid reservoir bottle (6) with sterile water, making sure that the large-bore tubing is closed off by the clamp; place reservoir bottle on reservoir bracket (7).

12. Open the clamp on the large-bore tubing; solution will now flow into nebulizer chamber.

13. Plug air supply module electrical cord to the rear receptacle in the nebulizer module.

14. Plug the nebulizer module cable to the two male receptacles on the power unit.

15. Plug in the power supply cable to the receptacle on the power unit (1), and plug into a 115-V ac 60-cycle power source.

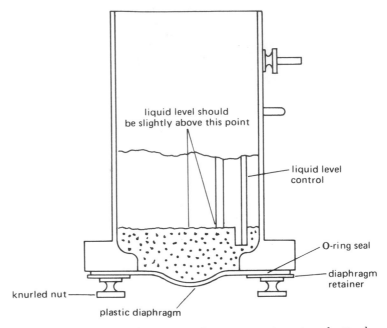

Figure 3-21. Nebulizer chamber, couplant compartment and attachments for DeVilbiss Ultrasonic Nebulizer.

Operation of Unit

1. Check solution level in couplant compartment and nebulizer chamber.
2. Adjust output control (13) to number 4 and switch power on (14).
3. If all is operating correctly the power light (15) will be on.
4. Adjust output control for proper aerosol output.
5. Administer aerosol to patient on attaching the apparatus.

DeVilbiss Model 35B Ultrasonic Nebulizer (Figure 3-22)

I. Introduction
    The Model 35B ultrasonic nebulizer is designed to provide the advantages of high-density, homogeneous ultrasonic aerosols to many types of medical equipment universally used for respiratory therapy, especially in those techniques where output volume of not more than 3 cm³ of aerosol per minute is indicated.

    In addition to the self-contained air supply, the carrier gas used to exhaust the aerosol droplets from the nebulizer

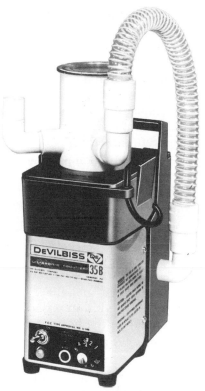

Figure 3-22.   DeVilbiss Model 35B Ultrasonic Nebulizer. (*Courtesy of the DeVilbiss Co., Somerset, Pa.*)

chamber can be the mainstream gas of an intermittent positive pressure machine, air from a compressor, or gases from a compressed gas cylinder and anesthesia machine. (Do not use flammable agents.) Central air and gas systems can also be utilized. As with other DeVilbiss ultrasonic nebulizers, it is also possible for the patient to withdraw aerosol from the chamber by his own respiration.

II. Assembly
   A. Bend back the rubber hold-down tabs and remove the two couplant compartment cover halves from the nebulizer, and check that no foreign material is in the couplant compartment.
   B. The unit can be operated while sitting on any convenient table. However, electronic cooling air enters through the nebulizer back. Therefore, it is important that the nebulizer air filter be kept clean and that the unit not be placed against

a wall or other object that could restrict air flow. A reversible bracket is provided on the back of the unit for attaching to other equipment (such as column of an IPPB machine or suitable stand).

C. Check the drain tube to make certain that it is inserted securely into the drain tube clip. Pour room-temperature water into couplant compartment until the water level reaches the fill line indicator in the front corner. The float should now be touching the retaining clip.

D. Place the two couplant compartment covers around the lower half of the nebulizer chamber (below the elbow outlets and above the bottom flange), and press together until the covers snap into place.

E. Insert the assembled nebulizer chamber and covers into the couplant compartment by pressing down until the two rubber hold-down tabs snap over the covers. Be sure that the longer cover is at the front of the nebulizer.

F. Remove cover from top of nebulizer chamber, and pour not more than 180 cm^3 of liquid into the chamber. Do not allow liquid level to go above the bottom of the elbow ports.

G. Check that both elbows are firmly installed in the nebulizer chamber.

H. There are various methods available to connect the carrier gas to the nebulizer chamber depending on the equipment being utilized.

I. Connect a suitable aerosol hose to the outlet elbow and lead to patient.

J. Connect the power cable to a 115-V ac 60-Hz power source. If a three-wire receptacle is not available, use a ground-type adapter with its ground wire secured to the electric ground. The Model 35B is now ready to operate.

K. If the continuous feed system (with the liquid level control in the nebulizer chamber, and liquid reservoir) is to be used, remove cap from the liquid reservoir. Connect the small-diameter tube between the smaller-diameter fitting on the cap and the smaller-diameter (lower) fitting projecting from side of the nebulizer chamber. Be sure that the tubing clamp is on the large-diameter tube; then connect this tube between the larger-diameter fitting on the cap and the larger-diameter (upper) fitting on side of nebulizer chamber.

L. Fill reservoir; check that tubing clamp is closing off large-diameter tube. Install filled reservoir in cap. Then hang reservoir on a suitable bracket near the unit.

M. Release tubing clamp; liquid will flow through the small-diameter tube to nebulizer chamber. Remove nebulizer chamber cover to observe liquid flow. When the liquid level in the chamber reaches the proper level, as sensed by the chamber liquid level control, the flow will stop. When liquid level in chamber falls, air flows through large-diameter tube into reservoir and allows more liquid through small-diameter tube. Replace nebulizer cover when satisfied that flow is proper.

N. For single-treatment use, using the continuous-feed nebulizer chamber, disconnect the large- and small-diameter tubes from the nebulizer chamber. It is not necessary to remove the liquid level control.

O. Remove cover from top of nebulizer chamber and pour not more than 180 cm^3 of liquid in the chamber. Do not allow liquid level to go above the bottom of the elbow ports.

P. Frequently it is desirable for aerosol to be administered to the patient on demand or by his own respiration. This technique eliminates any waste of nebulized solution. When utilized in this fashion, remove the air supply hose from the inlet elbow of the nebulizer chamber. This disconnects the air supply and prevents the aerosol from being continually delivered into the atmosphere and provides for better quantitative dosage control.

III. Operation

A. Recheck the water level in the couplant compartment. Be sure the water level reaches the fill level indicator. With the couplant compartment covers installed, the indicator windows will show black when water is at the proper level. If indicator window shows light, refill compartment. Periodically check indicator window during operation.

B. Check the liquid level within the nebulizer chamber; for single treatment, the level should be slightly below the ports. For continuous feed, the level should be slightly above the second surface of the liquid level control.

C. Set the output control knob of the nebulizer to no. 10 and turn the switch to *on* position.

D. If properly connected, the power pilot light will come on. Evidence of ultrasonic activity can be observed through the transparent cover of the nebulizer chamber.

E. Also turn output control knob to other visible positions to ensure operation on all ranges. No visible aerosol will be generated on the lower setting of no. 1.

F. If the unit appears to be operating satisfactorily, turn off the power, clean and prepare the liquid level reservoir, tubes, nebulizer chamber, and air and aerosol hoses to your specifications.

IV. Cleaning and Sterilization

A. Nebulizer couplant compartment—drain water from couplant compartment by removing drain tube from rubber clip. Hold the tube down, allowing the water to drain into a suitable container. Collect the remaining water with a soft damp cloth. Refill the compartment with fresh or distilled tap water.

B. Nebulizer chamber general cleaning—clean the nebulizer chamber following each treatment by using one of the following methods:

1. Autoclave.
2. Gas sterilization.
3. Wash in alcohol and air dry.
4. Wash in 2% acetic acid (white vinegar is 4% to 5% acetic acid); rinse with clear water and air dry.
5. Wash in hot detergent water or hot soap; rinse thoroughly and air dry.

C. Nebulizer chamber liquid level control—if desired, the liquid level control can be removed for periodic cleaning. Take off the knurled nut projecting through side of chamber and carefully pull control into chamber and out its top. Use a soft thin brush or pipe cleaner to clean the control passages. Reinstall, being sure that both O-ring seals are in place.

D. Nebulizer chamber diaphragm—periodically remove plastic diaphragm at bottom of chamber by loosening the four knurled nuts and rotating diaphragm retainer until it is free. Clean all loose parts in accordance with cleaning step B. Inspect diaphragm for pin holes or cracks. Replace diaphragm if pin holes or cracks are found. When reinstalling diaphragm, be sure it is centered on bottom of chamber with its concave (recessed) side facing interior of chamber. Be sure to install O-ring seal between diaphragm and chamber.

E. Air filter—under normal conditions, clean air filter weekly. Under adverse conditions or with heavy use, clean air filter daily.

F. Disassemble to clean nebulizer cooling fins and blower compartment.

G. Nebulizer cooling fins are cleaned by vacuuming or blowing out with compressed air. Remove all dust and foreign matter from between the fins.

H. Blower compartment—clean the following blower parts weekly by using one of the methods listed in step B.
   1. Filter retainer
   2. Filter frame
   3. Thumb screw
   4. Mounting and filter bracket
   5. Blower wheel
   6. Fan housing

I. Autoclave—the following parts can withstand a temperature of 250°F (121°C).
   1. Liquid reservoir
   2. Reservoir connecting tubes and clamp
   3. Aerosol hose
   4. Blower compartment parts
   5. Nebulizer chamber

J. Reassemble in the reverse order of disassembly.

Monaghan 670 Ultrasonic Humidifier (Figure 3-23)

I. Introduction
   The Monaghan 670 Ultrasonic Humidifier consists of two main components:

A. Power supply—converts ac power to low-voltage power for the transducer. The module contains the output controls and a fan that moves ambient air through an air filter to an orifice in the front of the unit, and thus provides a mode of transport for the aerosol.

B. Ultrasonic transducer assembly—contains four separate parts:
   1. Transducer—converts low-voltage power into high-frequency electronic waves that vibrate a Pyrex-coated crystal.
   2. Float assembly—regulates the flow of liquid to the crystal.
   3. Manifold—contains the aerosol until it is delivered to the patient by the output hose.
   4. Outer cylinder—connects the manifold to the transducer.

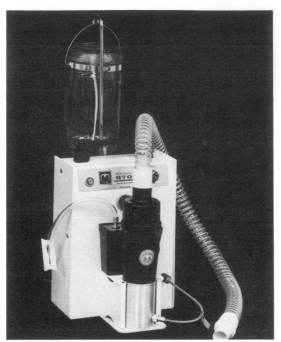

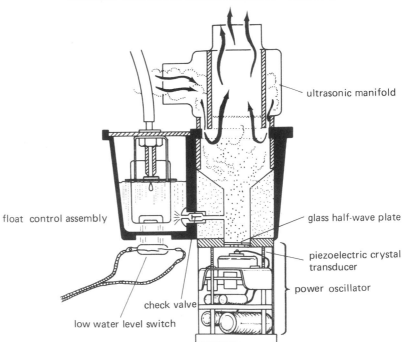

ultrasonic manifold

float control assembly

glass half-wave plate

piezoelectric crystal transducer

power oscillator

check valve

low water level switch

Figure 3-23. Monaghan 670 Ultrasonic Humidifier. (*Courtesy of Monaghan: a division of Sandoz-Wander, Inc., Littleton, Colo.*)

II. Assembly
   A. Slide the transducer assembly into the bracket on the power
      supply module.
   B. Insert the airflow inlet on the manifold into the blower air-
      flow orifice on the power supply module.
   C. Connect the power cable on the transducer to the power re-
      ceptacle on the front of the power supply module.
   D. Turn the ultrasonic *OUTPUT* control to the *off* position.
   E. Fill the water bottle with the desired solution and attach the
      cap. Slide clamp on the tubing so that liquid does not flow
      through tubing at this time. An alternative is to use one of
      the many prefilled units available. Invert the bottle and
      hang on the hanger stand on the back of the unit.
   F. Attach the supply tubing from the bottle or prefilled unit
      to the fitting on the float assembly. Release slide clamp on
      tubing. The liquid will flow into the float chamber until it
      reaches the most efficient operating level and then shuts
      off automatically.
   G. Connect the output hose (large-bore tubing approximately
      3 to 4 ft in length) to the top of the humidifier manifold.
      The free end may then be connected to a mask or directed
      into a tent.

III. Operating Procedure
   A. Orient the patient to the therapy.
   B. Assemble the unit as described above.
   C. Place the ultrasonic on a table or stand. Keep the manifold
      lower than the patient so that any condensation will flow
      away from the patient.
   D. Keep the fan outlet at least 3 in. from any obstruction to
      air input.
   E. Connect the power cord to a grounded 115-V ac receptacle.
   F. Turn the *OUTPUT* control to the right (clockwise). This
      activates the unit. The yellow indicator lamp should light
      and the blower motor start.
   G. Adjust the desired output of the humidifier by turning the
      OUTPUT control through a range from 0 to 10.
   H. If using a mask or a mouthpiece, position the patient in an
      upright but comfortable position. Adjust the equipment.
   I. For tent therapy, the end of the output hose may be placed
      into one of the openings in the tent canopy.

IV. Cleaning and Sterilization

    A. Disassemble all hoses and tubes. Remove transducer assembly from bracket; separate the float and manifold from the transducer assembly. Remove the power cable.

    B. The power supply module may be cleaned with a cloth moistened in a detergent and water solution. *Do not immerse.*

    C. Ultrasonic cleaners are available for use on the manifold, float chamber, crystal chamber, and the surface of the glass plate. The manifold and float assembly may be immersed in the solution but *do not immerse the transducer body.* The solution may be poured into the float and crystal chambers, and those areas scrubbed with a brush. Rinse and dry.

> *Note:* Never use soap on the ultrasonic as residue left in the crystal chamber reduces or eliminates fog output. Ultrasonic cleaner or 2% acetic acid may be used to clean a unit that has been contaminated with soap.

    D. After cleaning, the components may be cold or gas sterilized. *Do not autoclave.*

    E. The bottle, cap, and hose assembly may be washed in a detergent solution and rinsed in water. They may then be cold sterilized. Dry thoroughly.

    F. The air filter over the fan intake should be replaced frequently.

Bennett Model US-1 Ultrasonic Nebulizer (Figure 3-24)

The nebulizer of the US-1 converts liquid to aerosol by the application of high-frequency energy. Line-voltage alternating current (115 V, 60 Hz) is converted to a high frequency. This current is applied to a piezoelectric crystal. When energized, the crystal expands and contracts at the rate of approximately 1,350,000 times/second. The vibrations are transmitted through a coupling chamber, containing water, to a cup containing the liquid to be nebulized. These vibrations produce intense internal turbulence in the liquid. This turbulence overcomes surface tension and cohesive forces at the gas–liquid interface, reducing continuous disintegration of the liquid to a fine aerosol. The carrier gas used to exhaust the aerosol from the medication cup is provided by an adjustable blower, which draws in room air and passes it through the cup. A discriminator provides a baffling means to capture the larger aerosol particles. Use this ultrasonic nebulizer under the direction of a physician.

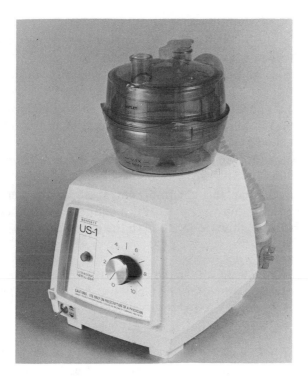

Figure 3-24. Bennett US-1. (*Courtesy of Puritan-Bennett Corp., Kansas City, Mo.*)

Assembly

1. Fit the crystal holder into the coupling chamber with a twisting motion. Be certain that it is firmly seated.
2. Lay the crystal cable into the slot at the rear of the module. Push the clamp (with tooth forward) onto two teeth inside of the seat. The clamp will snap into place and retain itself.
3. Fit the coupling chamber into the module, indexing the chamber keys to the module slots. Push the chamber down until the clamp engages its upper edge.
4. Fill the coupling chamber with water, using sterile distilled water, to a level between max–min.
5. Fit the seal into the groove around the medication cup. *Handle the cup with care.*
6. Pour the prescribed solution (sterile distilled water) into the cup (200 ml maximum). (If continuous liquid feed is to be used, bypass this step.)

7. Place the discriminator on the cup.

8. Position the discriminator to accept the cover feeder tubes. Push the cover over the medication cup.

9. Set the cup–discriminator–cover assembly in the coupling chamber.

10. Slide the edge of the cover under the two forward latches on the coupling chamber. Press the ridge of the clamp over the edge of the cover.

11. Secure the cap on the feed port over the two cover tubes. (if continuous liquid feed is to be used, bypass this step.)

12. Push the damper into the flow central elbow. Connect the elbow to the module blower outlet. Fit a connector to the elbow. Connect the 8-in. sidewinder tube to the connector and to the cover inlet.

Note: If oxygen is to be added, connect a tube from the oxygen flowmeter to the connector on the blower control. Oxygen analysis will be necessary to determine liter flow to be used if a specific FIO_2 is desired.

13. For continuous liquid feed, remove the cap from the feeder port, insert Add-A-Line secondary medication set into the sterile water for irrigation bag, and hang bag at a convenient level. Attach the other end of secondary medication set to the feeder part. The medication cup will fill automatically when on–off clamp of bag is released.

14. Connect the electrical cord to a wall outlet (the electrical circuit must be grounded).

15. Turn on the power switch (left front of machine) (amber pilot light will illuminate if machine is operating properly).

16. Set the output control (turn until adequate mist is present).

17. Set the blower control.

18. Begin treatment; readjust the controls as necessary.

19. For extended treatment, drape the tube or tubes so that condensate drains back into the nebulizer. During extended treatment, the medication cup and coupling chamber must be monitored (replenish solution as necessary).

Note: If the nebulizer is operated without water in the coupling chamber, the pilot lamp will flash to warn of this condition.

Delivery Procedure. In simplest use, a flexible main tube is connected to the nebulizer cover outlet. A mask or face tent (allowing free exhalation without removal) is connected to the tube and to the patient. Patient connection may be hand or strap held. If the patient is in a tent or canopy, the tube is inserted into the opening.

Cleaning and Sterilizing

1. Disassemble all parts. Remove the crystal holder from the coupling chamber.
2. Soak and wash all parts, *except the crystal holder*, in warm detergent solution. Rinse thoroughly with warm water. Air dry.
3. Make certain that the *nebulizer is turned off*; wipe the crystal clean with a soft cloth soaked in warm detergent solution. Remove all traces of detergent with a different damp soft cloth.

Note: All parts, including the nebulizer module, may be gas sterilized. If grossly contaminated, the ultrasonic nebulizer may be gas sterilized; otherwise, the exterior surface of the machine may be wiped off with 70% isopropyl alcohol and dried well. All parts that are sterilized using ethylene oxide must be aired for 7 days before use or placed in an aerator for the time suggested by the manufacturer.

4. Periodically, to remove water sediments and other impurities, clean the cup system as follows: use $1\frac{1}{2}$% acetic acid (white vinegar). Dilute 1 part vinegar with 2 parts water. Assemble ultrasonic nebulizer. Place vinegar solution in the coupling chamber and the medication cup. Set output at maximum. Turn on the switch. Adjust the blower for light aerosol delivery. Nebulize the solution for 10 min. Turn off nebulizer and disassemble. Rinse all parts thoroughly with warm water. Air dry.

Hydro-Sphere Nebulizer (Figure 3-25)

The Hydro-Sphere Nebulizer operates on the Babington principle whereby an aerosol is formed by rupturing a thin film of water with an air stream. No electronic or moving parts are required. Two aerosol generators are utilized to ensure maximal aerosol formation as well as complete humidification of all aspirated air flow.

The Hydro-Sphere Nebulizer is designed to operate from a source of compressed air or oxygen with a supply pressure of 20 psi. However, pressures ranging from 10 to 50 psi may be used successfully.

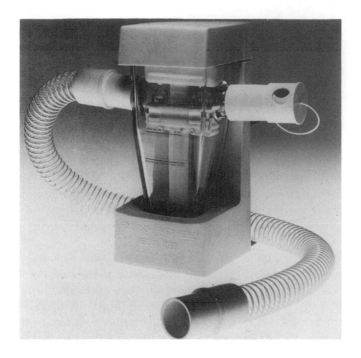

1. liquid supply

2. continuous thin liquid film

3. compressed gas supply

4. discharge orifice

5. impactor

6. run-off liquid for recirculation

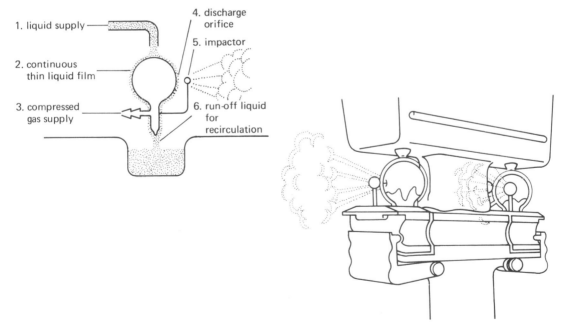

Figure 3-25.   Hydro-Sphere Nebulizer. (*Courtesy of Owens-Illinois Care Products, Toledo, Ohio*)

Assembly

Note: To maintain sterility, the manufacturer recommends wearing
sterile gloves while assembling the nebulizer.

1. Insert the pump plug into the manifold and turn counterclockwise to anchor in place. Some models have a threaded hole in
   the base into which the lift-pump plug is fitted and then tightened. (Check O-ring for wear; replace as necessary.)
2. Place the sphere assemblies into the manifold base and secure.
3. Place manifold cover on manifold. (Check O-ring for wear; replace as necessary.) The grooves in the manifold reservoir must
   connect with the lid latches.
4. Insert glass reservoir into base and place gasket on rim to form
   seal.
5. Insert manifold assembly into reservoir. Check gasket for
   proper positioning.
6. Slip front edge of cover under lip on reservoir. Lower cover
   and align.
7. With thumbs on front panel of the cover, squeeze cover with
   fingers to engage the lugs.

Operation

1. Attach the nebulizer to its mobile stand so that it is in an
   upright position.
2. If the nebulizer is to be used for continuous therapy, prefill the
   reservoir to the Maximum Prefill Level with sterile water,
   saline, or propylene glycol.
3. Fill feed bottle at least three-quarters full with desired solution. Tighten cap securely.
4. Connect feed bottle tubes to fittings on rear of unit and attach
   aspirator control and aerosol hose. When the bottle is inverted
   and elevated, the reservoir will automatically fill to its operating level.
5. Attach a high-pressure hose (either air or oxygen) to the inlet
   on the back of the unit. Attach the other end to a suitable flow-
   regulating device.
6. When maximum capacity and density are desired, use the
   Hydro-Sphere Nebulizer with both spheres in place. When low-
   capacity applications are required and the unit is to be used
   with a tent for maximum cooling but with a minimal oxygen
   concentration, the rear sphere may be removed.

7. Oxygen concentration of 100% may be obtained for either configuration by closing the aspirator control. Concentrations may be decreased by increasing the number on the aspirator through range from 1 to 3, or by removing the flow selector or filter housing. Although the manufacturer supplies a chart depicting settings and flows for use with both spheres and one sphere, the use of such a chart does not preclude the use of an oxygen analyzer to obtain an accurate FIO_2.

Cleaning and Sterilization

1. Disassemble all parts in reverse order of assembly.
2. Wash with a detergent solution and rinse well.
3. All parts may be cold sterilized or gas sterilized with ethylene oxide at 140°F. All but plastic parts may be autoclaved.

Maxi-Mist Aerosol Unit

I. Assembly and Preparation
   A. Parts
      1. Compressor
      2. Plastic air hose
      3. Finger valve
      4. Nebulizer (five parts)
         a. Outer shell
         b. Inner shell
         c. Capillary
         d. Body
         e. Gasket

   B. Assembly
      1. Plug the smaller end of the long air hose into the outlet at the base of the compressor.
      2. Assemble the nebulizer. See Figure 3-26.
         a. Push the inner shell into the outer shell as shown until you hear it snap.
         b. Fit the capillary over the tiny air jet inside the body; notice the position of the capillary and the legs of the body to see how they fit.
         c. Screw the outer shell to the body.
      3. The finger valve (Figure 3-27) fits between the large end of the long air hose and the nebulizer body.

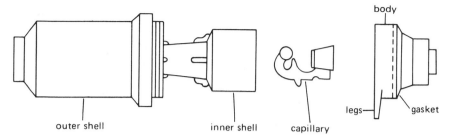

outer shell   inner shell   capillary

Figure 3-26. Assembly of the Maxi-Mist Aerosol Unit.

C. Preparation
   1. To fill the nebulizer, pour or drop the medicine through the open end of the barrel (the center of the inner shell).
   2. Slip finger valve into body of barrel.

   Note: When giving treatment be sure to have the legs on the body of the nebulizer pointing down or else no mist will be produced.

   3. Plug compressor into an electrical outlet.

II. Operation and Cleaning
   A. Operation
      1. Turn on compressor switch.
      2. Once the patient is comfortable, have him open his mouth wide.
      3. Have patient point the open end of the nebulizer into his mouth, but *not* touch it with his lips.
      4. Patient should first exhale completely.
      5. Then patient should close the finger valve by placing his finger over the hole.

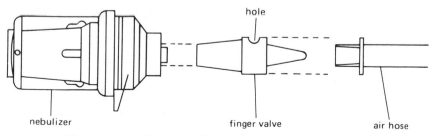

nebulizer   finger valve   air hose

Figure 3-27. Position of finger valve in aerosol unit.

6. Inhalation of the mist should be deep and rather slow; as soon as inspiration is completed, the patient should lift his finger from the finger valve to stop the mist while he exhales.

B. Cleaning
    1. Disassemble nebulizer.
    2. Rinse with warm (not hot) water.
    3. All pieces may be cold or gas sterilized.
    4. To clean jet, use stilette or cleaning needle.

III. Additional Information
    A. Just as in any breathing therapy treatment, the best position for the patient is sitting up.
    B. It is not necessary to remove the gasket when cleaning.

OXYGEN THERAPY DEVICES

Location of "No Smoking" Signs. As outlined in the National Fire Protection Association Manual No. 56B, *Respiratory Therapy 1973*, 56B-14-614, precautionary signs, readable from a distance of 5 ft, shall be conspicuously displayed at the site of administration and in aisles and walkways leading to the area. They shall be attached to adjacent doorways, to building walls, or supported by other appropriate means. Precautionary signs should be approximately 8 by 11 in. in size.

Nasal Cannula

The nasal cannula is a simple, relatively inexpensive means of administering oxygen at low concentrations of 22% to 30%, at liter flows of 1 to 5 liters/min. It consists of a flexible plastic tube with two pronglike extensions that fit into the nares (Figure 3-28).

  I. Equipment
    A. Plastic nasal cannula complete with tubing
    B. Humidifier
    C. Flowmeter for pipeline system, or regulator for oxygen cylinder
    D. Distilled water (sterile)
    E. "No Smoking" sign
    F. Department records

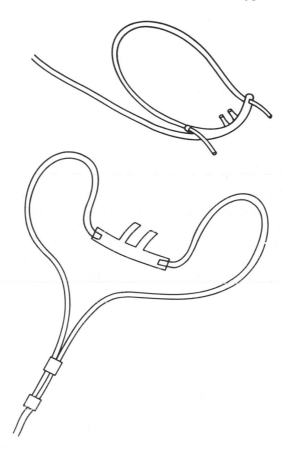

Figure 3-28.   Nasal cannula.

II. Procedure

A. A written order, signed by the physician, should be in the patient's chart specifying the liter flow desired. Although the oxygen concentration desired is the important factor, it is difficult to accurately establish a specific FIO_2. The patient's response to the therapy is the determining factor.

B. Orient the patient to this therapy.

C. Instruct the patient in oxygen safety rules.

D. Fill the humidifier with distilled water.

E. For central pipeline system:

1. Attach the humidifier to a pressure-compensated flow-meter having a suitable well-outlet adapter, and insert into an oxygen outlet.

2. Attach the cannula-tubing inlet to the humidifier outlet and adjust the flow by turning the pressure-compensated flowmeter needle valve to the desired flow, as indicated by the gauge; test to see that oxygen is flowing through the cannula by directing the flow onto your hand.

3. Enlarge the loop of the cannula so that it will slip easily over the patient's head, place the prongs into the nares, and tighten the loop; if the loop is too tight, the prongs will slide out of position and may cause damage to the mucous membranes of the nose.

4. Although it is not essential to tape the cannula in place, it is advisable to do so if the patient is particularly active; this may be done by placing a small piece of tape over the cannula on both sides of the face.

5. The patient should be instructed to breathe through his nose, as mouth-breathing would dilute the oxygen he is to receive.

6. To ensure proper functioning, the cannula should be changed every 8 hours, and at that time the condition of the nares should be examined; a water-soluable, nonoily lubricant may be used if the patient complains of crusting or irritation.

7. Place a "No Smoking" sign in the doorway.

8. Fill out department records.

9. When the liquid in the humidifier drops to the refill line, shut off the oxygen supply by closing the pressure-compensated flowmeter needle valve, empty out the remaining liquid, and refill the humidifier with sterile distilled water to the fill line; the jar should be replaced daily.

F. For cylinder and regulator:

1. Before connecting the regulator to a full cylinder of oxygen, crack (momentarily open and close) the cylinder valve to blow out any foreign particles from the outlet.

2. Attach the regulator to the cylinder-valve outlet, being sure you have a regulator that can be adjusted in liters per minute; the regulator-adjusting screw or needle valve should be in the *off* position.

3. Open the cylinder valve slowly so that the high-pressure content gauge will rise gradually to full pressure and turn the cylinder valve four to five times.

4. Attach the humidifier to the regulator outlet.

5. Attach the cannula-tubing inlet to the humidifier outlet, and adjust the flow by turning the regulator-adjusting

screw or needle valve to the desired flow as indicated by the gauge.

6. Proceed as for central pipeline system.

Nasal Catheter

The nasal catheter (Figure 3-29) is used to administer moderately high concentrations of oxygen, which may reach 30% to 35% at a liter flow of 1 to 5 liters/min.

I. Equipment
   A. Nasal catheter (sterile, plastic disposable catheter is preferable) in French catheter sizes 8 to 14 with six to eight holes at the tip
      1. For children, 8 to 10 F catheter
      2. For women, 10 to 12 F catheter
      3. For men, 12 to 14 F catheter
   B. Oxygen-connecting tubing
   C. Humidifier
   D. Flowmeter for pipeline system or regulator for oxygen cylinder
   E. Tongue depressor
   F. Water-soluble lubricating jelly
   G. Sterile distilled water
   H. Three-quarter-inch tape

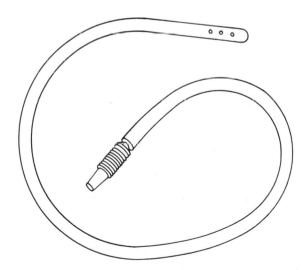

Figure 3-29. Nasal catheter.

    I. "No Smoking" sign

    J. Department records

II. Procedure

    A. A complete order, signed by the physician, should be in the patient's chart before the therapy is initiated; the order must include the desired liter flow.

    B. Orient the patient to this therapy.

    C. Stress oxygen safety rules.

    D. Fill the humidifier with sterile distilled water.

    E. For central pipeline system:

        1. Attach the humidifier to a pressure-compensated flowmeter having a suitable wall-outlet adapter, and insert into a wall outlet.

        2. Attach the catheter to the oxygen-supply tubing outlet.

        3. Measure the distance from the tip of the patient's nose (external naris) to the ear lobe with the catheter and mark this distance with tape or the finger; this is the approximate distance the catheter is to be inserted.

        4. Lubricate the catheter with water or a water-soluble nonoily surgical jelly; never use mineral oil or other oily lubricants, as even small quantities, if aspirated, could cause severe chronic irritation of the lung and even frank lipoid pneumonia.

        5. With the oxygen flow adjusted to approximately 3 liters/min, test to see that the oxygen flows freely through the catheter by placing the tip of the catheter into a glass of water and observing the bubbles.

        6. With the oxygen flowing, introduce the catheter slowly and gently into the naris to the previously marked distance.

        7. Observe the position of the catheter through the patient's open mouth (the tip should be visible at the level of the uvula), and withdraw the catheter slightly to prevent the patient from swallowing oxygen, which would result in abdominal distention; swallowed oxygen can obviously not be used for purposes of respiration and abdominal distention would eventually interfere with ventilation.

        8. Adjust the oxygen to the desired flow.

        9. Tape the catheter securely to the tip of the nose and then to either the forehead or the cheek.

10. A new catheter should be placed in the opposite naris every 8 hours.

11. When the water level in the humidifier reaches the refill line, dispose of any remaining fluid and add sterile distilled water to the fill line; also, the humidifier should be changed daily.

12. Place "No Smoking" sign in the doorway.

13. Fill out department records.

F. For cylinder and regulator:

1. Before connecting the regulator to a full cylinder of oxygen, crack (momentarily open and close) the cylinder valve to blow out any foreign particles from the outlet.

2. Attach the regulator to the cylinder-valve outlet, being sure that you have a regulator that can be adjusted in liters per minute; make sure that the regulator-adjusting screw or needle valve is in the *off* position.

3. Open the cylinder valve slowly so that the high-pressure content gauge will rise gradually to full pressure, and turn the cylinder valve four or five times.

4. Attach the humidifier to the regulator outlet.

5. Attach the catheter to the oxygen-supply tubing; attach the supply tubing to the humidifier outlet.

6. Proceed as for central pipeline system.

Rebreathing Versus Nonrebreathing Masks

The nonrebreathing mask is set aside from the partial rebreathing mask by the presence of a one-way inspiratory valve that closes during expiration, preventing any exhaled air from entering the reservoir bag and forcing it to leave through the expiratory valve on the face piece.

In the partial rebreathing mask, which has no valve, the earliest portion of exhaled air returns to the bag to be mixed with incoming air in the next breath. Expired air escapes through the mask exhalation ports.

Oxygen Mask with Partial Rebreathing Bag

This mask (Figure 3-30) may be used when an oxygen concentration of 60% to 90% is desired. Approximately the first third of the patient's expired air is directed into the reservoir bag for rebreathing. Since this air does not take part in gas exchange (dead space air), it is still

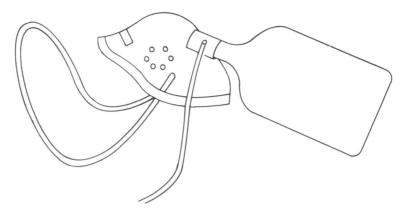

Figure 3-30. Oxygen mask with partial rebreathing bag.

high in oxygen, and together with the additional flow of oxygen from a cylinder or pipeline system it will provide relatively high concentrations to the patient. Sufficient exhalation ports are provided so that carbon dioxide levels remain negligible.

I. Equipment
    A. Oxygen mask with partial rebreathing bag (disposable ones are most convenient)
    B. Oxygen-connecting tubing
    C. Humidifier (optional but recommended)
    D. Flowmeter for pipeline system or regulator for oxygen cylinder
    E. Sterile distilled water
    F. "No Smoking" sign
    G. Department records

II. Procedure
    A. A complete order, specifying the oxygen concentration desired, should be in the patient's chart before initiating the therapy.
    B. Orient the patient to this therapy; since a mask is confining, the patient will require much psychological support.
    C. Stress oxygen safety rules.
    D. Fill the humidifier with sterile distilled water.
    E. For central pipeline system:
        1. Attach the humidifier to a pressure-compensated flowmeter having a suitable wall-outlet adapter, and insert into an oxygen outlet.

2. Attach the oxygen mask tubing to the humidifier outlet, and adjust the flow by turning the pressure-compensated flowmeter needle valve to the desired flow as indicated by the gauge.

3. Place the mask over the patient's face during expiration, fitting first the nose and then the mouth; if the mask can be molded to fit the contour of the face, do so at this time; adjust the strap.

4. When the patient inhales, the reservoir bag should not collapse completely; if it does, additional gas flow is required.

5. Place "No Smoking" sign in doorway.

6. Fill out department records.

7. When the water in the humidifier reaches the refill line, empty the remaining solution and refill with sterile distilled water; also, the humidifier should be replaced daily.

F. For cylinder and regulator:

1. Before connecting the regulator to a full cylinder of oxygen, be sure it is "cracked" to blow out any foreign particles from the outlet.

2. Attach the regulator to the cylinder-valve outlet (making sure you have a regulator in liters per minute), and make sure the regulator-adjusting screw or needle valve is completely off.

3. Open cylinder valve slowly so the high-pressure content gauge will rise gradually to full pressure; then turn the cylinder valve open four to five times.

4. Attach the humidifier to the regulator outlet.

5. Follow procedure for pipeline system.

Oxygen Mask Without Reservoir Bag

This mask (Figure 3-31) may be used to administer oxygen concentrations of 35% to 60% at liter flows of 8 to 12 liters/min.

I. Equipment
   A. Oxygen mask without reservoir bag
   B. Oxygen-supply tubing
   C. Humidifier
   D. Flowmeter for pipeline system or regulator for oxygen cylinder

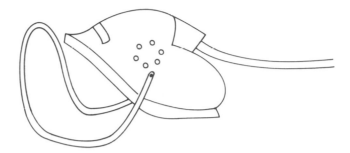

Figure 3-31. Oxygen mask without reservoir bag.

    E. Sterile distilled water

    F. "No Smoking" sign

    G. Department records

II. Procedure

    A. A complete order, specifying the oxygen concentration desired, should be in the patient's chart before initiating the therapy.

    B. Orient the patient to this therapy.

    C. Stress oxygen safety rules.

    D. Fill the humidifier with sterile distilled water.

    E. For central pipeline system:

        1. Attach the humidifier to a pressure-compensated flowmeter having a suitable wall-outlet adapter, and insert into an oxygen outlet.

        2. Attach the oxygen mask tubing to the humidifier outlet, and adjust the flow by turning the pressure-compensated flowmeter needle valve to the desired flow as indicated by the gauge.

        3. Place the oxygen mask on the patient (being sure to start from the nose downward), and adjust the nose clip and head strap.

        4. Fill out department records.

        5. When the liquid in the bottle drops to the refill line, refill with distilled water.

    F. For cylinder and regulator:

        1. Before connecting the regulator to a full cylinder of oxygen, be sure it is "cracked" to blow out any foreign particles from the outlet.

        2. Attach the regulator to the cylinder-valve outlet (making sure you have a regulator in liters per minute); make sure

the regulator-adjusting screw or needle valve is completely off.

3. Attach the humidifier to the regulator outlet.

4. Attach the oxygen mask tubing to the humidifier outlet,
   and adjust the flow by turning the needle valve or regulator-adjusting screw to the desired flow as indicated by
   the gauge.

5. Proceed as for pipeline system.

Venturi Mask

This mask (Figure 3-32) may be used when a carefully controlled
oxygen concentration is desired. Venturi masks are available in 24%,
28%, 35%, and 40% concentrations. Carbon dioxide buildup is minimal.

I. Equipment
   A. Venturi mask of desired concentration
   B. Oxygen-supply tubing
   C. Humidifier (optional)
   D. Flowmeter for pipeline system or regulator for oxygen
      cylinder
   E. Sterile distilled water
   F. "No Smoking" sign
   G. Department records

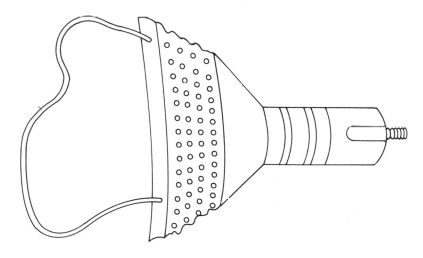

Figure 3-32.   Venturi mask.

II. Procedure
   A. A complete order, specifying the oxygen concentration desired, is necessary before initiating the therapy.
   B. Orient the patient to this therapy.
   C. Stress oxygen safety rules.
   D. Fill the humidifier with sterile distilled water.
   E. For central pipeline system:
      1. Attach the humidifier to a pressure-compensated flowmeter having a wall-outlet adapter, and insert into an oxygen outlet.
      2. Attach the oxygen-supply to the Venturi mask; then attach the supply-tubing outlet to the humidifier outlet and adjust the flow by turning the needle valve on the flowmeter to the desired flow as indicated on the Venturi mask body.
      3. Place the mask over the patient's face, molding the malleable band firmly around the bridge of the nose and the cheeks; depending on the manufacturer, some styles of mask fit snugly around the chin and some do not.
      4. Pull the elastic cord over the patient's head and into a comfortable position.
      5. The mask should be checked periodically for proper positioning.
      6. Discard mask after use.
      7. Place "No Smoking" sign in doorway.
      8. The humidifier should be changed daily; if the water level in the jar reaches the refill line, empty out the remaining fluid and refill with sterile water.
   F. For cylinder and regulator:
      1. Before connecting the regulator to a full cylinder of oxygen, be sure to "crack" it to blow out any foreign particles from the outlet.
      2. Attach the regulator to the cylinder-valve outlet (making sure you have a regulator in liters per minute); make sure the regulator-adjusting screw or needle valve is completely off.
      3. Open cylinder valve slowly so the high-pressure content gauge will rise gradually to full pressure; then turn cylinder valve open four to five times.
      4. Attach the humidifier to the regulator outlet.
      5. Attach the oxygen-supply tubing to the Venturi mask; then attach the supply tubing to the humidifier outlet and ad-

just the flow by turning the needle valve on the flow-meter or adjusting screw on the regulator to the desired flow as indicated on the Venturi mask body.

6. Follow procedure for pipeline system.

OEM Mix-O-Mask

I. Introduction

The OEM Mix-O-Mask (Figure 3-33) is another mask that utilizes a Venturi to deliver accurate concentrations of oxygen to those patients requiring precise FIO_2's.

II. Equipment
   A. Mix-O-Mask of desired concentration
   B. Humidity adapter (optional)
   C. Oxygen supply tubing
   D. Humidifier and nebulizer (optional)
   E. Oxygen flowmeter for cylinder or wall outlet
   F. Compressed air flowmeter if nebulizer is used for additional humidification

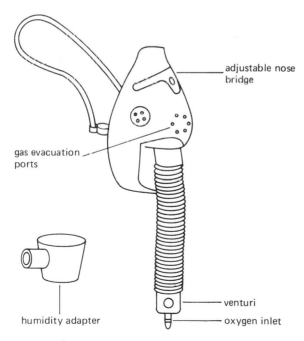

Figure 3-33. OEM Mix-O-Mask.

       G. Sterile water

       H. "No Smoking" sign

       I. Department records

III. Procedure

      A. A complete order in the patient's chart, specifying the oxygen concentration desired, is necessary before initiating the therapy.

      B. Orient the patient to the therapy.

      C. Stress oxygen safety rules.

      D. Fill humidifier and nebulizer (if used) with sterile water.

      E. Attach compressed-air flowmeter (if nebulizer is used) and oxygen flowmeter to cylinder or wall outlet.

      F. Attach suitable pressure tubing from compressed-air flowmeter to inlet of nebulizer. The nebulizer may be attached directly to the flowmeter, but this should be avoided if the nebulizer will be above the level of the bed.

      G. Attach large-bore tubing from outlet on nebulizer to humidity adapter. Adjust flow.

      H. Attach humidifier to oxygen flowmeter.

      I. Attach oxygen supply tubing from humidifier to inlet of mask.

      J. Adjust oxygen flow according to directions on each Mix-O-Mask.

      K. Adjust mask to patient's face, molding the adjustable nose bridge to fit the contours of the face. Position the elastic strap.

      L. The mask should be checked periodically for positioning.

      M. Place "No Smoking" sign in doorway or place assigned.

      N. Complete department records.

Positive Pressure Mask

This mask (Figure 3-34), sometimes referred to as a meter mask, is a device that applies positive pressure on expiration (IPPB/E). It is commonly used for the treatment of pulmonary edema.

Although diluter assemblies are available, it is preferable to use the mask without the diluter, thus delivering oxygen concentrations up to 95% (±5%). *No humidifier is used.*

    I. Equipment

      A. The mask consists of the following:

         1. Mask

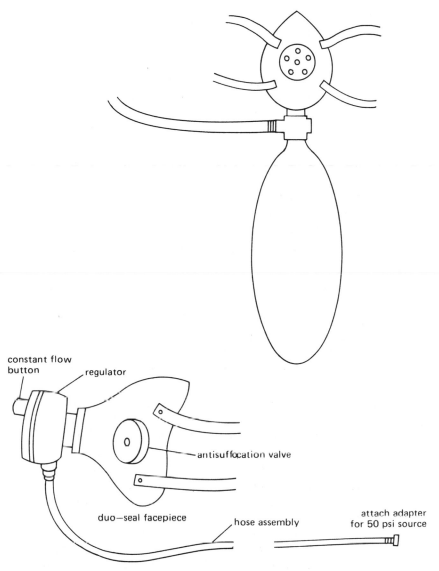

constant flow
button

regulator

antisuffocation valve

0

duo–seal facepiece

hose assembly

attach adapter
for 50 psi source

Figure 3-34. Positive pressure mask and Scott respirator mask.

2. Meter, calibrated from 0 to 4 cm of water pressure
3. Two head straps
4. One-way valve
5. Rubber bag
6. Large-bore rubber tubing.

B. Flowmeter for pipeline system or regulator for oxygen cylinder.

  C. "No Smoking" sign

  D. Department records.

 II. Procedure

  A. Since this mask is generally used in an emergency situation, a written order may not be available when the therapy is initiated. Check with the physician for specific orders until such time as they may become part of the patient's permanent record.

  B. Orient the patient to this therapy. Since he will be in respiratory distress, he will require much psychological support and should never be left without supervision.

  C. Observe oxygen safety rules.

  D. Set the calibrated meter on the mask at zero, the largest opening. At this setting there is no expiratory pressure.

  E. For central pipeline system:

   1. Attach the mask outlet tubing to the small-bore adapter on the flowmeter; *no humidifier is used;* set the liter flow by turning the needle valve to 10 (liters/min) at the start.

   2. Place the mask on the patient's face, and adjust the head strap carefully so there is no leakage of air.

   3. Readjust flow rate of oxygen so that the collecting bag never collapses fully.

   4. To increase the pressure of the mask, turn the calibrated knob until the amount of pressure determined by the physician's prescription has been reached, as follows:

    a. 0 to 1 cm H_2O: wait 5 min approximately

    b. 1 to 2 cm H_2O: wait 10 min approximately

    c. 2 to 3 cm H_2O: wait 15 min approximately

    d. 3 to 4 cm H_2O: wait 20 min approximately

    e. After the maximum pressure prescribed has been reached, the exhalation pressure valve should remain set at that pressure for about 20 min and then gradually return to zero using the above procedure in reverse order; interruption of the cycle, at a point when expiratory pressure is being applied, could result in return of the fluid to the alveoli.

   5. Place "No Smoking" sign in the doorway.

   6. Fill out department records.

  F. For cylinder and regulator:

   1. Before connecting the regulator to a full cylinder of oxygen, be sure it is "cracked" to blow out any foreign particles from the outlet.

2. Attach the regulator to the cylinder-valve outlet (making sure you have a regulator in liters per minute); make sure the regulator-adjusting screw or needle valve is completely off.

3. Open the cylinder valve slowly so that the high-pressure content gauge will rise gradually to full pressure; then turn the cylinder valve open four to five times.

Follow procedure for pipeline system.

Tracheostomy Collar

This collar (Figure 3-35) is used to administer high humidity to the tracheostomized patient. Oxygen concentration may be controlled by liter flow and the use of the dilution control on the Puritan All-Purpose Jar (nebulizer).

I. Equipment
   A. Tracheostomy collar
   B. Sixty inches of large-bore disposable tubing
   C. Puritan All-Purpose Jar (nebulizer)
   D. Immersion heater
   E. Two-psi safety relief valve
   F. Flowmeter for pipeline system or regulator with flowmeter for oxygen cylinder
   G. Sterile distilled water
   H. "No Smoking" sign
   I. Department records

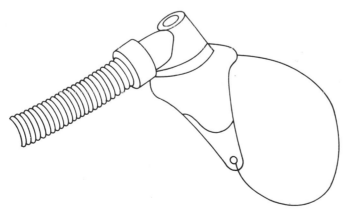

Figure 3-35.   Tracheostomy collar with tubing.

    J. Stand or pole

    K. Low-pressure oxygen tubing

II. Procedure

    A. A complete order, specifying the oxygen concentration desired, should be in the patient's chart before initiating therapy.

    B. Orient the patient to the therapy.

    C. Stress oxygen safety rules.

    D. Fill the Purital All-Purpose Jar (nebulizer) with sterile distilled water to the fill line on the jar.

    E. Place the immersion heater into one of the ports on the nebulizer head and plug into suitable wall outlet.

    F. Place a 2-psi safety relief valve into the port on the top of the nebulizer head.

    G. Set the dilution control on the nebulizer head to 40%, 70%, or 100% oxygen, depending on the oxygen concentration prescribed.

    H. For use with central pipeline system:

        1. Place the flowmeter into oxygen outlet, making certain the needle valve is in the *Off* position.

        2. Attach a low-pressure oxygen tube from the outlet of the flowmeter to the inlet connection on the nebulizer head, which has a standard oxygen thread; hand tighten only.

        3. Place the nebulizer on a stand or pole so that the nebulizer is below the level of the patient's bed; this will allow condensation from the large-bore tubing to drain back into the nebulizer and not into the patient's tracheostomy site.

        4. Attach the tracheostomy collar to one end of the large-bore tubing.

        5. Attach the remaining end of the large-bore tubing to the side port of the nebulizer jar.

        6. Fill nebulizer jar with sterile distilled water to the fill line.

        7. Plug in heating element to a suitable wall outlet.

        8. Adjust flowmeter to the liter flow prescribed by the physician.

        9. Set the dilution control and lock in place for the oxygen concentration ordered by the physician.

      10. Check the aerosol output; if it is not working properly, push up and down on the push-button orifice cleaner.

11. Place the tracheostomy collar over tracheostomy site and adjust the strap so that it will be comfortable for the patient.

12. Place "No Smoking" sign in doorway.

13. Complete necessary department records.

14. If the water level in the nebulizer falls below the fill line, refill with sterile distilled water.

15. Change entire setup at least once every 24 hours.

I. For compressed-gas cylinder with regulator with flowmeter:

1. Before connecting regulator with flowmeter to the compressed-gas cylinder, open the cylinder valve slowly, using both hands to blow out any foreign particles from the outlet; close cylinder valve.

2. Attach the regulator with flowmeter to the outlet of the compressed-gas cylinder valve, making certain that the regulator-adjusting screw or needle valve is completely off.

3. Connect a low-pressure oxygen tube from the outlet of the flowmeter to the oxygen-threaded connection on the nebulizer head.

4. Follow directions from 3 to 10 under outline entry II, H above, for assembly of nebulizer, and so on.

5. Open cylinder valve slowly until high-pressure gauge of cylinder rises to full pressure.

6. Follow directions from 11 to 15 under outline entry II, H above.

Aerosol Tee

The aerosol tee (Figure 3-36) is a T-shaped plastic adapter used to deliver oxygen and high humidity to those patients with endotracheal or tracheostomy tubes in place. It is also useful for weaning patients from mechanical ventilation.

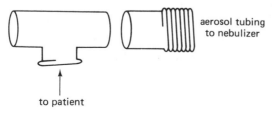

Figure 3-36. Aerosol tee.

1. For FIO_2's of 24%, 28%, 31%, 35%, and 40%, the tee is supplied with a Venturi, which accurately controls the FIO_2 delivered.
2. An aerosol tee may be run by compressed air only, if the major objective is to supply humidity.
3. FIO_2's above 40% may be obtained by mixing compressed air and oxygen; however, if the patient's minute volume changes, the initial reading may not remain stable.

I. Policies
   A. All respiratory therapy department personnel, after demonstration of competency to supervision, may apply this equipment.
   B. A written request (Oxygen/Humidity Request) signed by the physician must be submitted to the respiratory therapy department before therapy is initiated.
   C. Equipment is changed and the FIO_2 analyzed daily.
   D. A patient flow sheet is placed in the patient's chart at the time therapy is initiated. On this flow sheet the technician will indicate the FIO_2 ordered and analyzed, liter flow of gases used, times equipment is changed, and an assessment of the patient's response.
   E. Each patient on an aerosol tee must have his name added to the master O_2 sheet kept by the department.

II. Aerosol Tee at 21% O_2
   A. Equipment
      1. Aerosol tee
      2. Large-bore aerosol tubing
      3. Compressed-air flowmeter
      4. All-purpose nebulizer with stand and bracket and 2-psi relief valve
      5. Low-pressure tubing
      6. Immersion heater
      7. Sterile water
   B. Assembly and application
      1. Fill the all-purpose nebulizer with sterile water.
      2. Place the nebulizer in the bracket (on the stand).
      3. Insert the compressed-air flowmeter into the compressed air wall outlet.
      4. Connect one end of the low-pressure tubing to the outlet on the flowmeter and the other end to the inlet on the nebulizer. The nebulizer should be set on the 40% dilution.

5. Insert the immersion heater into one of the ports in the top of the nebulizer; plug into a grounded electrical outlet.

6. Attach one end of the aerosol tubing to the outlet port on the nebulizer, and the other end to the aerosol tee (see Figure 3-36).

7. Adjust the liter flow of gas until adequate nebulization is observed coming from the tee—usually about 8 liters/min.

8. Attach the patient port on the aerosol tee to the adapter of the endotracheal or tracheostomy tube.

9. Observe the patient's response to the therapy.

10. Fill out a patient flow sheet and place in chart.

Note: Although compressed air as such contains no more than 21% O_2, periodic analysis of the gas should still be done to assure that the gas in the pipeline system is correct.

III. Aerosol Tee: FIO_2 up to 40%

A. Equipment

1. Aerosol tee with Venturi of desired FIO_2 (with humidity adapter)

2. Large-bore aerosol tubing

3. All-purpose nebulizer with stand and bracket and 2-psi relief valve

4. Low-pressure tubing

5. O_2 humidity bottle

6. O_2 connecting tubing

7. Immersion heater

8. Sterile water

9. Compressed-air flowmeter

10. Oxygen flowmeter

B. Assembly and application

1. Fill the all-purpose nebulizer with sterile water.

2. Place the nebulizer in the bracket on the stand.

3. Insert the immersion heater into one of the ports in the top of the nebulizer; plug into a grounded electrical outlet.

4. Insert the compressed-air flowmeter into the compressed air wall outlet.

5. Connect one end of the low-pressure tubing to the outlet on the flowmeter and the other end to the inlet on the nebulizer.

6. The nebulizer should be set on the 40% dilution.

7. Attach one end of the aerosol tubing to the outlet port on the nebulizer, and the other end to the humidity adapter on the aerosol tee.

8. Insert the oxygen flowmeter into the oxygen wall outlet.

9. Fill the O_2 humidifier with sterile water; attach the humidifier to the outlet on the flowmeter.

10. Attach one end of the O_2 connecting tubing to the outlet port on the humidifier and the other end to the nipple on the venturi (see Figure 3-37).

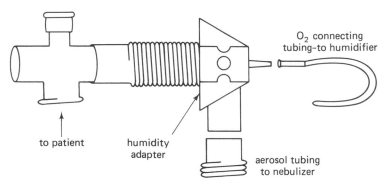

Figure 3-37. Aerosol tee: FIO_2 up to 40%.

11. Adjust O_2 liter flow to that indicated on the aerosol tee according to the FIO_2 being used.

12. Adjust the compressed-air flow until an adequate aerosol is seen (usually about 8 liters/min.).

13. Attach the patient port of the aerosol tee to the adapter on the patient's endotracheal or tracheostomy tube.

14. Analyze the FIO_2 as follows:
    a. Attach a *sterile* suction catheter to the sampling tube on the Beckman D2 oxygen analyzer.
    b. Insert the catheter through the aerosol tee into the endotracheal or tracheostomy tube, approximately 2 to 3 in.
    c. Analyze the FIO_2 in the usual manner.

15. Observe the patient's response to the therapy.

16. Fill out a patient flow sheet and place in chart.

17. Place a "No Smoking—Oxygen in Use" sign outside the patient's door.

IV. Aerosol Tee: FIO_2 over 40%

  A. Equipment

    1. Aerosol tee

    2. Large-bore aerosol tubing

    3. Oxygen flowmeter

    4. Compressed-air flowmeter

    5. All-purpose nebulizer with stand and bracket and 2-psi relief valve

    6. Low-pressure tubing

    7. Immersion heater

    8. Sterile water

    9. Black tee adapter

    10. O_2 connecting tubing

    11. O_2 humidifier

  B. Assembly and application

    1. Fill the all-purpose nebulizer with sterile water.

    2. Place the nebulizer on the bracket on the stand and attach the low-pressure tubing to the inlet on the nebulizer.

        Note: Experience will guide you in determining which gas source will be used to run the nebulizer. Usually, for FIO_2's close to 40%, you can run the nebulizer by compressed air and bleed in oxygen. However, you must be able to use high enough flows to ensure adequate humidity. Higher FIO_2's necessitate running the nebulizer on oxygen and bleeding in compressed air. The dilution on the nebulizer may also have to be changed to 70% in some instances.

    3. Insert the appropriate flowmeter into the wall outlet for the gas that is to run the nebulizer, and connect the other end of the low-pressure tubing to the outlet of the flowmeter.

    4. Insert the immersion heater in one of the ports on top of the nebulizer; plug into a grounded electrical outlet.

    5. Fill the humidifier with sterile water. Attach it to the flowmeter to be used for the secondary gas flow. Insert the flowmeter into the appropriate wall outlet.

    6. Attach connecting tubing to humidifier.

7. Attach black tee to outlet on nebulizer.

8. Attach other end of connecting tubing to nipple on black tee.

9. Connect aerosol tubing to black tee and then to aerosol tee (see Figure 3-38).

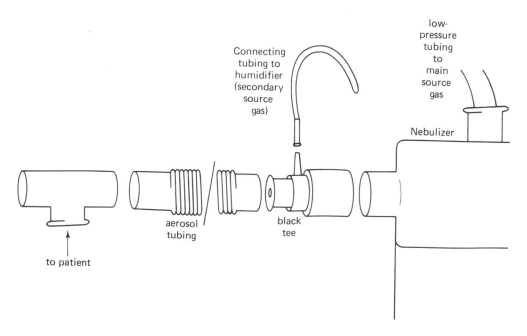

Figure 3-38.   Aerosol tee: FIO_2 over 40%.

10. Adjust liter flows of gases.

11. Attach aerosol tee to adapter on endotracheal or tracheostomy tube.

12. Analyze FIO_2 and adjust flows as necessary.

13. Chart on patient flow sheet.

14. Place "No Smoking—Oxygen in Use" sign in doorway.

V.   Special Notes

   A. *Dead space:* used to help raise Pa_{CO_2}; usually consists of a flex tube attached from the 15-mm port on the aerosol tee to the adapter on the trach tube (see Figure 3-39).

   B. *Reservoir:* used to increase FIO_2; consists of a flex tube attached to the expiratory port on the aerosol tee (see Figure 3-40).

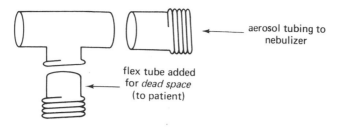

Figure 3-39. Dead space.

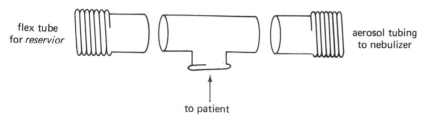

Figure 3-40. Reservoir.

VI. Cleaning and Sterilization
A. The large-bore aerosol tubing and connecting tubing are disposable. They are changed daily by the department.
B. The all-purpose nebulizer aerosol tee, humidifier, and black tee are changed daily, and are gas sterilized.

VII. Undesirable Side Effects
Side effects of this therapy are generally the result of requirements by the patient for a different FIO_2 to maintain adequate Pa_{O_2} levels. Therefore, it is essential to monitor arterial blood gases frequently. Any changes in the patient's behavior or state of consciousness should be reported to the physician immediately.

High humidity will mobilize secretions quite rapidly. For this reason, the nursing staff must suction the patient frequently.

OEM Tracheotomy Mix-O-Mask

I. Introduction
The OEM Tracheotomy Mix-O-Mask (Figure 3-41) is one of several on the market designed to incorporate the accuracy of the Venturi system with an aerosol tee for those patients with

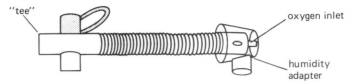

Figure 3-41.   OEM Tracheotomy Mix-O-Mask.

endotracheal or tracheotomy tubes. It is available in concentrations of 24%, 28%, 31%, 35%, and 40%.

II. Equipment
    A. Tracheotomy Mix-O-Mask of desired concentration with humidity adapter
    B. Oxygen supply tubing
    C. Large-bore tubing of 4- to 5-ft. length
    D. Humidifier (optional; however, if one is not used, there is no safety system in the event the oxygen supply tubing becomes occluded)
    E. Nebulizer with immersion heater, or ultrasonic nebulizer
    F. Compressed-air flowmeter (unless using ultrasonic)
    G. Oxygen flowmeter
    H. Sterile water
    I. "No Smoking" sign
    J. Department records

III. Procedure
    A. A complete order in the patient's chart, specifying the oxygen concentration desired, is necessary before initiating the therapy.
    B. Orient the patient to the therapy.
    C. Stress oxygen safety rules.
    D. Fill nebulizer with sterile water or assemble the ultrasonic nebulizer.
    E. Attach compressed-air flowmeter (if nebulizer is used) and oxygen-flowmeter to cylinder or wall outlet.
    F. Attach suitable pressure tubing from a compressed-air flowmeter to inlet on nebulizer. The nebulizer may be attached directly to the flowmeter, but this should be avoided if the nebulizer will be above the level of the bed.
    G. Attach large-bore tubing from outlet on nebulizer (or ultrasonic) to humidity adapter. Adjust flow.

H. Attach oxygen supply tubing from oxygen flowmeter to inlet of Tracheotomy Mix-O-Mask.

I. Adjust oxygen flow according to directions on each Tracheotomy Mix-O-Mask.

J. Place tee over endotracheal tube or tracheotomy tube adapter.

K. The unit should be periodically checked for positioning and the FIO_2 analyzed.

L. Place "No Smoking" sign in doorway or place assigned.

M. Complete department records.

Air-Shields Croupette

This tent may be used to provide an infant with an atmosphere of oxygen enrichment and humidity (see Figure 3-42).

I. Equipment
  A. Air-Shields croupette
  B. Flowmeter for pipeline system or regulator with flowmeter for oxygen or compressed-air cylinder
  C. Sterile distilled water
  D. Five feet of small-bore tubing
  E. Ice
  F. Pan
  G. Department records
  H. "No Smoking" sign

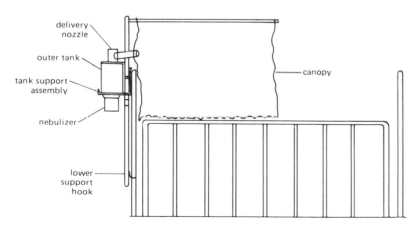

Figure 3-42. Air-Shields Universal Model Croupette.

II. Procedure

  A. A complete order should be in the patient's chart before initiating the therapy.

  B. Orient the patient or his family to the therapy.

  C. Attach flowmeter to suitable wall outlet or attach regulator to suitable cylinder of compressed gas.

  D. Set up croupette.

    1. Attach the end of the drain tubing that has no collar to the connection found on the bottom of the inner tank.

    2. Feed the drain tube through the hole in the bottom of the outer tank, as you place the inner tank in the outer tank.

    3. Slip the end of the drain tube with the collar into its retaining clip on the outer tank.

    4. Fit the delivery nozzle into the manifold tube located above the water jar.

    5. Fit the recirculation nozzle into the top of the other manifold tube.

    6. Place the atomizer in its base assembly.

    7. Attach the water jar to the base assembly of the atomizer.

    8. Attach the unit to the crib.

    9. Attach the canopy to the canopy frame.

  E. Fill atomizer unit with sterile distilled water.

  F. Fit the recirculation and delivery nozzles through their openings in the canopy.

  G. Attach one end of the small-bore tubing to the adapter on the flowmeter.

  H. Attach the other end to the atomizer unit.

  I. Set the flowmeter at 10 liters/min.

  J. Place the canopy over the patient.

  K. Tuck in all ends of the canopy securely.

  L. Place ice in the tank.

  M. Place "No Smoking" sign in doorway.

  N. Fill out department records.

Bunn Tent

This tent may be used to provide the patient with an environment in which the temperature, humidity, and oxygen concentration may be controlled (Figure 3-43).

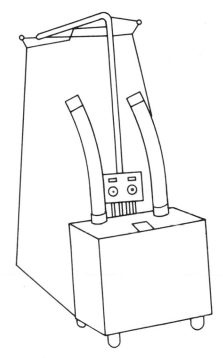

Figure 3-43. Oxygen tent.

I. Equipment
    A. Bunn Tent with canopy
    B. Nebulizer—ultrasonic or Micro-Mist models
    C. Flowmeter for pipeline system or regulator for oxygen or compressed-air cylinder (with flowmeter)
    D. Sterile distilled water
    E. "No Smoking" sign
    F. Department records

II. Procedure
    A. A complete order for the therapy should be in the patient's chart before initiating the therapy.
    B. Orient the patient to this therapy.
    C. Stress oxygen safety rules, if oxygen is to be used.
    D. Set up cylinder of oxygen or compressed air.
        1. Crack cylinder.
        2. Attach regulator with flowmeter.
        3. Turn cylinder valve several turns or connect pipeline flowmeter to suitable wall outlet.

E. Set up tent by attaching canopy.

F. Fill nebulizer with sterile water.

G. If using a nebulizer that runs by a secondary flow of gas (Micro-Sonic model), attach a length of small-bore tubing from the nipple on the regulator to the connector on the nebulizer; if using an ultrasonic nebulizer that operates independently, connect the tubing from the regulator to the connector on the tent.

H. Turn power switch on tent to the *on* position.

I. Set regulator on flush.

J. Place the canopy over the patient.

K. Tuck in all ends of the canopy.

L. Place aerosol tubing from nebulizer alongside of outlet stack. If aerosol from tent nebulizer is adequate, a secondary nebulizer may not be necessary.

M. Adjust temperature to about 70° to 72°F.

N. After allowing tent to fill, adjust regulator using a minimum of 10 liters/min (necessary to wash out carbon dioxide).

O. Place "No Smoking" sign in doorway.

P. Fill out department records.

Q. Oxygen concentrations in the tent should be monitored at least once every 4 hours.

R. When liquid in nebulizer drops to low level, refill with sterile water.

S. Each time the tent canopy is opened for patient care, the tent should be flushed if a specific oxygen concentration is desired.

Olympic Oxyhood

The Olympic Oxyhood is a controlled environment chamber for the administration of high concentrations of oxygen and aerosol to infants.

I. Equipment
   A. Olympic Oxyhood
      1. Small—6-in. diameter for infants under 2½ lb
      2. Medium—8-in. diameter for infants 2½ to 8 lb
      3. Large—10 in. diameter for infants 8 to 18 lb
   B. Puritan All-Purpose Nebulizer with immersion heater
   C. Four-foot large-bore tubing

D. Flowmeter for pipeline system or regulator for oxygen or compressed air

E. Sterile water

II. Procedure

A. A written order is required before initiating the therapy.

B. For the infant, Oxyhood using oxygen only for FIO_2 40% and over, refer to Figure 3-44.

C. For the infant, Oxyhood using compressed air and oxygen for FIO_2 under 40%, refer to Figure 3-45.

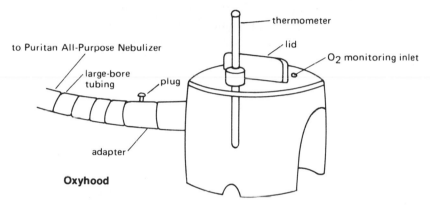

Figure 3-44. FIO_2 delivered depends on the diluter setting (40%, 70%, and 100%) and flowmeter setting.

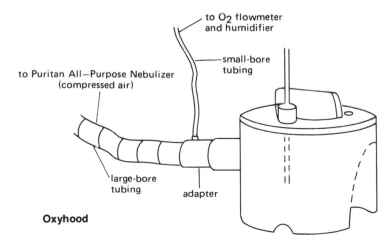

Figure 3-45. FIO_2 delivered depends on the oxygen flowmeter setting and the compressed-air flowmeter setting.

Note: 1. An oxygen analysis should be taken at least once every 2 hours.
2. The removable lid provides instant access to the infant's head, permitting suctioning of the infant without removing him from the hood.

Ohio-Armstrong Isolation Incubator

The Ohio-Armstrong Isolation Incubator is designed for use with the newborn infant. It consists of a transparent hood mounted on a main unit, which has a controlled heating unit, a heat-circulating system, a humidity system, and an air-filtering unit. It also has an infant bed, which when adjusted, will give you the Trendelenburg, Fowler's, and examination positions. The main unit is mounted on a cabinet with casters and has storage space for accessory equipment (Figure 3-46).

Operation of Incubator

1. Connect the electrical plug from the incubator to a 115- to 120-V ac electrical wall outlet.
2. Press main switch on.
3. Adjust temperature control to the start position.
4. With incubator in the start position, preheat until temperature stabilizes as observed on the thermometer.
5. To increase the temperature, turn the control clockwise; to decrease temperature, turn control counterclockwise.
6. Remember that the number on the control is for charting only; only the thermometer in the incubator will be correct.
7. Next, set the humidity control from a low to high position.
8. Pull out the water-fill indicator with your finger and fill water assembly with about 25 oz of setrile water.
9. The oxygen system is now set, if oxygen is to be used; the incubator is supplied with two oxygen inlets, one a 40% oxygen-limiting unit, the other a 100% screw-top unit; both units are located on the filter unit.
10. If oxygen is used, a pressure-compensated flowmeter should be used.
11. If oxygen is used at any concentration below 40%, you should use the 40%-limiting unit; for concentrations of 40% to 100%, the 100% unit should be used and the 40% unit capped.
12. *Remember:* Oxygen concentration should be taken with an oxy-

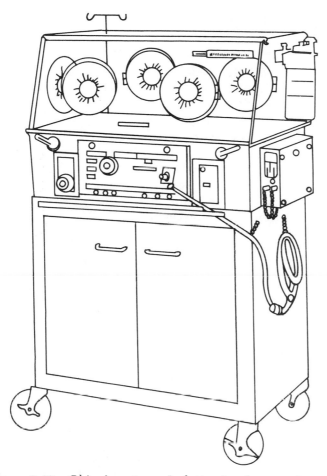

Figure 3-46. Ohio-Armstrong Isolation Incubator main unit.

gen analyzer, depending on the department procedure on time intervals.

13. Nebulization (if used)—attach Ohio nebulizer to unit and fill jar with sterile water to the fill line.

14. Adjust flowmeter for proper output of nebulizer; usually a flow of 3 to 5 liters/min should be used.

15. Be careful when administering nebulization, being sure that you use compressed air to power nebulizer or, if oxygen is used, remember about oxygen concentration.

16. Observation of infant in incubator should be constant; also, observation of temperature and oxygen concentration should be monitored and recorded.

Linde Walker and Reservoir

I. Reservoir (see Figures 3-47 and 3-48)

    A. Description—the Linde reservoir is a liquid-oxygen container. It may be used as an oxygen supply for an IPPB apparatus and for oxygen administration equipment, such as face masks and cannulae. The gas is provided at a pressure of 50 psi.

    B. Filling—the reservoir will, on an average, have to be refilled once a week. The indicator light, labeled "Refill reservoir when on," will light when the oxygen supply is getting low. When this light goes on, there will be enough oxygen for about three walker refills. The Linde representative will take care of refilling the reservoir.

> *Note:* The refill lamp will not go on if the reservoir is disconnected from the electrical outlet or if the power switch is off. The "Walker full" lamp will always be lighted when the power is on and the walker is not being filled. This indicator should be disregarded except when the walker is being filled.

    C. Connecting the reservoir—the reservoir has a power cord that may be plugged into a three-terminal outlet or a two-terminal outlet by means of an adapter.

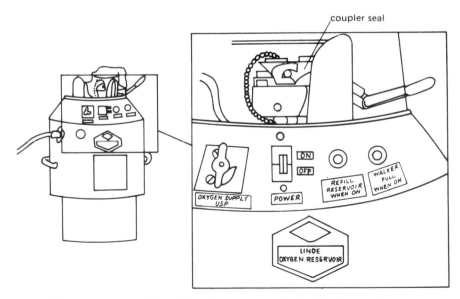

Figure 3-47. Linde Walker Reservoir and detail of control panel.

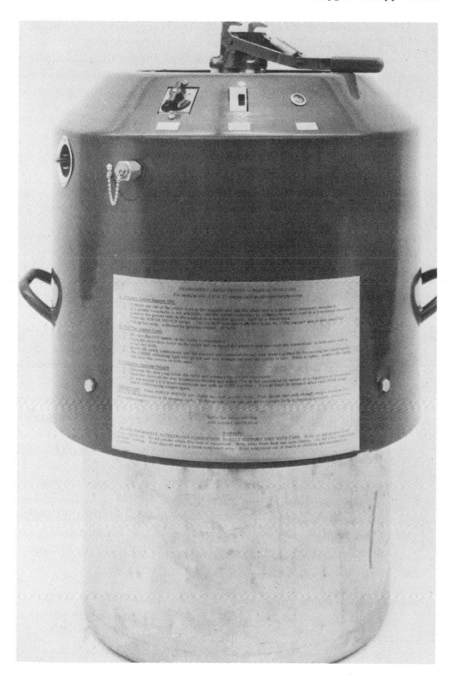

Figure 3-48. Linde Walker Reservoir. (*Courtesy of Union Carbide Corp., Linde Division, 270 Park Avenue, New York, N.Y. 10017*)

D. Use of reservoir for breathing—the reservoir can be connected directly to an IPPB machine or to another device, such as the flowmeter, for use with a mask. The reservoir will supply up to 15 liters/min. Electrical power is not needed, but it is wise to keep the power on so that the refill reservoir lamp will light when the reservoir reserve supply gets low.

The Walker may be filled while the reservoir is furnishing oxygen for breathing. The oxygen supply is controlled by a valve marked "oxygen supply."

II. The Walker
   A. Description—the Linde Walker is a liquid-oxygen container that affords a portable supply of oxygen.
   B. Filling the Walker
      1. Press the *off* switch on the walker to be sure the oxygen flow is shut off.
      2. Lift the latch handle on the reservoir and remove the coupler seal (see Figure 3-48).
      3. Open the coupler cover on the walker, and remove the walker coupler seal by lifting the handle straight up.
      4. Check that the reservoir is plugged in and that the power switch is turned *on*.
      5. Turn the walker upside down and guide it onto the reservoir so that the electrical pins of the walker engage the sockets of the reservoir [see Figure 3-49(1)].
      6. The latch handle is then pushed down [see Figures 3-49(2) and 3-50] to lock the couplers together.
      7. If the couplers are properly connected, the walker will begin to fill; the lamp marked "Walker full when on" will go off and will *relight* when the walker is full; filling the walker will take about 3 min and you should also watch as it is being filled.

      Warning: Due to the temperature of liquid oxygen (−300°F), *frost* may form on the couplings. Touching this will cause cold burns.

      8. If the "Walker full" lamp comes on and filling continues beyond the 3-min limit, and you observe a dense fog coming from the lower part of the reservoir, raise the latch handle to shut off the flow, and call the service representative.

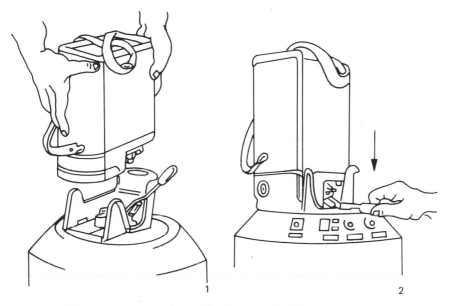

Figure 3-49. Linde Walker being filled from reservoir.

9. Replace the coupler seal on the walker, pressing the handles down to lock it.

10. Replace the coupler seal on the reservoir and lock it by pressing down the latch handle.

C. Use of the Walker

   1. The walker should always be used in the upright position, and there is a strap that facilitates carrying of the unit.

   2. The tubing on the breathing device may be attached to the outlet on the side of the walker.

   3. Open the selector cover and set the prescribed flow rate. There are buttons marked 1, 2, 4, and *off*, indicating liters per minute. The buttons are also color coded for convenience. To get 1, 2, or 4 liters, push only the button with the desired number until the button locks into place. For 3, 5, 6, or 7 liters/min, simultaneously press the two or three buttons that add up to the desired flow rate (the buttons *must* be pushed at the same time).

Color code

Off	Light blue	2	Yellow
1	Gray	4	Green

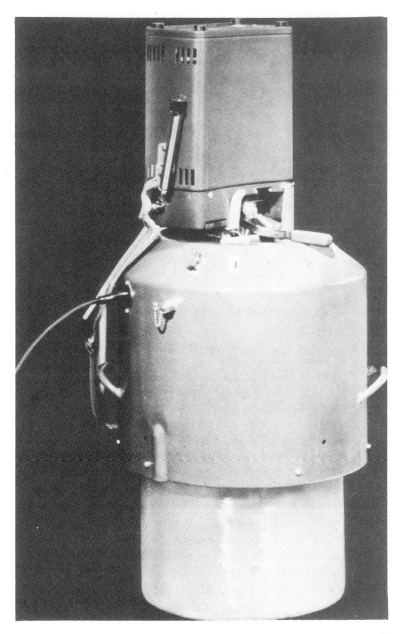

Figure 3-50.   Linde Walker being filled from reservoir. (*Courtesy of Union Carbide Corp., Linde Division, 270 Park Avenue, New York, N.Y. 10017*)

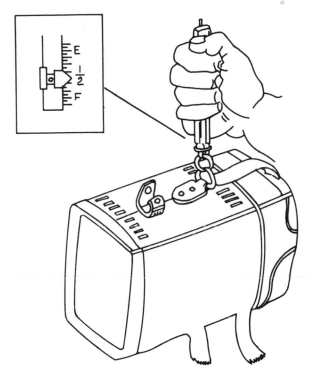

Figure 3-51. Checking Linde Walker contents by means of attached spring scale.

> *Note:* Do not block the ventilation slots of the case or the oxygen will be too cold for comfortable breathing.

    4. Press the *off* button to stop the oxygen flow.

  D. Checking walker contents—there is a spring scale on the side of the walker. Unfasten the holding strap and lift the walker by the barrel of the scale (see Figure 3-50). The scale is calibrated similarly to that of an automobile gas gauge; with *E* meaning empty and *F* meaning full.

> *Note:* The walker loses about one-fifth of its contents in a day through evaporation.

Linde Oxygen Walker System Mark II

  I. Introduction
    The Mark II, the newest of the Linde Oxygen Walker systems, consists of two parts.

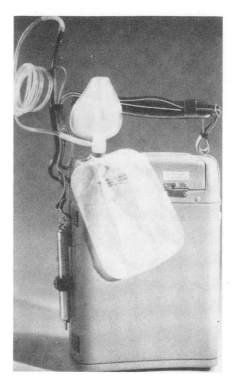

Figure 3-52.   Linde Walker and mask ready for use. (*Courtesy of Union Carbide Corp., Linde Division, 270 Park Avenue, New York, N.Y. 10017*)

    A. The Reservoir—holds approximately 40 lb of liquid oxygen.

    B. The Walker Unit—weighs approximately 11 lb when full and is equal to approximately 1025 liters of oxygen gas. The advantage of the walker unit is its portability. The reservoir, however, is multipurposed. It may be used to supply oxygen for use with a mask, cannula, or catheter, as well as for IPPB therapy.

  II. The Reservoir

    A. A flowmeter may be attached to the oxygen supply outlet fitting on the reservoir for use with those oxygen devices requiring careful flow adjustment. The reservoir will supply an uninterrupted flow up to 12 liters/min until empty.

    B. Contents—indicated on scale in special base

       1. *F* (full)—signifies that more than 15 lb of liquid oxygen remains in the reservoir. The area on the scale is *green*.

2. *R* (refill)—signifies on a *yellow* sector that between 10 and 15 lb of liquid oxygen remains.

3. *E* (empty)—signifies that 10 lb or less remains in the reservoir. The area on the scale is *red*.

4. Equipment attached to the reservoir or placed on top of it can cause the indicator scale to read inaccurately. However, the scale may be adjusted by a service representative to allow for this.

III. The Walker

A. The walker unit may be carried by its shoulder strap. It has a scale to indicate when it is full, three-quarters full, one-half full and empty. The flow selector valve provides five different flow rates and is located under the hinged cover on top of the unit. Oxygen therapy equipment tubing can be attached to the outlet on the side of the walker unit.

B. To fill the walker

1. Check reservoir contents—never refill walker if reservoir is on *E*.

2. To avoid wasting oxygen, do not refill walker if there is enough oxygen for its planned use.

3. The walker unit should be filled at room temperature only. Coupler fittings should be clean and dry.

4. Release and open the hinged cover on the walker unit and snap to the case to keep it open.

5. Turn the flow selection valve to the *off* position.

6. Raise the latch handle on the reservoir and swing the coupler seal away from the coupler.

7. Loosen and remove the coupler seal on the walker unit.

8. Using a clean, dry, oil-free cloth, wipe the coupler fitting on both units.

9. Invert the walker and lower it into position so that both coupler fittings fit together. There is only one correct way of doing so.

10. Push the latch handle down as far as possible to lock the couplers.

11. Push the *FILL* button to start. The unit should automatically stop when the fill is complete. If it fails to do so after 4 min, however, it is necessary to pull the *FILL* button manually. Therefore, one should always time the filling process.

12. When the walker is full, the *FILL* button should snap out

automatically and the hissing noise should stop. At this time, lift the latch handle and remove the walker.

13. Screw the cap onto the coupler of the walker and tighten. Close the walker cover.

14. Replace the coupler seal on the reservoir and lock in place.

C. If you encounter problems:

1. If the fill valve freezes open and the *FILL* button cannot be pulled out, lift the latch handle. Leave the walker inverted on the reservoir for 30 min or until it is possible to pull out the *FILL* button. Following this, it will be impossible to use the walker. Report such an occurrence to the service representative.

2. If, after a normal filling process, the walker sticks to the reservoir or if liquid is leaked from the connections, couple the two units immediately and wait until the frost has melted before lifting the walker off.

D. Operating times

It is frequently necessary to estimate the length of time a full walker unit will run. For example, at 2 liters/min, the oxygen supply will last approximately 8 hours.

$$\underset{\text{(flow)}}{2 \text{ liters/min}} \times \underset{\text{(1 hr)}}{60 \text{ min}} = 120 \text{ liters/hour}$$

$$\frac{1000 \text{ liters (approximate content of full walker)}}{120 \text{ (liters/hour)}} = \text{duration}$$

The Liberator/Stroller Oxygen System

The Liberator

The liberator (Figure 3-53) is the source from which the portable stroller can be filled; it may also be used as a direct source for oxygen therapy for those times when the patient is not ambulatory. The liberator holds approximately 50 lb of liquid oxygen; this is equal to approximately 17,000 liters of oxygen gas.

1. Liquid level indicator—shows the contents at all times. It is positioned on the top of the unit, and is labeled as to F (full), $\frac{1}{2}$, $\frac{1}{4}$, and E (empty). A red band in the indicator will move down as the level of the oxygen decreases. Use the *top* of the red band to determine the level of oxygen available in the liberator.

2. Flow rate selector—restricts flow of oxygen to the indicated rate. It is located on the top of the unit and is calibrated for flows of 1, 1.5, 2, 2.5, 3.0, 4, 5, 6, 8, 10, and 15 liters/min.

3. Supply outlet—located on the side of the unit near the top. It is the point at which the gas leaves the liberator. Attach the humidifier at this outlet.

4. Humidifier supply connector—the point at which connecting tubing is attached for the particular oxygen device being used (cannula, mask, etc.).

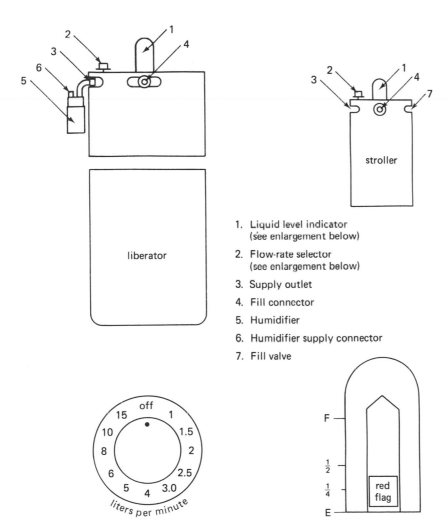

1. Liquid level indicator (see enlargement below)

2. Flow-rate selector (see enlargement below)

3. Supply outlet

4. Fill connector

5. Humidifier

6. Humidifier supply connector

7. Fill valve

Figure 3-53. Liberator/stroller oxygen system.

5. Fill connector—the point at which the portable stroller is connected for filling.

Use of the Liberator as a Direct Source of Oxygen

1. Fill the humidifier to the *Full* mark with sterile distilled water. Home patients who do not have this product available may use water that has been boiled for 20 minutes and stored in the refrigerator. However, they must be cautioned to allow the water to reach room temperature before using.
2. Attach the humidifier to the supply outlet.
3. Attach the connecting tubing for the oxygen device being used to the supply connector on the top of the humidifier.
4. Set the flow rate selector as prescribed by the physician. The liberator can only be set for those flows indicated on the selector; the knob will click into position. Flows other than those indicated cannot be set.
5. Adjust the oxygen device to the face.
6. At the time oxygen therapy is discontinued:
   a. Remove oxygen device from the face.
   b. Turn the flow rate selector to *off*.

The Stroller

The stroller is a portable oxygen supply unit weighing approximately 10 lb when full. Although it holds about 1100 liters of pure oxygen gas, the length of time between refills will vary, depending on the liter flows used.

1. Liquid level indicator—similar to that on the liberator. To read accurately, the unit must be in an upright position. Do not refill the stroller unless it is necessary, as doing so wastes oxygen through evaporation.
2. Flow rate selector—as on the liberator.
3. Supply outlet—for connection of the connecting tubing for the oxygen device. No humidifier is used with the stroller.
4. Fill connector (male) and fill valve—used for refilling the stroller.

To Fill the Stroller

1. Wipe the refill connectors on the liberator and stroller with a lint-free cloth to remove lint, moisture, and dirt.
2. Set the flow rate selector on the stroller to the *off* position.

3. Pick up the stroller and hold it with the refill connector positioned toward the liberator (away from your body).

4. Tilt the stroller at a 45° angle; insert the male fill connector on the stroller into the female fill connector on the liberator. (There is a pin on the male connector that must fit in a slot on the female connector.)

5. Rotate the stroller clockwise into a vertical position; this locks it into place.

6. Insert the T-handle wrench provided with the unit onto the fill valve on the side of the stroller. Turn the valve to the *on* position to start the filling process.

7. When the liquid level indicator on the stroller reaches the *Fill* mark (or at any other desired level), turn the fill valve to the *off* position using the T-handle wrench.

8. Wait a minimum of 15 to 30 sec before disengaging the stroller (turn it in a counterclockwise direction to a 45° angle and pull straight out from the liberator).

Special Notes

1. Filling will take from 1 to 2 min, depending on the internal temperature of the stroller.

2. Gas will escape from beneath the liberator cover during filling; this is normal.

3. Remain with the unit for the entire filling process.

4. If the refill connectors do not seal when disengaged, reengage the connectors, wait 30 sec, and disengage again. If this does not solve the problem, reengage the connectors and contact the service representative for the units.

5. Never touch exposed metal parts when they are frosted.

6. Instruct the patient and his family in oxygen safety rules, especially with regard to home use.

EXERCISES

1. Discuss the contraindications of ultrasonic nebulization.

2. Describe three methods of setting up a 35% aerosol tee.

3. List the advantages and disadvantages of prefilled humidifiers and nebulizers compared to reusables.

4. Compare the advantages and disadvantages of the Linde Walker/ Reservoir system to cylinder gas.

UNIT 4

INTERMITTENT POSITIVE PRESSURE BREATHING

This unit outlines the indications for use of IPPB therapy, the approach to the patient and medications commonly used, as well as the procedures for use of various types of equipment available for the administration of the therapy.

ADMINISTRATION OF INTERMITTENT POSITIVE PRESSURE BREATHING ON INSPIRATION (IPPB/I) TO ADULTS

Inspiratory Intermittent Positive Pressure Breathing—IPPB/I

Definition. Intermittent positive pressure breathing consists of a type of breathing pattern wherein the lungs are inflated by positive pressure (above atmospheric) during inspiration, and upon release of the pressure, expiration occurs passively.

Objectives of IPPB/I

1. Mobilize and liquefy secretions.
2. Relieve and/or prevent atelectasis.
3. Relieve bronchospasm.
4. Improve or promote cough.
5. Improve alveolar ventilation.
6. Sputum collection.

Indications for IPPB/I

1. Difficulty mobilizing secretions due to poor cough or tenacious secretions.
2. Strong clinical indication or x-ray evidence of atelectasis.
3. Conditions conducive to atelectasis or retention of secretions that are not preventable by simpler means, such as deep breathing or coughing techniques.
4. Evidence of bronchospasm.
5. Decreased alveolar ventilation as evidenced by arterial blood gases, tidal volume measurement, auscultation, respiratory rate, depth of breathing, x-ray, and/or pulmonary function studies.

Types of Equipment Used

1. Bennett Model PV-3P. May be used with compressed air or oxygen enrichment.
2. Bennett Model AP-4. Compressor model used to deliver 21% O_2.
3. Bennett Model TA-1. Compressor model designed for home use.
4. Ohio Model hand-E-vent. Compressor model designed for home use.

Medications Most Commonly Used

1. Isoproterenol (1:400): bronchodilator; usual dosage, 0.5 ml.
2. Isoetharine (1%): bronchodilator; usual dosage, 0.25 to 1.0 ml.
3. Racemic epinephrine (2.25%): bronchodilator; usual dosage, 0.5 ml.
4. Acetylcysteine (10%): mucolytic; usual dosage, 1.0 to 3.0 ml.
5. Sodium chloride (0.9%): physiologic saline; for humidity; usual dosage, 1.5 to 2.0 ml.
6. Distilled water: for humidity; usual dosage, 1.5 to 2.0 ml.

Duration of Treatment.   Treatment should be continued until medication is exhausted, usually 15 to 20 min (depends on amount of medication ordered).

Pressure Ordered.   Pressure for an IPPB machine is ordered and delivered in centimeters of water (cm H_2O). Usual pressure is 10 to 20 cm of water. However, the patient's tolerance of the pressure must be taken into consideration. The technician *may not* administer more pressure than is ordered, but if in his estimation the patient cannot tolerate as much pressure, he may administer less.

Considerations to Be Observed for the Successful Administration of IPPB

1. Orientation of the patient: A *simple* explanation of the IPPB apparatus and treatment is given when the patient receives the initial treatment. (See detailed explanation that follows.)
2. Never administer a dry gas. There must always be some medication in the nebulizer. Always make certain that the medication is nebulizing properly.
3. The IPPB unit should follow the patient's breathing cycle. The patient should not experience more difficulty breathing.
4. All equipment must be clean; follow established procedure for changing main air hoses and setups.

Specific Instruction and Preparation of the Patient

1. Identify your patient. Check wrist band to determine that it is the patient for whom the order was written. If the patient does not have a wrist band, do not administer the treatment until properly identified (notify the nursing staff).
2. Identify yourself and the department.
3. Explain the treatment and what effect is desired (based on the physician's objectives of therapy). The patient may be told that the machine will exert a regulated, gentle pressure on his lungs when he breathes in, helping him to breathe deeply. As he breathes in, a fine mist of medication will be delivered to his lungs. Explain that he may breathe out at any time he wishes, although more benefit will be derived if he is able to take a deep, slow breath and hold it for a few seconds.
4. Instruct the patient to breathe in deeply enough to turn the machine on, but then to let the machine do the work of filling his lungs. (If you tell most patients to take a deep breath, at least initially they use their accessory muscles and thus ventilation is inefficient.)
5. Once the patient has become accustomed to the pattern of breathing on the IPPB machine, instruct him in the technique of diaphragmatic breathing; this will make the treatment more effective.
6. Relate the objectives of the therapy to the patient's condition. He will be more cooperative if he can understand the relevance to him.

7. Explain the use of the nose clip if one is used.

8. Explain the duration and frequency of the therapy.

9. Position the patient for effective therapy:
    a. In bed: roll the head of the bed as high as is comfortable for the patient. Be sure that the patient's buttocks are at the bend in the bed, not his back.
    b. Out of bed: have the patient sit in a straight-backed chair with his feet flat on the floor and his arms resting comfortably.
    c. Unless the patient has had spinal surgery, or there is some other medical indication, no IPPB treatment should be administered with the patient lying flat on his back or on his side.

Undesirable Side Effects

1. To identify undesirable side effects of therapy, it is first necessary to ascertain the patient's condition before initiating the therapy.
    a. Observe patient's color; is it cyanotic (degree), flushed, pale?
    b. Observe patient's pulse and respiratory rates.
    c. Observe patient's state of consciousness.
    d. Observe patient for physical symptoms: apparent wheezing, productive cough, visible bleeding from any source, open tracheostomy site, and so on.

2. Potential undesirable side effects of IPPB therapy:
    a. The respiratory therapy personnel administering IPPB therapy must know the side effects of each medication being used.
    b. All personnel must be cognizant of the effects of oxygen therapy, particularly in regards to the chronic obstructive pulmonary disease patient.
    c. Although rare, positive pressure on inspiration could cause rupture of emphysematous blebs.

3. All patients receiving IPPB therapy must be observed closely. Therefore, it is essential that personnel remain with the patient for the duration of the treatment.
    a. Note any changes in the color of the patient's skin. If he becomes cyanotic, or cyanosis present becomes more pronounced, discontinue the therapy and notify the physician.
    b. The patient's breathing should not become more difficult. If it does, discontinue the therapy and notify the physician.
    c. Medications that act as bronchodilators generally also act as cardiac stimulants. Recording the patient's pulse rate before, during, and after the administration of such drugs will

give an indication of this undesirable side effect. Report such occurrences to the physician for evaluation.

d. Medications such as acetylcysteine may precipitate bronchospasm, particularly in those patients with chronic obstructive pulmonary disease. Observe the patient closely for increased wheezing or respiratory difficulty. Stop the therapy and notify the physician immediately. If severe, resuscitation methods may have to be instituted.

e. If the patient experiences chest pain or hemoptysis, discontinue the therapy and notify the physician for evaluation.

f. If a patient becomes very lethargic while receiving an IPPB treatment, particularly when on oxygen, stop the treatment and notify the physician.

g. Respiratory therapy personnel must be able to judge circumstances as they arise, and decide at which point the physician must be notified. If a patient's complaint *could* be directly related to the therapy, it is best to stop the treatment until the respiratory therapist can consult with the patient's physician.

Proceed with the record work of your individual department.

ADMINISTRATION OF INTERMITTENT POSITIVE PRESSURE BREATHING TO CHILDREN

I. Introduction

Only flow-sensitive or flow-adjustable equipment should be used for the administration of IPPB/*I* to children and infants.

II. Policies

A. The medication dosage will vary from patient to patient, mostly depending on the age and particularly the size of the child.

B. A written order with all specific instructions, signed by a *physician*, is necessary before initiation of this therapy. The indication and purpose of treatment should be outlined.

III. Undesirable Side Effects

A. The side effects of IPPB/*I* therapy are usually related to the mechanical effect of positive pressure breathing and/or medications. Instances of sudden death have been reported due to pneumothorax in asthmatic children. For this reason, some physicians prefer not to administer the desired medications by positive pressure.

B. Any deterioration of the patient's condition while receiving treatment is an indication for its discontinuation. Report to the physician any such occurrences.

C. Because children have a tendency to hyperventilate, causing light-headedness, it is best to have them remain in bed for a few minutes directly following the therapy.

IV. Preparation of the Patient

A. The older child should be sitting up as straight as possible.

B. The infant or young child should be held in the lap; if a parent is present, they might hold the child or, if necessary have the nursing staff help.

C. Instruct the child when possible in the treatment procedure. The parents should also be instructed, as their cooperation may be required in order to provide effective therapy to the very young child.

D. Making a game of the treatment will often gain the child's interest and cooperation. He can watch the dials on the machine and pretend he is a jet pilot or astronaut breathing oxygen.

V. Equipment for the Infant

A. Minimum dead space manifold

B. Plastic connector

C. Nebulizer manifold

D. Twin-jet nebulizer (10 cc)

E. Infant mask

VI. Assembly and Operation of Infant Equipment

A. Treatment with mask

1. Place the medication in the nebulizer

2. Place the nebulizer into the bottom opening of the manifold.

3. Connect the manifold to the support arm of the unit.

4. Using the plastic connector, attach the minimum dead space manifold to the nebulizer manifold.

5. Attach the mask to the minimum dead space manifold. Both of these parts may be turned to provide easier access to the patient. Attach tubings.

6. Adjust the IPPB unit as required. Inspiratory pressures

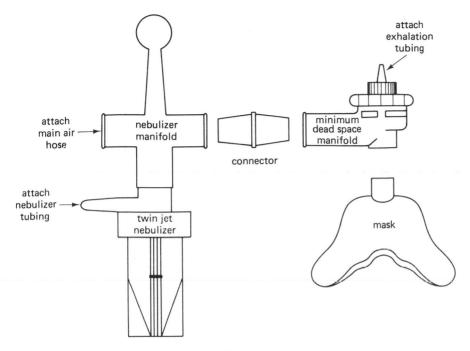

Figure 4-1. Pediatric IPPB/*I* set-up.

required to deliver the medication may appear high, compared to the size of the infant. However, due to the smaller size of the airways, this pressure is required to overcome resistance. See Figure 4-1.

B. Treatment when infant is intubated or tracheostomized.

1. The unit is set up as described above, omitting the mask.

2. In most instances, the opening on the minimum dead space manifold will fit directly onto the tracheostomy or endotracheal tube adapter. In the event an adapter is needed, it will be provided by the respiratory therapy department. See Figure 4-2.

VII. Assembly and Operation of Equipment for the Older Child

A. The older child can probably use an adult patient setup.

B. In the event the child requires a mask rather than a mouthpiece, the mask is attached to the flex tube.

C. If the child is tracheostomized or intubated, the adult setup may be used with a tube adapter in place of the mouthpiece. See Figure 4-3.

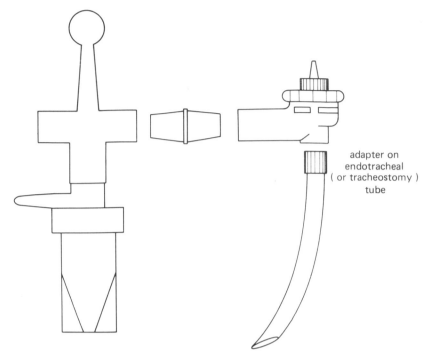

Figure 4-2.   Pediatric IPPB/*I* set-up for use with endotracheal tube.

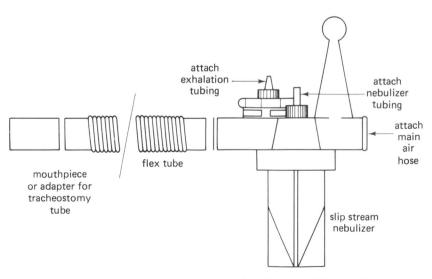

Figure 4-3.   IPPB/*I* set-up for the adult or older child.

MEDICATIONS USED IN RESPIRATORY THERAPY

This discussion is designed to familiarize the therapist with some of the medications available for treatment of respiratory problems. The list of medications, as well as the information provided, is by no means intended to be complete, and reference should be made to product literature before administration. The therapist may not be involved with the administration of some of these drugs; however, because of their interaction with medications that he may deliver to the patient, it is important that he be aware of their action.

I. Bronchodilators
   A. Isoproterenol hydrochloride 1:200, 1:400
      1. *Action*—relaxes bronchial spasm and facilitates expectoration of pulmonary secretions; a sympathomimetic amine that is an almost pure beta stimulator, with resultant bronchodilitation, increased heart rate, increased heart force.

      2. *Indications*—for symptomatic relief of bronchial asthma, chronic pulmonary emphysema, bronchitis, and other chronic bronchopulmonary disorders in which bronchospasm is a complicating factor, such as bronchiectasis, pulmonary fibrosis, and pneumoconiosis; may also be useful in preventing postoperative pulmonary complications in patients with acute or chronic bronchopulmonary disease.

      3. *Contraindications*—use in patients with preexisting cardiac arrhythmias associated with tachycardia is generally considered contraindicated because the cardiac stimulant effect of the drug may aggravate such disorders.

      4. *Warnings*
         a. Excessive use of adrenergic aerosol should be discouraged as it may lose its effectiveness.
         b. In patients with status asthmaticus and abnormal blood gas tensions, improvement in vital capacity and in blood gas tensions may not accompany apparent relief of bronchospasm; therefore, administration of oxygen mixtures and ventilatory assistance may be necessary.
         c. Severe paradoxical airway resistance, cardiac arrest, and death have been reported as a result of excessive use.

5. *Precautions*
   a. Should not be administered with other sympathomi-metic amines, as these drugs are cardiac stimulants and their combined effects may induce serious arrhythmia.
   b. Use with caution in patients with cardiovascular disease, diabetes, hyperthyroidism, pregnancy, and in those individuals sensitive to sympathomimetic amines.
6. *Adverse reactions*—by inhalation few untoward reactions are experienced, and those that do result usually disappear quickly; generally, they do not inconvenience the patient to the extent that the drug must be discontinued; sometimes may produce tachycardia, palpitation, headache, and nausea.
7. *Dosage*—usual dosage for inhalation: 0.3 to 0.5 ml of 1:200; 0.5 to 1.0 ml of 1:400. May be used alone in the nebulizer, but is generally administered in a mixture with normal saline or sterile water.

B. Racemic epinephrine, 2.25%
1. *Action*—relaxes bronchial smooth muscles by acting on the muscle and reduces bronchial edema by vasoconstriction.
2. *Indications*—provides temporary relief of asthmatic attacks.
3. *Precautions*
   a. No prescription is necessary; should not be used without the advice of a physician. Use with caution in patients with hypertension, heart disease, diabetes, thyroid disease, or for children under 12 years of age.
   b. This drug should not be administered with other drugs having similar actions.
4. *Side effects*—excessive dosage may cause bronchial irritation, nervousness, restlessness, or sleeplessness.
5. *Dosage*—usual dosage is 0.3 to 0.5 ml.; may be used alone in the nebulizer, but is generally administered in a mixture of normal saline or sterile water.

C. Isoetharine, 1.0%
1. *Action*—provides rapidly effective and relatively long-acting potent bronchodilation; produces a synergistic relaxation of bronchospasm, shrinkage of swollen mucosal membranes and the diminishing of mucus secretion; as a result, vital capacity may significantly increase. Has a

somewhat higher beta-2 effect than beta-1, so cardiac effects are less.

2. *Indications*—for rapid relief of bronchial asthma and other conditions in which bronchospasm is a complicating factor.

3. *Warnings*—should not be administered along with epinephrine or other sympathomimetic amines, as such drugs are direct cardiac stimulants and may cause excessive tachycardia.

4. *Precautions*—use carefully in patients with hyperthyroidism, hypertension, acute coronary disease, cardiac asthma, limited cardiac reserve, and in those persons sensitive to sympathomimetic amines.

5. *Adverse reactions*—relatively free of toxic effects; excessive use may result in tachycardia, palpitation, nausea, headache, changes in blood pressure, anxiety, tension, and restlessness, as is the case with other sympathomimetic amines.

6. *Dosage*—usual dosage is 0.25 to 1.0 ml.

D. Metaproterenol sulfate

1. *Action*—a potent beta-adrenergic stimulator with rapid onset of action; decreases reversible bronchospasm; increases FEV_1; increases maximum expiratory flow rate; increases forced vital capacity and/or decreases airway resistance.

2. *Indications*—bronchial asthma and reversible bronchospasm associated with bronchitis and emphysema.

3. *Contraindications*—cardiac arrhythmias associated with tachycardia, as this drug may aggravate such a condition.

4. *Warnings*—cardiac arrest following excessive use has been reported. Paradoxical bronchoconstriction has been reported following repeated excessive use of other sympathomimetic amines, so that it is conceivable that this could happen with metaproterenol sulfate.

5. *Precautions*—use with caution for patients with hypertension, coronary artery disease, congestive heart failure, hyperthyroid, diabetes, and if sensitive to the drug. Safety in pregnancy has not been established.

6. *Adverse reactions*—tachycardia, hypertension, palpitations, nervousness, tremor, nausea, and vomiting.

7. *Dosage*—metered inhalor: 2 to 3 inhalations, not to exceed 12 inhalations per day; also provided as syrup for

pediatric use, as well as an oral preparation for adult use.

E. Terbutaline sulfate
1. *Action*—synthetic sympathomimetic amine; beta-adrenergic agonist.
2. *Indications*—for treatment of acute bronchospasm of asthma and reversible bronchospasm associated with bronchitis and emphysema.
3. *Contraindications*—hypersensitivity to the drug.
4. *Precautions*—use with caution in diabetes, hypertension, hyperthyroid conditions, and cardiac patients with arrhythmias. Should not be administered with other sympathomimetic amines.
5. *Adverse reactions*—increased heart rate, nervousness, tremor, palpitations, dizziness, headache, nausea, and vomiting.
6. *Dosage*—usual dosage, 5 mg, 6 hours apart, 3 times daily, usually during waking hours; not to exceed 15 mg in 24 hours.

II. Mucolytics
A. Acetylcysteine
1. *Action*—the mucolytic action probably "opens" disulfide linkages in mucus, thereby lowering the viscosity.
2. *Indications*—as adjuvant therapy for patients with abnormal, viscid, or inspissated mucous secretions in such conditions as acute and chronic bronchopulmonary disease, pulmonary complications, posttraumatic chest conditions, and atelectasis due to mucous obstruction.
3. *Contraindications*—in those patients who are sensitive or who have developed a sensitivity to it.
4. *Warnings*
   a. Administration may result in an increased volume of liquefied bronchial secretions; therefore, provisions must be made to maintain patency of airways.
   b. Asthmatics should be watched carefully for progression of bronchospasm.
   c. Should never be added directly to a heated nebulizer.
5. *Adverse effects*—stomatitis, nausea, and rhinorrhea; varying degrees of bronchospasm.
6. *Dosage*—3.0 to 5.0 ml of either the 10% or 20% solution.
7. Compatibility (see Table 4-1).

TABLE 4-1　In Vitro Compatibilities of Acetylcysteine

| PRODUCT AND/OR AGENT(S) | MANUFACTURER (TRADEMARK) | COMPATI-BILITY RATING* | RATIO TESTED** | |
			ACETYL-CYSTEINE	PRODUCT OR AGENT
ANESTHETIC, GAS				
Halothane U.S.P.	Ayerst (Halothane)	Compatible	20%	Infinite
Nitrous Oxide U.S.P.	National Cylinder Gas Company	Compatible	20%	Infinite
ANESTHETIC, LOCAL				
Cocaine HCl	Merck	Compatible	10%	5%
Lidocaine HCl	Astra (Xylocaine HCl)	Compatible	10%	2%
Tetracaine HCl	Winthrop (Pontocaine HCl)	Compatible	10%	1%
ANTIBACTERIALS				
Neomycin Sulfate	Upjohn (Mycifradin Sulfate)	Compatible	10%	100 mg/ml
Streptomycin Sulfate	Merck	Compatible	10%	200 mg/ml
Penicillin G Potassium (mix and use at once)	Lilly	Compatible	10%	100,000 U/ml
Bacitracin (mix and use at once)	Upjohn	Compatible	10%	5,000 U/ml
Polymyxin B Sulfate	Burroughs Wellcome (Aerosporin)	Compatible	10%	50,000 U/ml
Methicillin Sodium	Bristol (Staphcillin)	Compatible	10%	500 mg/ml
Novobiocin Sodium	Upjohn (Albamycin)	Compatible	10%	25 mg/ml
Dihydrostreptomycin Sulfate	Upjohn	Compatible	10%	50 mg/ml
Kanamycin Sulfate	Bristol (Kantrex)	Compatible	17%	85 mg/ml
Chloramphenicol Sodium Succinate	Parke, Davis (Chloromycetin)	Compatible	20%	20 mg/ml
Oleandomycin Phosphate (mix and use at once)	Roerig	Compatible	10%	25 mg/ml
Lincomycin HCl	Upjohn (Lincocin)	Compatible	10%	150 mg/ml
Chlortetracycline HCl	Lederle (Aureomycin)	Incompatible	10%	12.5 mg/ml
Sodium ampicillin	Bristol (Polycillin-N)	Incompatible	10%	50 mg/ml
Amphotericin B	Squibb (Fungizone Intravenous)	Incompatible	4-15%	1.0-4.0 mg/ml
Erythromycin Lactobionate	Abbott (Erythrocin)	Incompatible	10%	15 mg/ml
Oxytetracycline HCl	Pfizer (Terramycin HCl)	Incompatible	10%	12.5 mg/ml
Tetracycline HCl	Lederle (Achromycin)	Incompatible	10%	12.5 mg/ml
BRONCHODILATORS				
Isoproterenol HCl	—	Compatible	3.0%	0.5%
Isoproterenol HCl	—	Compatible	10%	0.06%
Isoproterenol HCl	—	Compatible	20%	0.06%
Isoproterenol HCl	Winthrop (Isuprel 1%)	Compatible	13.3% (2 parts)	33% (1 part)
Epinephrine HCl	Parke, Davis (Adrenalin HCl 1:100)	Compatible	13.3% (2 parts)	33% (1 part)
Bronkospray	Breon	Compatible	13.3% (2 parts)	(1 part)
Aerolone Compound	Lilly	Compatible	13.3% (2 parts)	(1 part)
CONTRAST MEDIA				
Propyliodone Suspension	Glaxo (Dionosil)	Compatible	10%	28% (W/V)
Iodized Oil USP	Fougera (Lipiodol)	Incompatible	20%/20 ml	40%/10 ml
DECONGESTANTS				
Phenylephrine HCl	—	Compatible	3.0%	25%
Phenylephrine HCl	Winthrop (Neo-Synephrine)	Compatible	13.3% (2 parts)	10% (1 part)
DETERGENTS				
Alevaire	Breon	Compatible	13.3% (2 parts)	(1 part)
Tergemist	Abbott	Compatible	13.3% (2 parts)	(1 part)
ENZYMES				
Pancreatic Dornase (mix and use at once)	Merck (Dornavac)	Compatible	16.7%	8,000 U/ml
Chymotrypsin	Armour	Incompatible	5%	400 γ/ml
Trypsin	Armour	Incompatible	5%	400 γ/ml
SOLVENTS				
Propylene Glycol		Compatible	3%	10%
Alcohol		Compatible	12%	10-20%
STEROIDS				
Prednisolone 21-Phosphate	Merck (Hydeltrasol)	Compatible	16.7%	3.3 mg/ml
Dexamethasone 21-Phosphate	Merck (Decadron Phosphate)	Compatible	16%	0.8 mg/ml
OTHER AGENTS				
Hydrogen Peroxide		Incompatible	(All ratios)	

P-23

Date of Printing June 1970

*The rating **COMPATIBLE** means that there was no visible physical change in the admixture and that there was no predicted chemical incompatibility. All of the mixtures have been tested for short term chemical compatibility by assaying for the concentration of acetylcysteine after mixing.

The rating **INCOMPATIBLE** is based on the formation of a precipitate, a change in color, clarity or odor or other physical chemical alteration.

**Entries are final concentrations. Values in parentheses relate volumes of like-control solutions to volumes of test solutions.

III. Steroid Preparations

A. Dexamethasone sodium phosphate

1. *Action*—is an effective, versatile adrenocortical hormone preparation with potent antiinflammatory and antifibrogenic effects.

2. *Indications*—relative to respiratory therapy
   a. Acute bronchial asthma
   b. Status asthmaticus
   c. Laryngeal edema
   d. Acute, life-threatening infections
   e. Croup

3. *Contraindications*
   a. Tuberculosis, whether active or healed, is usually an absolute contraindication to steroid therapy; however, employment of dexamethasone may be a lifesaving measure to control the acute toxicity associated with overwhelming tuberculosis infection; it must be accompanied by appropriate specific antituberculosis therapy.
   b. Ocular herpes simplex and acute psychoses also are usually absolute contraindications to steroid therapy.
   c. Relative contraindications include diverticulitis, fresh intestinal anastomoses, active or latent peptic ulcer, renal insufficiency, hypertension, thromboembolic tendencies, osteoporosis, acute or chronic infections including fungus and viral diseases, especially chickenpox and vaccinia, myasthenia gravis, and pregnancy, particularly during the first trimester.

4. *Precautions*—corticosteroids may mask signs of infections and enhance the dissemination of the infecting organism.

5. *Adverse reactions*—are somewhat less pronounced when administered by inhalation than when the drug is administered by other routes; may result in Cushing's syndrome with diabetes, osteoporosis, moon facies, lowering of body's resistance, increase of gastric acidity, and elevation of blood pressure.

6. *Dosage*—2 to 4 mg by inhalation.

B. Beclomethasone dipropionate

1. *Action*—an antiinflammatory steroid.

2. *Indications*—only for patients who require chronic treatment with corticosteroids for control of symptoms of bronchial asthma.

3. *Contraindications*
   a. If bronchodilators and other nonsteroid preparations will control disease process.
   b. Patients who require systemic corticosteroids for treatment.
   c. Nonasthmatic bronchitis.
   d. Hypersensitivity to the drug.
   e. If the primary treatment of status asthmaticus or other acute episodes requires intensive measures.
4. *Precautions*
   a. This drug is *not* a bronchodilator.
   b. Withdrawal from systemic steroids may cause adrenal insufficiency.
5. *Adverse reactions*
   a. Localized infections of the mouth, pharynx, and occasionally the larynx by *Candida albicans* or *Aspergillus niger* may occur, requiring treatment.
   b. Death due to adrenal insufficiency during and after transfer from systemic corticosteroids has been reported.
6. *Dosage*—provided as metered inhaler; usual dosage is 2 inhalations (100 mcg) 3 to 4 times daily, not to exceed 20 inhalations. If a bronchodilator is to be used, it should be administered prior to use of the inhalator.

IV. Miscellaneous Medications
   A. Cromolyn sodium
      1. *Action*—inhibits degranulation of sensitized mast cells, which occurs after exposure to specific antigens. Bronchial asthma induced by inhalation of specific antigens can be inhibited to varying degrees by pretreatment with the drug. Has no intrinsic bronchodilator, antihistamic, or antiinflammatory activity. Is meant for prophylactic action, not for acute asthma.
      2. *Contraindications*—sensitivity to the drug.
      3. *Warnings*—renal or hepatic insufficiency may result.
      4. *Adverse reactions*—maculopapular rash and urticaria; cough and/or bronchospasm.
      5. *Dosage*—provided as a powder in a capsule; the capsule is placed in a Spinhaler, which punctures it; when the patient inhales, he inhales the powder, which he later swallows. Usual dosage for adults and children over 5 years is 1 capsule (20 mg), 4 times daily.

B. *Antibiotics*—several antibiotic preparations are available that may be used for inhalation. Their actions may be either bacteriostatic or bactericidal. However, because of the possibility of sensitizing the patient to such drugs, and the large incidence of adverse reactions, some physicians are hesitant to use them. It would be advisable to consult your hospital pharmacy before administering any such preparations.

Unit Doses of Medications

Many pharmaceutical manufacturers are now packaging 3–5-ml sterile solutions of normal saline and water. These may be used for one treatment and then discarded. Other manufacturers are also packaging bronchodilators in appropriate doses in this manner. See Figure 4-4.

The advantages of using such solutions are that no syringes are required for measurement (each vial is calibrated in milliliters) and also that contamination of the medication is avoided.

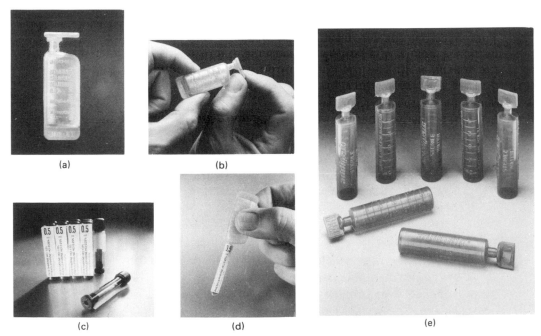

(a)   (b)

(c)   (d)   (e)

Figure 4-4.   (a–d) Warner-Chilcott Dispo-sa-med and Dispos-a-vial System. (*Courtesy of Warner-Chilcott Labs, Morris Plains, N.J.*) (e) Other Disposable Vials. (*Courtesy of Respiratory Care, Inc., Arlington Heights, Ill.*)

PATIENT ORIENTATION TO AN IPPB TREATMENT

Hello—I am _____ from the Respiratory Therapy Department, here to give you a breathing treatment ordered by your doctor to help you breathe better and easier. These breathing treatments, using specific medication, are also designed to help you bring up sputum or phlegm from your throat and lungs.

These treatments also help patients who are short of breath. In addition, these treatments aid in preventing pneumonia and aid in obtaining samples of sputum for your doctor to study and analyze.

It's easy: Taking an IPPB (intermittent positive pressure breathing treatment) is relatively simple. The machine used in giving you this treatment is plugged into a wall outlet of oxygen or air. This gas aids in transporting the medication used to your lungs.

To start: You should be sitting up as straight as possible when taking this treatment. The therapist will turn on the machine for you. Take the mouthpiece and put it in your mouth, being sure to close your lips around it as tight as you can. All we want you to do is to breathe slowly and deeply. When you exhale, blow out as slowly and as far as you can.

This treatment does not hurt: When you inhale or breathe in, there will be a slight pressure in your mouth as the compressed gas and medication enter; however, be sure to keep your lips closed tightly.

How long does the treatment last: Medication that your doctor has ordered is in the nebulizer; as the compressed gas enters the nebulizer, it breaks up the medicine into a fine mist, which you breathe. The treatment lasts until you have used up all the medicine. This usually takes 10 to 20 minutes.

Important: If at any time during your treatment, you should feel sick to your stomach, dizzy, or have any chest pain, please tell the therapist immediately. He will let you rest or he will stop the treatment.

We want to help you to recover and feel better: So please listen to your therapist's instruction and follow his instructions.

Thank you.
The Respiratory Therapy Department

Any questions? We have tried to tell you some things about your IPPB treatment on this sheet. If you have any other questions, the therapist will gladly answer them.

Be seein' you!

PROCEDURE FOR ASSEMBLY AND OPERATION OF THE BENNETT PRESSURE BREATHING THERAPY UNIT: IPPB THERAPY FOR ADULTS

Model TV-2P

I. Assembly

    A. Attach the unit to the compressed gas cylinder after the cylinder valve has been "cracked" to blow out any possible dust particles; support the unit with one hand and with the other hand start the nut on the threads of the cylinder valve; continue to support the unit vertically and proceed to tighten the nut on the valve with a wrench.

    B. Screw the support arm into the threaded hole on the unit head; tighten or loosen the adjusting knobs to the desired positions; do not force any section of the arm into place without first adjusting the wing nuts.

    C. Attach the manifold (with exhalation valve) to the end of the support arm and tighten the manifold ball into the socket using the wing nut; make certain the exhalation port is facing the patient.

    D. Attach one end of the large main air tube to the port under the Bennett valve.

    E. Attach the remaining end of the main air tube to the bottom port of the manifold if a horizontal nebulizer is being used; when using a vertical nebulizer, the main air hose is connected to the port on the back of the manifold.

    F. Connect the smaller-diameter tubing to the exhalation port on the manifold and the other end to the small connector below the Bennett valve (to the left as you are facing the machine).

    G. Connect the large-diameter tubing to the nebulizer tailpiece and the remaining end to the nebulizer control at the top of the unit head.

    H. Attach the flex tube and mouthpiece and/or mask to the end of the manifold nearest the exhalation valve.

II. Operation

    A. Using both hands, open the cylinder valve all the way; it is best to stand behind the unit when doing this as a safety measure.

    B. Move the shutoff lever on the unit head downward; this lever must be in a vertical position to activate the unit. When

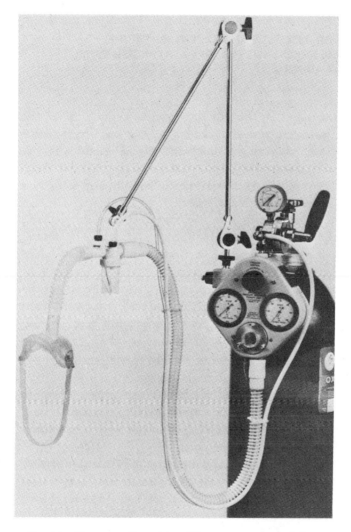

Figure 4-5. Bennett Pressure Breathing Therapy Unit Model TV-2P. (*Courtesy of Puritan-Bennett Corp., Kansas City, Mo.*)

the handle is all the way up, it is in an *off* position; when all the way down, it is in the *on* position.

C. Turn the pressure control clockwise until the gauge registers the pressure prescribed by the physician (usually 10 to 20 cm of water pressure).

D. Set the dilution control prescribed by the physician to either the 100% oxygen setting or the air–oxygen setting (usually for the chronic chest patient, the air–oxygen mixture will be used).

E. Place the medication order by the physician in the nebulizer; always be certain there is medication, distilled water, or physiological saline in the nebulizer to provide humidity to the patient—never administer dry gas to the patient.

F. Open the nebulizer control outlet until a slight mist or fog is produced.

> Note: Do not set the fog or mist by the visual activity observed in the nebulizer. This may result in excess flow from the needle valve, which will cause either a waste of medication or popping off the nebulizer tubing from the nebulizer.

G. See previous discussion for administration of this treatment.

III. Conclusion of therapy

A. Remove the face mask or mouthpiece during the exhalation phase: if they are removed during the inhalation phase, gas under pressure will continue to flow through the unit. If this should occur accidentally, you may pinch off the flex tube tightly to stop the flow.

B. Shut off the nebulizer control (needle valve).

C. Move the shutoff lever to the off position.

D. Turn the pressure control until the pressure gauge registers zero.

E. Using both hands, close the cylinder valve.

> Note: To reduce the pressure in the high-pressure regulator, move the shutoff lever to the on position. Open the nebulizer control slowly and watch the needle on the high-pressure regulator gauge return to zero. Return the shutoff lever to the off position. Close the nebulizer needle valve. This removes all pressure in the unit and will prolong the life of this device.

IV. Clean all the accessories according to established procedures.

V. Emergency use as a manual resuscitator

A. Follow the preceding instructions using a Bennett mask and/or Bennett seal with nose clips. In addition:

1. Remove the dust cover from the Bennett valve.

2. Move the drum pin gently up and down with the tip of the fingers (moving the pin upward causes the inspira-

tory phase, the downward movement initiates the expiratory phase).

3. Establish a steady rhythm, allowing a longer period for exhalation than for inspiration.

4. Do not cycle too rapidly; keep time with your own rate of breathing.

5. Do not push the drum pin hard against the rubber stops, as excessive pressure could cause a change in the mechanics of the entire Bennett valve.

Model PV-3P

Model PV-3P (Figure 4-6) is a pedestal-mounted unit designed for use with piped oxygen or air from wall outlets, from a cylinder using a high-pressure regulator, or from a Bennett MC-1 compressor. This procedure is related to use of the PV-3P with piped oxygen or air.

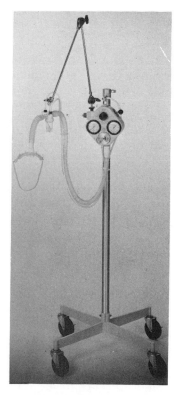

Figure 4-6. Bennett Pressure Breathing Therapy Unit Model PV-3P. (*Courtesy of Puritan-Bennett Corp., Kansas City, Mo.*)

Assembly

1. Set the pedestal base on the floor. Insert the column into the collar of the base and tighten the clamping bolt to a snug fit.
2. Mount the unit in the pedestal column by inserting the filter housing.
3. Attach the high-pressure hose to the filter housing of the unit.
4. Connect the other end to the wall outlet of the piping system.

Treatment Procedure

1. Turn the pressure control knob clockwise until the control pressure gauge indicates the pressure prescribed by the physician (usually 10 to 20 cm of H_2O).
2. Set the dilution control as prescribed by the physician (the air–oxygen setting is usually used, approximately 40% O_2).
    a. *Air–oxygen*—push dilution control *all the way in* to the stop position.
    b. *100% oxygen*—pull dilution control *all the way out* to the stop position.
3. Unscrew the nebulizer vial and place the medication ordered by the physician into same. If no medication is ordered by the physician, place sterile distilled water in the nebulizer vial to add humidity. Never administer a dry gas to a patient.
4. Open the nebulizer control until a very light fog is produced.

Patient Position

1. Sit directly in front of and facing the unit in a straight-backed chair.
2. Have patient place both feet firmly on the floor and sit upright, keeping the back straight. This position will improve ventilation and use of the diaphragm.
3. Position the support arm so that the manifold points directly at the nose, approximately 4 to 5 in. away.
    a. *Tube mouthpiece*—instruct the patient to bite gently on the mouthpiece and seal the tube with his lips. Instruct the patient to breathe in through his mouth only (nose clips may be used to occlude the nose until the patient is more familiar with mouth breathing).
    b. *Bennett seal mouthpiece*—place it in the mouth with the flange between the teeth and bite down lightly. Bring the strap around the neck and clip it to the plastic. The strap

should be adjusted for a comfortable fit and to prevent leakage.

c. *Mask fitting*—fit the mask over the bridge of the nose, high on the nose and close to the eyes, with the lower position of the mask away from the chin. Rotate the mask downward over the nose and mouth, sliding the mask downward until it conforms to the contour of the nose bridge. Then press it firmly against the cheeks. While holding the mask in position, center the mask harness on the back of the head, and attach the top strap to the upper fasteners on the plastic facepiece. Do not make this upper strap too tight. Attach the lower strap to the lower fastener on the plastic facepiece. Make this strap somewhat tighter than the upper strap. If the mask leaks around the nose, tighten the lower straps to pull the mask farther down the face.

Treatment Procedure

1. Instruct the patient to breathe slowly and deeply during treatment. Instruct him to relax and let the machine do the work. He must allow his lungs to fill completely; when his lungs are full, relax, and exhale completely. If the patient experiences difficulty in starting inhalation or exhalation, check the mouthpiece and/or mask for leaks. If there are no leaks in the system, the patient should experience no difficulty on inspiration or expiration.

2. Instruct the patient to watch the mask pressure gauge as he breathes in, and instruct him to try to keep the needle of this gauge at pressure longer by continuing to inflate the lungs slowly. This type of practice will provide more effective ventilation of the lungs, and also the greatest treatment value.

3. Instruct the patient that the treatment will last 15 to 20 min, or until the medication vial is depleted.

Safety Precaution. Always instruct the patient *not to smoke* near the PV-3P when it is turned on or in use. In the hospital setting, a *No Smoking* sign must be placed on the door to alert the patient's visitors and other hospital personnel that oxygen is in use.

Cleaning and Sterilizing

1. Wash the mouthpiece and/or mask and flex tube in warm detergent solution. Rinse thoroughly with clear warm water.

2. Disassemble the nebulizer manifold. Unscrew the nebulizer vial. Unscrew the nut, and remove the jet. Remove the suction tube from the jet. Unscrew the expiration manifold cap. Then loosen the nut and remove the expiration diaphragm. Wash all parts in warm detergent solution and rinse well in clear warm water. *Before washing, place a cap over the expiration diaphragm connector to keep water from entering the diaphragm.*

3. Replace the blue tube on the jet suction connector. Slip the nebulizer tube over the jet, turn on the nebulizer control, and blow gas through. If there is evidence of obstruction, clean with the metal cleaner.

4. All parts may then be cold sterilized with a solution such as 2% Cidex. Follow carefully any manufacturer's recommended time for immersion of the accessories in the solution. Rinse all parts thoroughly, flushing tubes carefully, drain, and let accessories dry well.

5. All accessories in the patient system may be gas sterilized. All parts must be aired for at least 7 days to dissipate residual ethylene oxide, or accessories must be placed in an aerator for the manufacturer's recommended time period.

Routine Maintenance. Periodically the air–oxygen diluter at the side of the unit must be removed and cleaned (refer to *Bennett Operating Instruction Model PV-3P*).

The Model PV-3P has a metal filter in the round housing at the back of the unit to trap particles sometimes found in air–oxygen piping systems. Remove the screws and cap on top of the housing. Then remove the O-ring and filter disc. Clean the disc in warm detergent solution, rinse, dry, and reassemble in order.

The Bennett valve should be cleaned occasionally or when the need is evidenced by sticky action (refer to Bennett operating instructions for the Model PV-3P).

Model AP-4 (Figure 4-7)

I. Assembly

Note: The Bennett Model AP-4 self-stores all parts necessary for use. Open both the front and rear doors of the unit. Allow them to turn back against the handle on the top of the unit. The main air tubing stores in the front compartment. (Place inside carefully so as not to disturb the Bennett valve.) The electrical cord, manifold, flex tube,

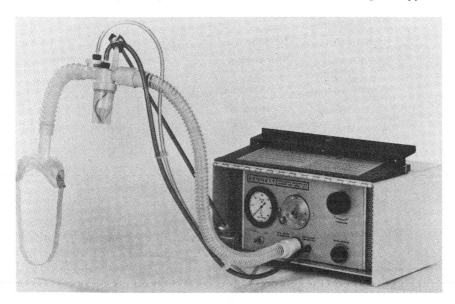

Figure 4-7. Bennett Pressure Breathing Therapy Unit Model AP-4. (*Courtesy of Puritan-Bennett Corp., Kansas City, Mo.*)

mouthpiece, nose clip, nebulizer, support arm, and the small tubing assembly store in the rear compartment. Remove and assemble as follows:

A. Connect the main air tubing to the large outlet directly beneath the Bennett valve.

B. Connect the smaller tubing assembly as follows:

    1. Place the blue tubing (the larger-diameter tubing) into the nebulizer outlet on the front of the unit (to the right of the main air tubing).

    2. Place the clear tubing (the smaller-diameter tubing) into the outlet on the front of the unit (to the left of the main air tubing).

    3. Attach the support arm to its holder in the extreme left-hand corner of the front of the unit.

    4. Attach the manifold securely to the ball socket at the end of the support arm.

    5. Attach the remaining end of the main air tube to the bottom port of the manifold if a horizontal nebulizer is being used; when using a vertical nebulizer, the main air tube is connected to the port on the back of the manifold.

6. Connect the clear smaller-diameter tubing to the exhalation port on the manifold.

7. Connect the blue larger-diameter tubing to the nebulizer tailpiece.

8. Connect the flex tube with mask, Bennett seal, or mouthpiece to the opening of the manifold facing the patient (make certain that the flex tube with patient attachment is connected to the end of the manifold nearest the exhalation valve).

Note: Make certain all connections fit securely.

9. Remove the electrical cord from the rear compartment of the unit and connect to a wall outlet; Model AP-4 may be used *only* with 110- to 120-V, 50- or 60-cycle; as a safety measure, the electrical circuit must be grounded.

Note: The Model AP-4 therapy unit compresses and delivers room air to the patient. However, it does provide means of administering oxygen enrichment of the room air if the physician prescribes same (see Part III of this outline). The unit may be placed on a table or desk; however, select a surface that will allow the manifold to be at the mouth level of the seated patient.

II. Treatment Procedure
A. Follow the physician's orders carefully regarding the following:
1. Amount of specific medication to be used
2. Amount of pressure ordered
3. Oxygen enrichment if ordered
4. Duration and frequency of the treatment
B. Remove the nebulizer from the manifold and place the medication ordered into the vial.
C. Turn on power.
D. Open the nebulizer control until a slight mist is produced.
E. Position your patient and adjust the support arm so that the manifold is at the mouth level of the patient.
F. Turn the pressure control to a low setting, attach the nose clips on the patient's nose, place the mouthpiece in the patient's mouth, and have him begin to inhale; on inspiration, turn the control pressure gauge until the control pressure

gauge reaches the prescribed pressure ordered by the physician.

G. Breathe in slowly and deeply during the treatment, then relax and exhale as much as possible.

H. At the completion of the treatment, remove the mouthpiece.

I. Turn off the power switch.

J. Clean all the accessory parts according to established procedure.

III. Oxygen Enrichment

A. Oxygen is added to power the nebulizer.

B. The nebulizer tubing (blue) is connected to an oxygen supply source instead of to the unit; this supply source may be an oxygen cylinder with a regulator and liter flow-measuring mechanism or piped-in oxygen administered from a flowmeter. The following demonstrates the *approximate* oxygen concentrations for various values of oxygen flow rates for adults: to obtain 25% to 35% of oxygen, set the oxygen flow rate on 5 liters/min; 7 liters/min will give approximately 30% to 40% oxygen; and 9 liters/min will give about 35% to 45% oxygen.

Note: In children who have lower air flow rates, the oxygen percentage will be increased. Consult the physician for liter flow for the child.

C. Procedure

1. Turn the nebulizer control to the *off* position.

2. Remove the nebulizer tubing (blue) from the nebulizer outlet and connect this tubing to the oxygen regulator or flowmeter outlet.

3. Turn on power.

4. Open the cylinder valve slowly.

5. Turn the regulator control knob until the prescribed liter flow registers on the liter flow gauge or, if using a flowmeter, turn this control on until the prescribed liter flow registers in the tube of the flowmeter.

6. Proceed with treatment.

7. At completion of treatment, clean all the accessory parts according to established procedure.

8. Store equipment as described in the note in part I of this outline.

IV. Emergency Use

Note: This Bennett unit can be used to give artificial respiration similarly to the Bennett TV-2P. It is primarily a therapy unit for patient-controlled breathing; however, it can be used effectively in an emergency as a manually activated resuscitator.

A. Procedure

1. Turn on the power.
2. The nebulizer must be in the manifold; however, the nebulizer need not be turned on.
3. Remove the dust cover from the Bennett valve.
4. Position the mask (or mouthpiece and nose clip) firmly and tightly and support with your hand to prevent leakage; position the patient's chin upward and the head extended slightly backward.
5. Move the drum pin on the Bennett valve up and turn the pressure control knob until the gauge registers about 15 to 20 cm of water pressure; do not use more pressure than necessary to maintain breathing.
6. Move the drum pin gently up and down, keeping time with your own rate of breathing; do not cycle too rapidly; establish a steady rhythm; allow a longer period of time for expiration than for inspiration.
7. Sterilize all accessory parts after this procedure and store all parts in their proper compartments.

Model TA-1

The Bennett Model TA-1 unit (Figure 4-8) operates by compressing room air and is used for the administration of intermittent positive pressure breathing treatments (IPPB). It is also equipped to provide additional oxygen if required. This unit must be prescribed by a physician and used under his direction.

I. Assembly

A. Place the Bennett Model TA-1 unit on a desk or table that will be convenient for patient use.
B. Connect one end of the white supply tube to the unit outlet.
C. Connect the other end of the white supply tube to the jet on the handpiece.

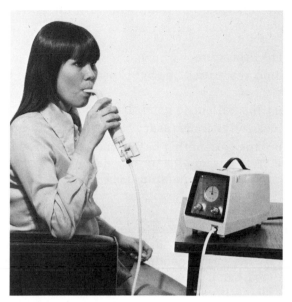

Figure 4-8. Bennett TA-1. (*Courtesy of Bennett Respiration Products, Santa Monica, Calif.*)

    D. Remove the medication vial from the handpiece, carefully insert the prescribed amount of medication, and replace. Be certain that the suction tube in the medication vial reaches the bottom of the vial.

II. Patient Instruction to Begin Treatment
    A. Turn the power knob to the *on* position.
    B. Turn the pressure control knob until the gauge indicates the pressure prescribed by the physician.
    C. Hold the handpiece and bite the mouthpiece gently, sealing the mouthpiece with the lips.
    D. Press thumb or finger on the button on the handpiece. This will seal the exhalation port and direct the flow through the mouthpiece.
    E. Breathe in slowly, allowing the machine to do the work. Allow the lungs to fill completely. At this time the pressure gauge will register the prescribed pressure.
    F. At the end of inspiration, remove the thumb or finger from the button, this opens the exhalation port. Relax and breathe out completely.

G. At the conclusion of treatment, turn the power knob to the *off* position.

III. Treatment Procedure
   A. Position the patient upright, preferably in a straight-back chair.
   B. Orient the patient to good therapy.
   C. Use nose clips if necessary to ensure mouth breathing only.
   D. Assure the patient that he does not have to remove the handpiece from his mouth on exhalation. His expired air will escape from the exhalation port.

IV. Sterilization
   A. Home care sterilization—after each treatment, discard any medication that was not used from the vial and rinse. Preferably, the entire handpiece should be disassembled after each treatment. Wash all parts in a warm detergent solution. Use a brush to be certain that all small holes in the body are clear. Use the jet cleaner if necessary and rinse all parts thoroughly. Dry all parts thoroughly. Approximately twice weekly, the entire handpiece and tubing should be disassembled and soaked in a disinfectant solution for about 15 min. Rinse all parts in clear water and dry well. (Two tablespoons of white vinegar to one quart of water is effective as a disinfecting solution.)
   B. Hospital use sterilization—after each patient treatment, the tubing and handpiece should be disassembled. Wash in a warm detergent solution using a brush and jet cleaners. Rinse well and then cold sterilize (Cidex) or gas sterilize.

   Note: Allow sufficient aeration time for all parts.

V. Oxygen Enrichment
   If the physician prescribes oxygen enrichment of the room air, it may be entrained at the handpiece elbow inlet or, if the Cascade Junior Humidifier is used, at the humidifier inlet.

   Note: The percentage of oxygen in the mixture delivered to the patient will depend on the oxygen flow rate and the average flow rate of the air. The following demonstrates the *approximate* oxygen concentration for the various values of oxygen flow rate.

5 liters/min = 25–35%

$$7 \text{ liters/min} = 28\text{–}38\%$$

$$9 \text{ liters/min} = 30\text{–}40\%$$

A. Follow these steps if adding oxygen at the handpiece elbow unit:

1. Place a No Smoking sign in use.
2. Instruct the patient, his visitors, and his family that no smoking will be permitted when oxygen is turned on. The oxygen cylinders must be well supported in a case on a base or in a cart or strapped or chained to a firm support. Oxygen should not be used near an open flame or heater. Inspect the cylinder carefully, i.e., for correct gas, and "crack" the cylinder valve to blow out any airborne contaminants.
3. Connect a supply tube to the elbow of the handpiece.
4. Connect the other end of the supply tube to the oxygen regulator or flowmeter outlet.
5. Open the cylinder valve.
6. Turn the regulator control until the desired flow registers on the liter flow gauge, or turn the flowmeter control until the desired flow registers on the flowmeter.

B. When adding oxygen via the Cascade Junior Humidifier, follow these steps:

1. Connect the supply tubing to a black tee adapter placed on the cascade cover.
2. Attach the other end to an oxygen regulator or flowmeter outlet. Follow above procedure.

   Note: The extra supply tubing and the black tee adapter are not supplied with the Bennett Therapy Unit Model TA-1.

BIRD MARK 1 VENTILATOR

The Bird Mark 1 (Figure 4-9) is an intermittent positive pressure device that is designed for treating patients with a variety of respiratory diseases. It is classified as a flow-variable, pressure-limited assistor.

The Bird Mark 1 will cycle on when the patient makes an inspiratory effort. The inspiratory effort that triggers the machine on may be adjusted by means of a sensitivity control. The machine also employs a flow rate control to adjust the speed at which the flow

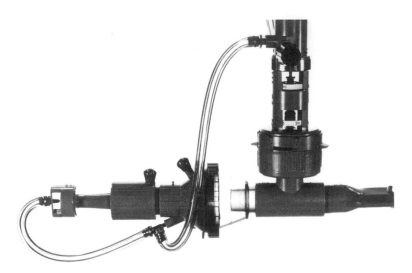

Figure 4-9.   Bird Mark 1 Ventilator. (*Courtesy of Bird Corp., Palm Springs, Calif.*)

of gas enters the patient's lungs. Next, the pressure control adjusts the volume of gas the patient is to receive. Remember that the higher the pressure, the greater the volume; the lower the pressure, the less will be the volume. This, of course, depends on the compliance of the patient's lung. Generally, pressures of 10 to 20 cm of water pressure are used for IPPB therapy.

Medication is administered by means of the Bird Micro-Nebulizer, which nebulizes on inspiration only. The Bird Mark 1 is powered by a small air compressor or regulation device attached to a cylinder.

Set up Assembly and Operation for the Bird Mark 1

1. Attach the inlet power line to the nipple on the outside of the air compressor
2. Plug the compressor cord into a 115-V ac outlet.
3. Set sensitivity calibration wheel until 10 appears in the window.
4. Set pressure calibration wheel until 10 appears in the window.
5. Place proper medication into Micro-Nebulizer.

6. Turn flow rate control to the *off* position; then turn one full turn.
7. Turn compressor on.
8. Place mouthpiece between lips and blow out slowly; inspiration will start the machine automatically.
9. Readjust sensitivity calibration wheel if too much inspiratory effort is needed to start machine.
10. Readjust pressure calibration wheel for proper volume.
11. Readjust flow rate control for proper inspiratory rate and depth.

Disassembly of the Bird Mark 1.   Refer to Figure 4-10.

1. Disconnect (1) from (2).
2. Remove (2) from (6).
3. Disconnect (9) from (8).
4. Remove (10) and separate the two units.
5. Remove (8) and disassemble.
6. Remove (7) from (6).
7. Remove (11) from (2).
8. Disassemble servo units.
    a. Remove bell housing.
    b. Pull out post nut and expose diaphragm.

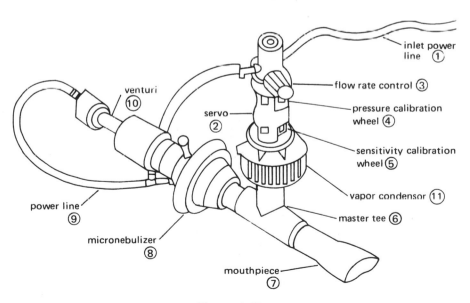

Figure 4-10.

After each treatment the unused medication should be discarded, and the nebulizer should be rinsed in warm water. Sterilization should be done by means of gas or chemical agents.

OHIO hand-E-vent II BREATHING UNIT

The Ohio hand-E-vent II (Figure 4-11) is an intermittent positive pressure breathing device that is designed for treating patients with various respiratory diseases. This convenient, easily hand-held unit can deliver medication prescribed by the physician by means of an aerosol nebulizer that is a part of the unit. It is powered by a simple compressor pump that has an adjustable needle valve and gauge. The compressor allows adjustment from 0 to 25 cm of water pressure at the mouthpiece. However, pressures of more than 20 cm of water pressure are rarely necessary.

    I. Assembly

        A. Connect the in-line filter to nipple on the front of the compressor. (This filters the air as it comes from the compressor;

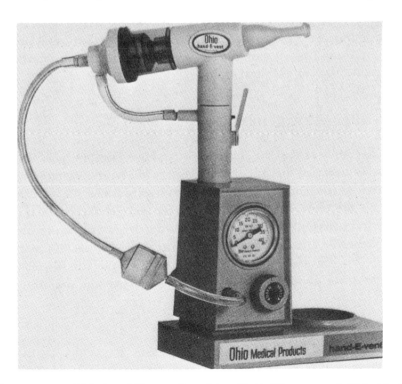

Figure 4-11. Ohio hand-E-vent Breathing Unit. (*Courtesy of Ohio Medical Products, a division of Airco, Inc., Madison, Wisc.*)

this in-line filter should be checked frequently and replaced when it becomes dirty.)

B. Attach the supply tubing to the in-line filter.

C. Attach the remaining end of the supply tubing to the tailpiece on the back of the nebulizer.

D. Attach the small piece of tubing from the tailpiece under the nebulizer.

E. Connect the remaining end to the tailpiece on the handle of the unit (see Figure 4-11 for details).

F. Remove the nebulizer from the nebulizer housing and carefully insert the prescribed amount of medication, then replace.

G. Insert electrical plug into a suitable wall outlet.

H. Turn on *on–off* switch.

I. Open needle valve (lower right front of unit) approximately one-half to one full turn counterclockwise.

J. Close thumb valve on the handle of the unit.

K. Adjust needle valve slowly until the pressure ordered is indicated on the pressure gauge.

> Note: It is necessary that the thumb valve be depressed while adjusting the needle valve.

II. Treatment Procedure

A. Position the patient and remove entire handle from unit; use nose clips if necessary.

B. Orient the patient to the therapy as follows:

1. Instruct the patient to insert the mouthpiece in his mouth and seal his lips tightly about same.

2. Teach him to depress the thumb valve on the handle when he inhales; he will release the thumb valve when exhaling.

> Note: It is not necessary for the patient to remove the mouthpiece on exhalation; his expired air will escape from the bottom of the handle.

3. Instruct him to breathe in slowly and deeply; exhalation should be longer so as to empty his lungs as much as possible.

> Note: If the patient is receiving oxygen via nasal cannula therapy, this therapy does not have to be discontinued while he is receiving an IPPB treatment with the hand-E-vent.

III. Sterilization
    A. Home care sterilization—after each treatment, if there is unused medication in the nebulizer, discard and rinse the entire nebulizer and mouthpiece in warm water. Approximately twice a week, the nebulizer, mouthpiece, handle, and tubing should be soaked in a disinfectant solution for about 15 min. Rinse all parts in clear water and dry well. (Two tablespoons of white vinegar to one quart of water is effective as a disinfecting solution.)
    B. Hospital use sterilization—after each patient treatment, the nebulizer, mouthpiece, tubing, and handle should be completely disassembled; all parts may be cold sterilized (Cidex) or gas sterilized.

    Note: Remember to allow sufficient aeration time for all parts.

EXERCISES

1. List the criteria that you would use to define an effective IPPB treatment.
2. What factors should be considered by the physician when ordering IPPB therapy?
3. Why is it important that IPPB should be administered by a qualified individual?
4. Compare the use of IPPB, CO_2 rebreathing devices, and incentive spirometers.
5. Design a chart for the medications used in your department for IPPB showing:
    a. Classification
    b. Generic name
    c. Brand name
    d. Strength
    e. Action
    f. Dosage
    g. Side effects

UNIT 5

ARTIFICIAL MECHANICAL VENTILATION

This unit presents the basic classifications of lung ventilators, details the procedures for the various types of ventilators on the market today, and outlines the technique for weaning a patient from the ventilator.

The following procedures are designed as a guide for the therapist in setting up the ventilators discussed. It is impossible to include all information contained in each manufacturer's instruction manual; therefore, it is essential that the therapist study each manual thoroughly before using the ventilator.

CLASSIFICATION OF LUNG VENTILATORS

Classification

Lung Ventilator: A device that is connected to the patient's airway and is designed to augment or replace the patient's ventilation automatically. A lung ventilator is employed with a mask or endotracheal or tracheostomy tube. The performance of a lung ventilator is identified as follows:

I. Types of Lung Ventilators
   Controller—A ventilator that controls. A lung ventilator that operates independently of the patient's inspiratory effort.
   Assistor—A lung ventilator that assists. A lung ventilator that augments inspiration of the spontaneously breathing patient

243

by operating in response to the patient's inspiratory effort.
Assist–Controller—A lung ventilator that may assist and/or control. A lung ventilator that combines both controller and assistor functions.

II. Modes of Action
Certain lung ventilators can be adjusted to give more than one of the alternate modes of action.

III. Ventilator Characteristics
   A. Pressure Preset
   B. Volume Preset
      1. Tidal volume
      2. Minute volume

IV. Cycling Control
   A. Inspiratory to expiratory
      1. Volume
      2. Pressure
      3. Time
      4. Combined
      5. Other
   B. Expiratory to inspiratory
      1. Pressure
      2. Time
      3. Combined
      4. Patient
      5. Manual override
      6. Other

V. Types of Safety Limit
   A. Volume limit
   B. Pressure limit
   C. Time limit
   D. Other

VI. Types of Pressure Pattern
   A. Positive-atmospheric
   B. Positive-negative
   C. Positive-positive

VII. Source of Power
    A. Pneumatically powered
    B. Electrically powered
    C. Other

Note: A given ventilator may be difficult to characterize as volume preset or pressure preset just by considering its construction or assumed function. Its functional characteristics are often modified as a result of pressure, volume, flow, or cycle duration.

Evaluation of the performance characteristics of different ventilators should be made using standard lung models. A full range of impedance and leaks that can occur in clinical usage should be imposed as test conditions, and the ability of ventilators to compensate should be used to characterize the ventilators as volume or pressure preset.

Detailed discussions on classification of various types of ventilators may be found in W. W. Mushin, L. Randall Baker, P. W. Thompson, and W. W. Mapleson, *Automatic Ventilation of the Lungs*, F. F. Davis Co., Philadelphia, 1969.

PRESSURE-CYCLED OR PRESSURE-LIMITED VENTILATORS. This includes those which will continue to inflate the patient's lungs until a preset pressure has been reached, at which time the inspiratory phase stops and expiration begins. Effect of moderate airway obstruction or decrease in compliance due to twisted endotracheal tubes, secretion, or bronchospasm will cause patient ventilation and machine volume to decrease. Thus a pressure-preset ventilator maintains its ventilation with small leaks in the system but compensates poorly for obstruction.

VOLUME-CONTROLLED OR VOLUME-LIMITED VENTILATORS. This includes those which permit maintenance of constant minute and tidal ventilation regardless of the changes in pulmonary compliance and airway resistance. A volume-limited ventilator should have incorporated in it a safety valve that will bleed the system when a preset ceiling pressure has been reached. Effect of moderate airway obstruction or decrease in compliance due to twisted endotracheal tubes, secretion, or bronchospasm will cause ventilation to be maintained with a rise in pressure to compensate for the obstruction. Thus a volume-preset ventilator maintains its tidal volume with partial obstruction but compensates poorly for leaks in the system.

TABLE 5-1   Monitoring of Ventilator

Condition		Volume Preset	Pressure Preset
Normal function	Volume	Fixed	Varies
	Flow	Fixed	Varies
	Pressure	Varies	Fixed
Obstruction	Volume	Fixed	Decreased
	Flow	Fixed	Decreased
	Pressure	Increased	Unchanged
Leaks	Volume	Fixed	Increased
	Flow	Varies	Varies
	Pressure	Decreased	Unchanged

TABLE 5-2   Ventilatory Compensation

Condition		Volume Preset	Pressure Preset
Normal function	Volume	Fixed	Variable
	Pressure	Variable	Fixed
Partial obstruction	Volume	Unchanged	Decreased
	Pressure	Increased	Unchanged
	Compensation	Good	Poor
Leaks	Volume	Decreased	Unchanged
	Pressure	Decreased	Unchanged
	Compensation	Poor	Good

Tables 5-1 and 5-2 compare volume-preset and pressure-preset ventilator function.

EXAMPLES OF PRESSURE-LIMITED MACHINES

Bennett PR-1, PR-2
Bird Mark 7, 8, 10, 14

EXAMPLES OF VOLUME-LIMITED MACHINES

Emerson   Ohio 560
Engstrom   Searles
Morch   Monaghan 225
Bennett MA-1   Bourns
Bennett MA-2   Gill I

BIRD MARK 7 VENTILATOR

The Bird Mark 7 is a positive-pressure, pressure-cycled, assistor-controller (pneumatic) ventilator. The system pressure is adjusted by the operator, and the volume delivered to the patient is variable depending on lung compliance.

Examples of Use

1. Patient with apnea
2. Assisted ventilation
3. Patient with airway resistance

I. Assembly (see Figures 5-1 and 5-2)
   A. Attach breathing tubing to inlet of micronebulizer.

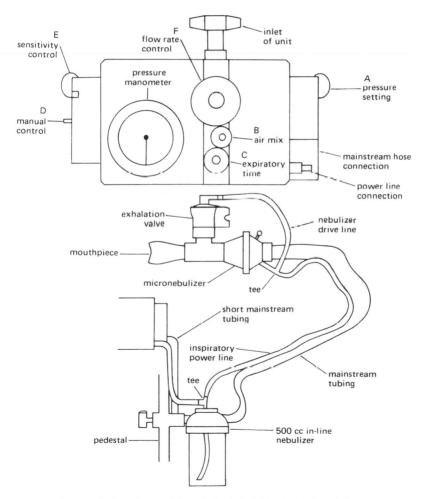

Figure 5-1. Assembly of the Bird Mark 7 Ventilator.

B. Attach nebulizer drive line to exhalation valve cap.

C. Attach nebulizer pressure line first to exhalation valve cap and then to micronebulizer inlet below capillary tube.

D. Attach micronebulizer to exhalation valve assembly.

E. Attach mouthpiece or proper ventilation connection.

F. Attach Bird Mark 7 to pedestal; screw on tightly.

G. Attach support arm assembly.

H. Attach 500 cc nebulizer; mount on bracket.

I. Attach 500 cc in-line nebulizer.

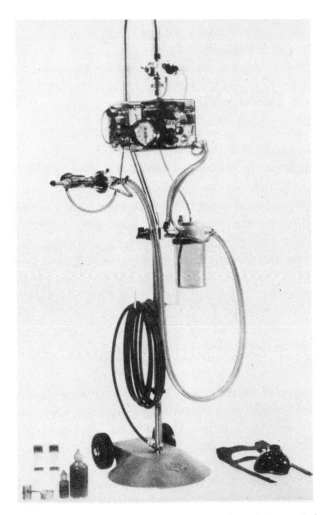

Figure 5-2. Bird Mark 7 Ventilator. (*Courtesy of Bird Corp., Palm Springs, Calif.*)

J. Attach short mainstream tubing from mounting bracket to outlet of pressure compartment.

K. Attach power drive line to nipple projecting from pressure compartment side.

L. Attach other end of power drive line to the top of the 500 cc in-line nebulizer top.

M. Attach mainstream breathing line to outlet of 500 cc in-line nebulizer.

N. Attach inspiratory power line to tee on top of 500 cc in-line nebulizer.

O. Attach high-pressure tubing, either 50-psi pipeline system or 50-psi gas regulator assembly.

II. Operation of the Bird Mark 7

A. Pressure setting—determines the pressure generated by the ventilator, 0 to 60 cm of water pressure at 50 psi; usually, start pressure at 15 to 20 cm of water pressure, check tidal volume, and reset pressure accordingly.

B. Air-mix plunger—pulled out and with spacer ring in place will give you air dilution; plunger pushed in all the way will give you 100% gas supply by means of bypassing the Venturi.

C. Expiration time—cycles automatically when set for patient in apnea or assist ventilation; set expiration time slightly below patient's own rate if on assist ventilation or set rate for patient in apnea; set expiration time in *off* position for manual IPPB therapy.

D. Manual control—when pushed in, cycles the ventilator on; mostly used in manual IPPB therapy to check unit before applying to patient.

E. Sensitivity control—is used to adjust patient's effort under ventilation; set control for best patient effort so patient does not have to tug on ventilator.

F. Flow rate control—adjusts the inspiratory time and turns the ventilator from *off* to *on*; set flow rate for best patient needs; remember, the higher the flow rate, the more turbulent the flow becomes.

BIRD MARK 8 VENTILATOR

The Bird Mark 8 (Figure 5-3) is a positive-pressure, pressure-cycled, assistor-controller (pneumatic) ventilator. The system pressure is

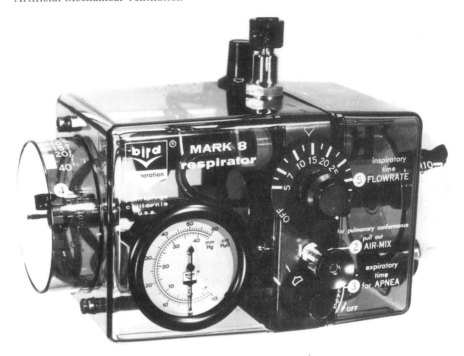

Figure 5-3.   Bird Mark 8 Ventilator. (*Courtesy of Bird Corp., Palm Springs, Calif.*)

adjusted by the operator and the volume delivered to the patient is variable depending on lung compliance.

The Bird Mark 8 differs from the Mark 7 by the incorporation of a Venturi in the breathing head. The mechanism that regulates the breathing head Venturi is built into the center body of the Mark 8 and is controlled by turning the calibrator knob located on top of the center body behind the $\frac{9}{16}$-in. swivel inlet.

Attach tubing the same as for Bird Mark 7, except attach negative tubing to Venturi breathing head and negative flow line on pressure compartment side.

Operation.   Same as for Bird Mark 7, *except negativity knob.* To create subambient pressure during expiration, cycle the respirator off and manually pull and hold the hand timer off. Then turn the negativity knob counterclockwise to a degree that generates 2 to 3 cm of negative pressure as registered by the manometer point in the red segment of the dial. Now rotate the sensitivity arm onto the red negative scale to match the manometer reading and then release the hand timer rod.

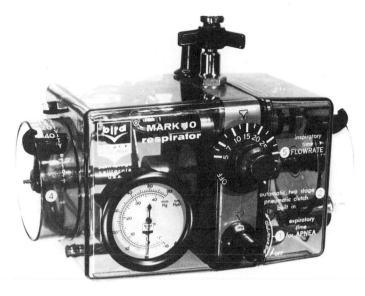

Figure 5-4. Bird Mark 10 Ventilator. (*Courtesy of Bird Corp., Palm Springs, Calif.*)

BIRD MARK 10 VENTILATOR

The Bird Mark 10 (Figure 5-4) leak-compensated positive phase respirator has all the characteristics of the Bird Mark 7 plus the additional feature of terminal inspiratory flow acceleration.

BIRD MARK 14 VENTILATOR

The Bird Mark 14 (Figure 5-5) positive phase ventilator with automatic flow accelerator has all the combined characteristics of the Mark 7 and Mark 10 with extended function providing for airway pressure up to 140 mm Hg and flow rate up to 160 liters/min.

For detailed operating instructions of all the Bird mechanical ventilators refer to the instruction manuals supplied by the manufacturer.

BABY BIRD VENTILATOR

The Baby Bird Ventilator (Figure 5-6) operates as a pneumatically powered, time cycled, pressure limited, constant flow controller. Its clinical capabilities include the delivery of continuous positive

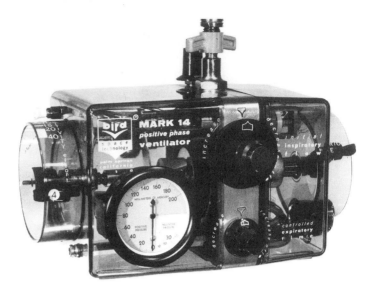

Figure 5-5. Bird Mark 14 Ventilator. (*Courtesy of Bird Corp., Palm Springs, Calif.*)

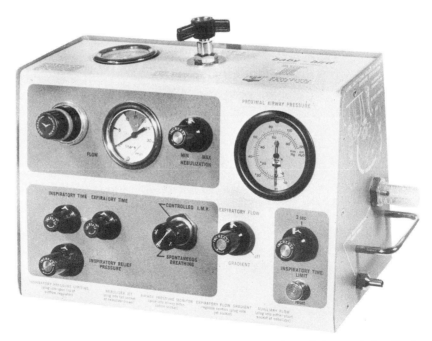

Figure 5-6. Baby Bird Ventilator. (*Courtesy of Bird Corp., Palm Springs, Calif.*)

airway pressure (CPAP), intermittent mandatory ventilation (IMV), and controlled mechanical ventilation (CMV). All modes may be used with or without elevated baselines by simple operation of a single outflow valve.

Assembly

1. Install 50-in. post into stand base.
2. Place collar hanger on the post. Tighten 13 in. from top of stand base.
3. Place utility tray on post down to collar hanger.
4. Install a dovetail mount bracket at the top of post.
5. Place the Baby Bird Respirator on the mount bracket. Install Bird Oxygen Blender to Baby Bird inlet.
6. (a) Install a 12-in. post into the bracket mounting flange under the respirator and tighten two set screws.
   (b) Place the mount bracket on post.

Patient Breathing Circuit Assembly

1. Insert the keyed adapter of the fused shuttle valve assembly into the mount bracket until spring loaded pin engages hole in adapter, securing fused shuttle valve assembly in proper position.
2. Into the tee fitting atop the shuttle valve, insert the intake relief valve into the rear post and the 500 cc micronebulizer into the front port.
3. Install tee into the outlet of the 500 cc nebulizer.
4. Place small therapy micronebulizer in the backside of the tee with its stopper in place.
5. Install the Air Bird Valve assembly on the Air Bird Bag and install into the open end of the master tee.
6. Mount the outflow valve atop the Air Bird Valve with the red PEEP control lever in front.
7. Mount BOOM arm bracket on 50-in. post and install BOOM arm.
8. To connect tubing, read instructions across lower front of Baby Bird, starting at left. Connect large-diameter green tube to inspiratory pressure limiting socket on respirator and top of outflow regulator.
9. Connect small green tube to nebulizer jet outlet and tall socket of 500 cc nebulizer.

10. Connect small-diameter green tubing from bifurcation to airway pressure monitor outlet.
11. Connect small red tube from expiratory flow gradient outlet to negative Venturi jet socket on shuttle valve assembly.
12. Connect remaining small clear tube to auxiliary flow socket on respirator and either short socket of the 500 cc nebulizer.
13. Assemble breathing circuit according to diagram on the side of the respirator cabinet, and connect green inspiratory tube to open end of the tee connected to the 500 cc micronebulizer outlet.
14. Connect red expiratory tube of breathing circuit to bottom port of the shuttle valve assembly.

Operation

1. Connect airway bifurcation to test lung.
2. Select desired oxygen concentration and turn gas supply on. Check operating pressure gauge (minimum 45 to 55 psi). If alarm sounds continuously, push reset.
3. Switch to spontaneous breathing.
4. Set flow at 10 liters/min.
5. Select minimum nebulization.
6. Select desired level of end expiratory positive pressure by adjusting control lever.
7. With end expiratory positive pressure in *off* position, any remaining positive airway pressure may be reduced by adjusting expiratory flow gradient.
8. Set inspiratory time limit at 3 sec.
9. Open expiratory time, inspiratory time, and inspiratory relief pressure control knobs fully counterclockwise.
10. Switch to ventilator *on*.
11. Lengthen expiratory time clockwise as desired.
12. Lengthen inspiratory time clockwise as desired.
13. Adjust inspiratory relief pressure as desired.
14. Tidal volume may be controlled by adjusting inspiratory time and flow or adjusting inspiratory relief pressure.
15. Adjust nebulization to desired level. Connect airway bifurcation to patient.
16. All further adjustments should be accomplished while visually monitoring chest motion and clinical signs.

IMV BIRD VENTILATOR

The IMV Bird (Figure 5-7) is a pneumatically powered, flow controlled, pressure limited, time cycled ventilator for delivery of continuous positive airway pressure (CPAP), intermittent mandatory ventilation (IMV), and controlled mechanical ventilation (CMV) with or without elevated baselines (PEEP).

Assembly

1. Slide utility tray onto tapered (bottom) end of crookneck pole followed by dual collar hanger. Position latter approximately 14 in. from tapered end and tighten Allen set screw.
2. Insert pole in base and secure grounding chain with screw into end of pole.
3. Slide collar hanger onto top end of pole and secure with set screw at top of first bend.
4. Insert pole extension into top of pole.
5. Clamp pole mounting bracket on pole, resting on collar.
6. Mount ventilator on pole bracket.

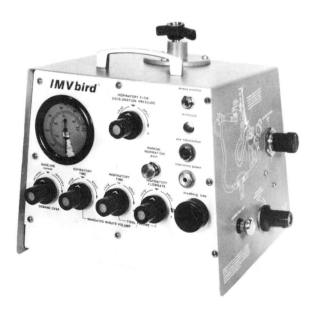

Figure 5-7. IMV Bird Ventilator. (*Courtesy of Bird Corp., Palm Springs, Calif.*)

7. Slide oxygen blender mount into pole, and couple blender to ventilator with wing nut.

8. Attach air and oxygen supply hoses to oxygen blender inlet fittings, and attach to 50-psi air and oxygen sources.

9. Install extension arm on top of main pole assembly.

10. Mount nebulizer mounting bracket on vertical segment of pole just below bend with winged knob to your left as you face the ventilator.

11. Install 500-ml nebulizer in mounting bracket.

12. Connect multichanneled breathing tube harness with auxillary nebulizer and inspiratory power lines to breathing tube outlet and color-coded sockets on front panel of ventilator.

13. Connect male end of therapy bifurcation to female outlet of 500-ml nebulizer.

14. Attach male outlet of 5-ml micronebulizer to female outlet of bifurcation.

15. Connect male connector of inspiratory power line to female connector of inspiratory power line. Plug metal tapered tee of inspiratory power line into either mating socket of 500-ml nebulizer dual-jet crown.

16. Plug line from auxiliary nebulizer socket into remaining mating socket of 500-ml nebulizer dual-jet crown.

17. Insert end of main breathing hose into female outlet of bifurcation.

18. Install water trap in the open section of the main breathing hose near the middle.

19. Connect distal end of main breathing hose to one of the female inlets of the airway connector.

20. Connect short length of main breathing hose, with exhalation valve attached to the remaining female inlet of the airway connector.

21. Connect distal end of inspiratory power line to exhalation valve.

22. Check all connections for tightness of fit.

Operation

1. Check all external tubing connections for tightness and proper matching. Remove 500-ml nebulizer crown; fill reservoir with sterile distilled water or other prescribed solution and replace.

2. Master switch (located on right of ventilator cabinet) *off*.

3. Power source connected and *on* (ventilator operates from a source pressure of 50 psi).

4. All control knobs to 12 o'clock.

5. Set oxygen blender to prescribed concentration.

6. Master switch *on* (this switch must be turned to the *on* position before the ventilator will function).

7. Manual inspiration, push for flow.

8. Connect ventilator breathing circuit to unobstructed patient airway.

9. Baseline: PEEP or CPAP is determined by adjusting the baseline/demand flow control from 12 o'clock position to any point between ambient and a maximum pressure of 35 cm of water.

10. Set rate (IMV); establish rate by turning expiratory time knob.

11. Set tidal volume; establish volume by:
    a. Inspiratory time—turn knob to obtain desired time.
    b. Inspiratory flow rate; turn until adequate chest excursion is observed.
    c. Auscultate patient's chest and set inspiratory flow deceleration pressure to achieve optimal bilateral distribution of inspired gas.

12. Whenever the ventilator is to be used for pediatric purposes, the initial setting for the expiratory time, inspiratory time, and inspiratory flow rate should be initially at the 9 o'clock position instead of the 12 o'clock position as for adults.

13. Monitoring of patient:
    a. Check for bilateral distribution of tidal volume.
    b. Arterial blood gases should be measured to determine effectiveness of ventilation.

14. Weaning the patient from the ventilator: IMV can be used to wean a patient from a mechanical ventilator by gradually slowing the controlled cycling rate of the ventilator until the patient assumes a spontaneous breathing pattern on his own.

Cleaning and Sterilization.   Ventilators manufactured by Bird Corporation are compatible with ethylene oxide gas sterilization. Breathing circuits are compatible with ethylene oxide gas sterilization and liquid agents, glutaraldehyde, and quaternary ammonium agents, used according to manufacturer's instructions. For cleaning, use only detergents compatible with plastic materials.

Phenols must *not* be used. All plastics must not be abused by excessive thermal stress or incompletely vaporized (liquid phase) droplets of ethylene oxide. *Do not* steam, autoclave or otherwise subject ventilators or components manufactured by Bird Corporation to temperatures over 60°C (140°F).

BENNETT RESPIRATION UNIT

Model PR-1

The Bennett Respiration Unit Model PR-1 is classified as a positive-pressure pneumatic ventilator. It operates as an assistor or controller, depending on the patient's ability to initiate inspiration. If he has an inspiratory effort of at least $\frac{1}{2}$ cm of negative pressure, the ventilator will supplement his efforts and assist him. If the patient is apneic, the PR-1 may be set to cycle automatically and thus control his ventilation. However, a patient may override the controls at any time.

Assembly

1. Place the column inside the base and tighten securely.
2. Place the ventilator unit into the top of the column.
3. Slip the support arm into its housing and tighten screw.
4. Adjust all sections of the support arm to the desired tension and tighten the wing nuts.
5. Attach the spirometer condensation pole and bracket to the ventilator column, and tighten securely.
6. Attach the heating element for the cascade humidifier to the ventilator column and tighten securely.
7. Attach a spirometer adapter to the port below the Bennett valve.
8. Slip the cover of the cascade humidifier over its heating element and lock securely.
9. Fill the cascade jar with sterile water and attach onto the cover; it must be aligned correctly or a leak in the patient system will result.
10. Plug the black cord on the humidifier into an electrical outlet, making certain that it is properly grounded.
11. Set the inspired gas temperature by rotating the knob on the humidifier to the desired number (see Bennett Cascade Humidifier in Unit 3).
12. Attach one end of a 12-in. flex tube to the spirometer adapter and attach the other end to the inlet port on the cascade.
13. Assemble the Bennett Monitoring Spirometer according to the procedure given in Unit 6.
14. Attach a short piece of small-bore tubing to the nipple on the black valve, located on the bottom of the spirometer, place the spirometer on the metal condensation tube, and attach the

other end of the small-bore tubing to the nipple on the spirometer adapter.

15. Assemble the spirometer condensation vial and adapter; slip the adapter onto the metal condensation tube.

16. Attach a slipstream manifold to the flex arm; in place of the usual manifold cap and mushroom, attach a gas collector head, which directs gas into the spirometer for measurement of expired volumes.

17. Insert a probe thermometer and its elbow into the back of the slipstream manifold; this thermometer records the temperature of the gas being delivered to the patient and should be used whenever a heated humidifier is used.

18. Attach a flex tube with the proper-sized adapter to the manifold; the flex tube is always attached as near the exhalation port as possible in order to keep mechanical dead space to a minimum.

19. The main air hose consists of three parts: a large-bore tube that carries the main flow of gas to the patient, a smaller nebulizer tubing through which a secondary flow of gas is directed to power the medication nebulizer, and the smallest tubing, which allows for alternate opening and closing of the exhalation port.

20. Connect one end of the large-bore tube to the outlet port on the cascade humidifier.

21. Connect one end of the nebulizer tubing to the nebulizer nipple on the unit.

22. Connect the exhalation tubing to the nipple on the ventilator (to the bottom left as you face the unit).

23. Connect the other end of the main tube to the thermometer elbow on the manifold.

24. Connect the exhalation tubing to the exhalation mushroom.

25. Connect the nebulizer tubing to the top of the nebulizer.

26. Attach one end of the large-bore spirometer tube to the spirometer condensation vial.

27. Attach the other end to the collector head on the manifold.

28. A high-pressure source of 50 psi is needed to power the PR-1; this may be delivered through high-pressure tubing connected to a standard wall outlet, by the Veriflo MR-1 Respirator Oxygen Controller, or by a high-pressure regulator attached to a cylinder of compressed gas (see Unit 6).

29. A high-pressure hose attached to any of these devices carries the gas to the gas inlet on the back of the unit.

Setting of Controls

1. To activate the unit, the gas source must be in operation.
2. The prescribed pressure is adjusted by the pressure control knob on the front of the unit; when this knob is rotated, the pressure is recorded on the control pressure gauge (to the right as you face the unit); the PR-1 is capable of delivering 0 to 45 cm of water pressure.
3. The gauge to your left records the system pressure, or the pressure being delivered to the patient's tube; it may be read on the inspiratory phase of the respiratory cycle.
4. The rate control, on the left front of the unit, controls the rate of automatic cycling; it is adjustable from 0 to 50 cycles per minute; if a patient is being assisted, set the unit rate slightly below his own rate, but if he is being controlled, the rate may be set precisely.
5. *Turn the unit to the side.*
6. The sensitivity control adjusts the amount of inspiratory effort needed to initiate inspiration. To set it at its most sensitive point:
   a. Turn off rate.
   b. Attach a test lung to the flex tube adapter.
   c. Rotate sensitivity knob until unit begins to cycle automatically.
   d. Turn knob back slightly; the unit is now at its most sensitive point.
7. The dilution control allows for delivery of 100% oxygen in the out position, or an air–oxygen mixture when pushed in.
8. The nebulization controls power the medication nebulizer for delivery of aerosol therapy.

Operation

1. After activating the unit and setting the controls, the ventilator may be attached to the patient.
2. Set the Bennett Monitoring Spirometer Alarm (see procedure in Unit 6).
3. Check for leaks in the patient system, as evidenced by a long inspiratory phase and unequal control and system pressure gauge readings.
4. Make any adjustments in settings.

Model PR-2

The Bennett Respiration Unit Model PR-2 (Figure 5-8) is a mobile unit designed for the clinical application of intermittent positive pressure breathing in therapy, as a respiratory assistant, and, in the complete absence of respiration, as a respiratory controller.

Note: The controls on the PR-2 are noninteracting. In other words,

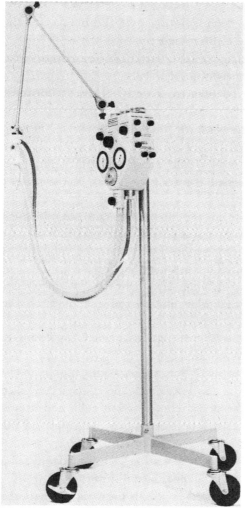

Figure 5-8.   Bennett Respiration Unit Model PR-2. (*Courtesy of Puritan-Bennett Corp., Kansas City, Mo.*)

a change in one parameter does not generally necessitate a change in another.

Cycling

1. Inspiration and expiration are time cycled by a pneumatic mechanism, which allows for an inspiration–expiration ratio of approximately $1:1\frac{1}{2}$, regardless of rate, pressure, or leaks in the system.
2. Inspiration may be patient cycled as well; a negative pressure equivalent to approximately $-\frac{1}{2}$ cm of water pressure allows the Bennett valve to open, delivering a variable flow, depending on circumstances of compliance and resistance; the patient may override these settings at any time; however, should his respiratory rate decrease to a point below the rate setting, or should he become apneic, the time-cycling mechanism takes over.
3. Expiration may also be initiated by a low terminal flow; the variable flow decreases to a point (terminal flow point) of approximately 1 liter/min, at which time the Bennett valve closes.

Assembly

1. Place the column inside the base and tighten securely.
2. Place the ventilator unit into the top of the column.
3. Slip the support arm into its housing and tighten screw.
4. Adjust all sections of the support arm to the desired tension and tighten the wing nuts.
5. Attach the spirometer condensation pole and bracket to the ventilator column and tighten securely.
6. Attach the heating element for the cascade humidifier to the ventilator column and tighten securely.
7. Attach a spirometer adapter to the port below the Bennett valve.
8. Slip the cover of the cascade humidifier over its heating element and lock securely.
9. Fill the cascade jar with sterile water and attach onto the cover; it must be aligned correctly or a leak in the patient system will result.
10. Plug the black cord on the humidifier into an electrical outlet, making certain that it is properly grounded.
11. Set the inspired gas temperature by rotating the knob on the humidifier to the desired number (see Unit 3).

12. Attach one end of a 12-in. flex tube to the spirometer adapter and attach the other end to the inlet port on the cascade.

13. Assemble the Bennett Monitoring Spirometer according to the procedure in Unit 6.

14. Attach a short piece of small-bore tubing to the nipple on the black valve, located on the bottom of the spirometer; place the spirometer on the metal condensation tube and attach the other end of the small-bore tubing to the nipple on the spirometer adapter.

15. Assemble the spirometer condensation vial and adapter; slip the adapter onto the metal condensation tube.

16. Attach a slipstream manifold to the flex arm; in place of the usual manifold cap and mushroom, attach a gas-collector head, which directs gas into the spirometer for measurement of expired volumes.

17. Insert a probe thermometer and its elbow into the back of the slipstream manifold; this thermometer records the temperature of the gas being delivered to the patient and should be used whenever a heated humidifier is used.

18. Attach a flex tube with the proper-sized adapter to the manifold; the flex tube is always attached as near the exhalation port as possible in order to keep mechanical dead space to a minimum.

19. The main air hose consists of three parts: a large-bore tube that carries the main flow of gas to the patient, a smaller nebulizer tubing through which a secondary flow of gas is directed to power the medication nebulizer, and the smallest tubing, which allows for alternate opening and closing of the exhalation port.

20. Connect one end of the large-bore tube to the outlet port on the cascade humidifier.

21. Connect one end of the nebulizer tubing to the nebulizer nipple on the unit.

22. Connect the exhalation tubing to the nipple on the ventilator (to the bottom left as you face the unit).

23. Connect the other end of the main tube to the thermometer elbow on the manifold.

24. Connect the exhalation tubing to the exhalation mushroom.

25. Connect the nebulizer tubing to the top of the nebulizer.

26. Attach one end of the large-bore spirometer tube to the spirometer condensation vial.

27. Attach the other end to the collector head on the manifold.

28. A high-pressure source of 50 psi is needed to power the PR-2; this may be delivered through high-pressure tubing connected to a standard wall outlet, by the Veriflo MR-1 Respirator Oxygen Controller, or by a high-pressure regulator attached to a cylinder of compressed gas.

29. A high-pressure hose attached to any of these devices carries the gas to the gas inlet on the back of the unit.

Setting of Controls

1. To activate the unit, the gas source must be in operation.

2. The prescribed pressure is adjusted by the pressure control knob on the front of the unit; when this knob is rotated, the pressure is recorded on the control pressure gauge (to the right as you face the unit); the PR-2 is capable of delivering 0 to 45 cm of water pressure.

3. The gauge to your left records the system pressure or the pressure being delivered to the patient's tube; it may be read on the inspiratory phase of the respiratory cycle.

4. The expiration-time control is used to increase the time of expiration; the knob is located on the front of the unit in the top right-hand corner; it may be used or not.

5. The peak flow control, located below the Bennett valve, provides a slower rise to the control pressure and thus increases inspiration time.

6. The rate control, on the left front of the unit, controls the rate of automatic cycling; it is adjustable from 0 to 50 cycles per minute; if a patient is being assisted, set the unit rate slightly below his own rate, but if he is being controlled, the rate may be set precisely.

7. Turn the unit to the side.

8. The terminal flow control adjusts the point at which the valve closes; it may be used to compensate for a leak in the system, but care must be taken to ensure that the patient is still being ventilated adequately; many units require that the terminal flow control be opened one-quarter-turn at all times.

9. The sensitivity control adjusts the amount of inspiratory effort needed to initiate inspiration. To set it at its most sensitive point:
   a. Turn off rate.
   b. Attach a test lung to the flex tube adapter.
   c. Rotate sensitivity knob until unit begins to cycle automatically.

d. Turn knob back slightly; the unit is now at its most sensitive point.

10. The dilution control allows for delivery of 100% oxygen in the out position, or an air–oxygen mixture when pushed in.

11. The nebulization controls power the medication nebulizer for delivery of aerosol therapy.

Operation

1. After activating the unit and setting the controls, the ventilator may be attached to the patient.

2. Set the Bennett Monitoring Spirometer Alarm (see Unit 6 for procedure).

3. Check for leaks in the patient system, as evidenced by a long inspiratory phase and unequal control and system pressure guage readings.

4. Make any adjustments in settings.

Model MA-1

The Bennett Respiration Unit Model MA-1 (Figure 5-9) is an electrically powered device that uses ambient air as the principal gas. However, oxygen enrichment or 100% oxygen may be provided.

The MA-1 may be used as a controller, where inspiration is initiated by a timing mechanism. Inspiration may also be patient initiated, at which time the unit acts as an assistor. The unit should be adjusted, however, so that if the patient should become apneic the ventilator will take over control of his respiration.

Assembly

1. Slip the spirometer condenser tube into its bracket on the side of the unit and tighten securely.

2. Mount the spirometer on the top of the condenser tube.

3. Connect one end of a small-bore tube to the nipple on the black valve on the base of the spirometer.

4. Connect the other end to the spirometer outlet on the left side of the MA-1.

5. Assemble the condensation vial and adapter.

6. Slip the adapter onto the bottom of the condenser tube.

7. Fit the cover of the cascade humidifier over the heating element and lock securely.

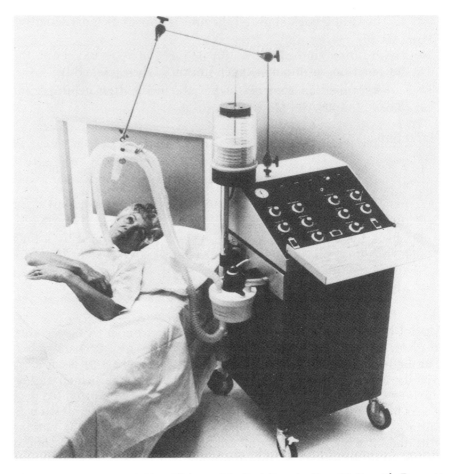

Figure 5-9. Bennett MA-1 Volume-Limited Respiration Unit with Bennett Monitoring Spirometer. (*Courtesy of Puritan-Bennett Corp., Kansas City, Mo.*)

8. Fill the cascade jar with sterile distilled water; align the jar with the threads on the cascade cover and tighten securely.

9. Plug in the electrical cord of the cascade and set the desired temperature (see Bennett Cascade Humidifier, Unit 3).

10. Open the door of the unit and secure the micro bacteria filter through the hole in the upper left with the clamp and thumb nut.

11. Fit the angled connector from the machine outlet to the cascade inlet.

12. Fit a 12-in. flex tube from the filter inlet to the unit outlet, inside the machine.

13. Screw the support arm into its bracket and tighten securely.

14. Attach the manifold assembly to the support arm, with the large openings facing the unit.

15. Fit the nebulizer bacteria filter with adapter to the jet connector on the manifold.

16. Connect the main air hose from the cascade outlet to the manifold inlet.

17. Connect the nebulizer tubing to the nebulizer bacteria filter and to the nebulizer connector on the side of the unit.

18. Fit the large-bore spirometer tubing from the exhalation port on the manifold to the spirometer vial adapter.

19. Fit the exhalation tubing (small bore) from the mushroom on the exhalation valve on the manifold to the exhalation connector on the side of the unit.

20. Insert a probe thermometer with rubber adapter into its port on the inspiration side of the manifold.

21. Connect the two circle tubes to the small openings on the manifold, opposite the inhalation and exhalation tubes.

22. Connect both these tubes to a suitable wye.

Description and Setting of Controls

1. Plug electrical cord into suitable wall outlet.

2. Turn on switch marked *Power.*

3. Set normal volume for the desired tidal volume; the control is calibrated from 0 to 2200 ml.

4. Set normal pressure limit; the control is calibrated for 20 to 80 cm of water pressure; while excessive pressure need not be used, be certain to allow enough to deliver the tidal volume you have set. If the normal pressure limit is reached, the pressure light will light and a buzzer will sound.

5. The rate control may be adjusted for 6 to 60 respirations per minute; respiration rates from 60 to 100 per minute are possible, but are not calibrated on the control.

6. Set the desired oxygen percentage, which is calibrated from 21% to 100% in 5% increments; if concentrations over 21% are used, the high-pressure oxygen hose on the back of the unit must be connected to a 50-psi source.

7. Set sigh volume for an automatic deep breath; it is calibrated from 0 to 2200 ml.

8. Sigh pressure limit must be set sufficiently high to accommodate the sigh volume; inspiration ends when this pressure,

which is calibrated from 20 to 80 cm of water pressure, is reached. If the sigh pressure limit is reached, the pressure light will light and a buzzer will sound.

9. Sighs per hour may be adjusted for 4 to 15 deep breaths per hour.
10. The multisigh control sets the number of sighs per interval: 1, 2, or 3.
11. The sigh indicator will light each time a deep breath is delivered.
12. Set the sensitivity control; this determines the amount of patient effort needed to initiate inspiration; the unit may be set so that the patient is unable to trigger inspiration (turned completely counterclockwise) or so that the unit will respond to from approximately −10.0 cm to 0.1 cm of water pressure. However, care must be taken not to set the unit so it becomes oversensitive and self-cycling.
13. The assist indicator lights each time the patient initiates inspiration or when the unit is oversensitive.
14. Other controls
    a. Manual normal or sigh inspiration—may be used to initiate a single inspiration.
    b. System pressure gauge—calibrated from −10 to +80 cm of water pressure; indicates pressure in the tubing.
    c. Nebulizer control—for aerosolization of medication on inspiration.
    d. Expiratory resistance control—for retardation of expiratory flow.
    e. Ratio warner—indicates when inspiration time exceeds expiration time.
    f. Oxygen signals—a green light indicates oxygen enrichment; a red light and audible alarm indicate that the present oxygen concentration is not being met owing to low source pressure.
    g. All lights may be pressed to test the lamp—will light if functioning.
    h. Pressure limit warning buzzer—may be set for loud to soft and off.

Operation

1. After setting controls, the ventilator may be attached to the patient.
2. Check for any leaks in the patient system.
3. Make any adjustments according to the needs of the patient.

Note: An IMV circuit board is now available for use with the MA-1 Ventilator.

Bennett MA-2 Ventilator

The MA-2 Ventilator (Figures 5-10 and 5-11) is an electrically powered volume lung ventilator, which provides machine-delivered breaths for patients who cannot sustain breathing on their own. It operates in three modes: continuous mandatory ventilation (CMV), intermittent mandatory ventilation (IMV), and continuous positive airway pressure (CPAP).

The principal gas is room air drawn into the unit during expiration and delivered to the patient during inspiration. The air may be enriched to any desired O_2 concentration. It may also be enriched

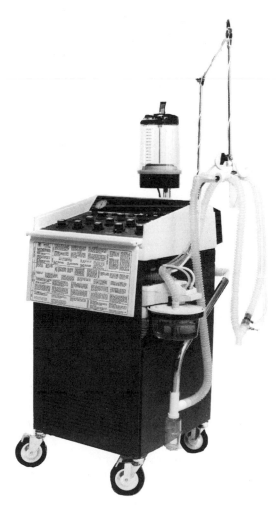

Figure 5-10.   MA-2 Ventilator. (*Courtesy of Puritan-Bennett Corp., Kansas City, Mo.*)

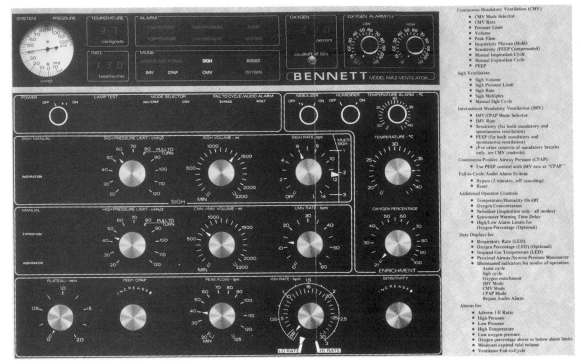

Figure 5-11. MA-2 Ventilator. (*Courtesy of Puritan-Bennett Corp., Kansas City, Mo.*)

with aerosol medicament from the nebulizer, as well as warmed and humidified by the humidifier. A complement of audible and visible alarms provides monitoring capability in all modes of ventilator operation.

Assembly

1. Slip condenser column into condenser tube bracket.
2. Attach the bracket to either of two mounting brackets located on the left and right sides of the ventilator.
3. Attach cap to bottom of condenser column and screw vial into cap.
4. Attach flex arm to attachment point on top left or right side of unit.
5. Attach spirometer alarm on spirometer dome by turning alarm clockwise. Flag switch should be in the *off* position.

Note: The spirometer alarm should be checked prior to each use.

6. Insert smaller end of metal spirometer mounting tube into bottom of mounting tube bracket and tighten knob. Mount spirometer on mounting tube being sure tidal volume indexes face toward front of ventilator and spirometer is as far forward as possible.

7. Attach black tube to black connector underneath the spirometer base and to the spirometer connection at the back of unit.

8. Open top front door. Swing humidifier mount out. Install main-flow bacteria filter in its slot, with flow direction arrow on filter pointing up.

9. Attach connector tube to filter inlet port and ventilator outlet port.

10. Check that (a) clear connector tube and blue umbilical tube are connected to the humidifier mount and ventilator, (b) both tubes are routed properly without kinks or twists, and (c) blue rubber grommets are properly positioned in brackets.

11. The blue umbilical tube is not part of the patient system tubing and should not be detached from the humidifier mount or the ventilator outlet.

12. Attach the jar and cover to the humidifier mount; first position the cover front marking below the front of the mount and align the electrical connection on the cover with the receptacle in the bottom of the mount. Then raise the jar and cover until the blue latches engage.

13. Attach flex tube to the outlet of the main-flow filter and to the inlet port of the humidifier.

14. Swing and slide humidifier mount to either the left or the right side of the ventilator. Secure humidifier mount to cabinet by engaging stud with latch.

15. Attach manifold assembly to flex arm, with the large openings in manifold facing the unit. Connect nebulizer filter coupling to outlet side of nebulizer bacteria filter. Connect the coupling to the white jet connector on the manifold. Attach the patient pressure bacteria filter to the patient pressure connection on the manifold, with inlet side of filter facing away from manifold.

16. Connect main tube to the humidifier outlet and to the manifold inlet.

17. Connect clear expiration valve tube and blue patient pressure tube and white nebulizer tube to their respective connectors, so labeled on the humidifier mount. Connect the opposite ends of the clear expiration valve tube and the blue patient pressure tube to their respective connectors on the manifold. Connect

the opposite end of the white nebulizer tube to the inlet side of the nebulizer bacteria filter, which is attached to the white jet connector on the manifold.

18. Attach collector tube to the manifold outlet and to the cap.

19. Attach elbow connector to the back port of the condenser column. Position the condenser column and tighten clamp on bracket. Connect condenser tube to the lower, inlet end of the spirometer.

20. Attach the two circle tubes to the inspiratory side and expiratory side of the manifold. Attach connector and coupling to the inspiratory side of the tube. Join the two circle tubes with a straight wye or with an angled wye. These wyes have 15-mm female and 22-mm male connections.

21. Attach patient pressure tube to connector and to filter, which is attached to the manifold patient pressure fitting.

22. Push and twist temperature sensor probe into socket of cable. Insert probe into coupling. Route cable around flex arm and connect socket on other end of cable to temperature sensor connection.

23. If oxygen is to be used, connect oxygen pressure hose to the oxygen inlet port at the rear of the ventilator. If external compressed air is to be used, connect a small water trap to the air inlet port at the rear of the ventilator. Using the high-pressure air hose, connect the water trap to an external air source.

24. If optional oxygen monitor is to be used with the ventilator, install oxygen monitor sensor probe at ventilator outlet port.

25. Open top front door. Disconnect connector tube from ventilator out port. Connect flex adaptor and plastic tee manifold to ventilator outlet port with tee manifold in the vertical position. Connect connector tube to tee manifold.

26. Insert oxygen sensor in the tee manifold. Align the largest hole in the plug on sensor cable with the largest-diameter pin in the connector on the ventilator. Push the plug straight onto the connector.

Operation. The MA-2 control panel is divided into two major sections, (1) the top section for displays and indications, and (2) the lower section for control settings, as shown in Figure 5-10.

1. Set power switch to *off* position. Connect ventilator electrical cord to a properly grounded 115-V, ac, 60-cycle electrical outlet.

2. If oxygen enrichment is desired, connect the high-pressure oxygen hose to a 40- to 100-psi oxygen source. If external com-

pressed air is to be used, connect the high-pressure air hose to a 35- to 100-psi dry air source.

3. Ensure that all tubes in the patient system are properly connected.

4. If medication is desired, place the specified amount in the nebulizer vial.

5. Fill humidifier jar with sterile distilled water to the full mark. Secure humidifier assembly to left or right side of ventilator. A continuous water feed system also may be used if desired.

6. Set humidifier power switch at *off* position.

7. Set temperature control at 37°C position or as desired. After temperature has stabilized, readjust the control as necessary.

8. Set the temperature alarm at a desired setting. Recommended is 3°C above temperature control set point.

9. Set sensitivity at extreme counterclockwise position (*off*).

10. Set peak flow at approximately 40 liters/min. After start-up, readjust if necessary.

11. Set CMV pressure limit at maximum pressure limit; readjust after start-up.

12. Set CMV volume at desired volume; after start-up, readjust for proper Tidal Volume.

13. Set CMV rate as desired for operation in CMV mode or for backup to operation in IMV mode.

14. Set straight pressure limit at minimum pressure limit.

15. Set sigh volume at minimum volume, the extreme counterclockwise position.

16. Set sigh rate at *off* position, with multiple sigh lever at 1 position.

17. Set oxygen percentage at desired concentration.

18. If the ventilator is equipped with the oxygen monitor, set the high oxygen alarm limit as desired and set the low alarm to the *off* position.

19. Set nebulizer switch to the *off* position.

20. Set plateau at extreme counterclockwise position (0).

21. Set PEEP/CPAP at extreme counterclockwise position, zero PEEP.

22. If the ventilator is to be operated in the IMV mode, set the IMV rate at desired setting. If the ventilator is to be operated in CMV mode only, set this control at the same rate as the CMV rate setting.

23. Set the audio alarm volume switch as desired (located inside the front door on left-hand side).

24. Set the spirometer alarm warning time control calibrated in seconds to accord with the IMV and CMV rate settings. Readjust later, if necessary, to accord with patient spontaneous rate indicated on the rate display.

25. Attach a test lung to the patient wye. Turn ventilator power switch *on*, cycle the ventilator, and check manual controls.

26. Check the following: system pressure gauge, temperature display, rate (breaths per minute), oxygen percent display, and spirometer (tidal volume).

27. Turn ventilator power switch *off*.

28. Ventilator may now be readjusted to CMV, controlled or assistor, IMV, or CPAP mode of operation.

Cleaning and Sterilization

1. Following each patient use, or more frequently if necessary, disassemble and clean all the components in the patient system.

2. Before disassembly for cleaning, turn ventilator Power Switch *off* and disconnect the power cord. If the humidifier has been turned on, allow sufficient time for it to cool off before disconnecting the heater.

3. *Note:* Do not remove blue umbilical tube for cleaning. This tube is not in the patient system. Do not wash or sterilize cable.

4. See Table 5-3 for recommended procedures broken down by ventilator parts.

Maintenance

1. Check System Pressure gauge with ventilator power switch *off* and patient pressure tube disconnected from humidifier; verify that system pressure gauge reads zero. If it does not, recalibrate gauge.

2. Lamp replacement: each visual alarm or mode indicator is equipped with two bulbs to assure continued display when a bulb burns out. If any indicator appears dim, one of its two bulbs will need replacing.

3. After each sterilization of the oxygen sensor, or anytime that the oxygen percent display fails to respond to the calibration adjustment, service will be needed on sensor.

4. Apart from sterilization, maintenance of the three bacteria filters, (a) main-flow bacteria filter, (b) nebulizer bacteria filter, and (c) patient pressure bacteria filter, is limited to replace-

TABLE 5-3 Cleaning and Sterilization Chart

Part	Recommended Action	Cautions
Ventilator exterior	Wipe clean with alcohol or a bactericidal agent	Do not allow liquid to penetrate the inside of the ventilator or control panel; do not gas sterilize the entire ventilator
Heater assembly: Autoclavable model	Steam autoclave	"Autoclavable" marking clearly appears on heaters that are autoclavable
Nonautoclavable model	Gas sterilize or cold sterilize	Connector end of heater should not be immersed in solution
Temperature sensor	Steam autoclave, gas sterilize, or cold sterilize	Connector end should not be immersed in solution
Oxygen sensor	Gas sterilize or cold sterilize	Cable end should not be immersed in solution
Bacteria filters: Nebulizer Main flow Patient pressure	Steam autoclave Steam autoclave Steam autoclave	Check filter resistance before use
Patient system tubing and connectors	Wash and steam autoclave	Inspect for nicks and cuts on diaphragm
Humidifier system parts (except heater)	Wash and steam autoclave	
Spirometer parts (except black valve)	Wash and steam autoclave	Inspect for nicks and cuts on spirometer bellows
Spirometer black valve	Dry wipe clean	Do not autoclave or immerse in solution
Spirometer alarm	Dry wipe clean	Do not autoclave or immerse in solution
Control tubing: Spirometer tube (black) Nebulizer tube (white) Patient pressure tube (blue) Exhalation valve tube (translucent) Nebulizer coupling (white) Patient pressure coupling (blue) Patient pressure adapter tube (translucent)	Dry wipe clean	If washed or cold sterilized, blow out all moisture from internal bore before use with pressurized air
Manifold assembly	Disassemble, wash, and steam autoclave	Inspect for leaks on 0705 exhalation diaphragm before assembly and use

ment of a filter if it becomes damaged or so loaded with particles that it offers excessive resistance to the flow of gas.

5. The cooling air filter screens dust and lint from room air drawn into the motor pump chamber. Open the door located at the front lower half of the ventilator by prying with a screwdriver at the top sides of the door. Pull out and examine the filter. If it has accumulated lint or dust, wash the filter element in warm detergent solution, rinse well, and dry; replace filter.

6. The air inlet filter intercepts air drawn into the internal bellows by the compressor. It is located in the front compartment of the ventilator. Examine the filter. If it has accumulated dirt or other clogging, wash the filter in warm detergent solution, rinse well, and dry. Reinstall the filter. Inspect and clean the filter periodically, at least once every 500 hours.

7. The high-pressure oxygen inlet filter intercepts pressurized oxygen that is delivered from an external gas source to the oxygen accumulator bag to be drawn into the bellows. It is located at the oxygen inlet port at the rear of the ventilator. Remove screws, fitting, filter, and O-ring. Wash the filter in warm detergent solution, rinse well, and dry. Reinstall in reverse order. Inspect and clean this filter periodically, at least once every 1000 hours.

8. The high-pressure air inlet filter intercepts pressurized air that is delivered from an external gas source to power the ventilator. It is located at the air inlet port at the rear of the ventilator. Remove screws, fitting, filter, and O-ring. Wash the filter in warm detergent, rinse well, and dry. Reinstall in reverse order. Inspect and clean this filter periodically, at least once every 1000 hours.

9. After every 10,000 hours of operation, the entire ventilator should be returned to the factory or a Puritan Bennett service center for a complete check, preventive maintenance, and replacement of limited life components.

EMERSON POSTOPERATIVE VENTILATOR

The Emerson Postoperative Ventilator is a constant-volume, pressure-variable ventilator, with assisted or controlled ventilation of the patient. (A simple assistor attachment can now be used for patients who are able to make spontaneous breathing efforts.) This means that the ventilator will deliver a preset volume in spite of the changes in lung compliance. Ceiling pressure (in centimeters of water) should be set depending on lung compliance and an additional

10 to 20 cm of water pressure should be set for changes in compliance and sighing.

Examples of Use

1. Patient with apnea
2. Spontaneous ventilatory movements are paradoxical
3. Assisted ventilation is ineffective

Assembly (refer to Figures 5-12 through 5-15)

1. Attach clear tubing, approximately 14 in. in length, to the reducing elbow of the inhalation tubing outlet and secure with screw clamp.
2. Attach the other end of the tygon tubing to the inlet of the condensation trap bottle and secure with screw clamp.

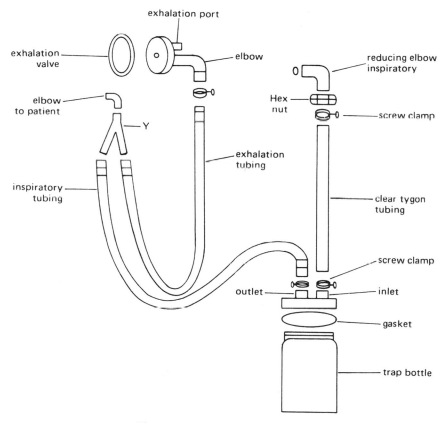

Figure 5-12. External tubing.

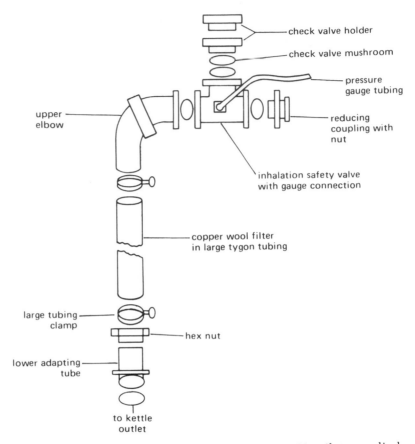

Figure 5-13. Assembly of Emerson Postoperative Ventilator: cylinder to humidifier tubing.

3. Attach corrugated inspiratory tubing, approximately 60 in. in length, to the condensation trap bottle and secure with screw clamp.

4. Attach the other end of the corrugated inspiratory tubing to the **Y**-piece with 15-mm elbow.

5. Attach corrugated expiratory tubing, approximately 50 in. in length, to **Y**-piece with 15-mm elbow.

6. Attach the other end of the corrugated expiratory tubing to the exhalation valve metal tubing elbow and secure with screw clamps.

7. Attach corrugated tubing, approximately 50 in. in length, to the exhalation port elbow.

8. Attach the other end of the corrugated tubing to the inlet of the spirometer.

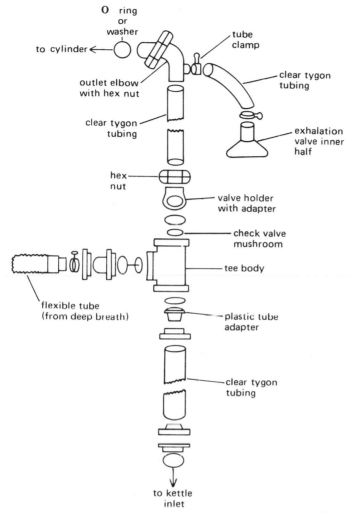

Figure 5-14. Delivery tubing humidifier to cabinet wall.

Table of Controls

1. Pressure gauge—shows pressure in system in centimeters of water; set the pressure ceiling by turning the knob of the safety valve located on the filling cap of the kettle.

2. Volume adjustment—the inspiratory volume limit ranges from 0 to 2000 cc.

3. Volume scale—shows volume for which machine is set.

4. Dilution—machine delivers room air (21% oxygen); oxygen enrichment may be added through the oxygen inlet in the top back of the unit.

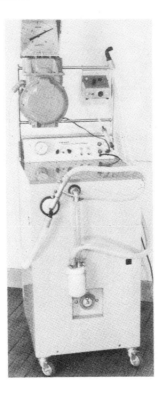

Figure 5-15.   Emerson Postoperative Ventilator. (*Courtesy of J. H. Emerson Co.*)

To calculate the liters per minute of oxygen to add, the two quantities that must be known are the percentage of oxygen desired and the minute volume (MV) in liters for which the machine is set. Use the following formula:

$$\frac{(\% \ O_2 - 21) \times MV}{79} = \text{liters per minute of } O_2$$

Example: How many liters per minute of oxygen must be supplied to a ventilator with MV of 4 liters in order to deliver 60% O_2 to the patient?

$$\frac{(60 - 21) \times 4}{79} = \text{liters/min } \dot{O}_2$$

$$\frac{39 \times 4}{79} = \frac{156}{79} = 1.97 \quad \text{or} \quad 2 \text{ liters/min } O_2$$

It is still necessary to check the O_2 concentration being delivered to the patient by means of an oxgen analyzer.

5. Inhalation time control and exhalation time control—the duration of the inspiratory and expiratory phases can be independently adjusted to from 12 to 70 respirations per minute.
6. Trim screw—adjustments permit speed compensation if the ventilator is operated on abnormal line voltages.
7. Pump switch—turns unit on or off.
8. Humidity switch—adjusts temperature of heater to high or low.
9. Fuse light—if lighted, indicates fuse needs changing (mda 10 fuse).
10. Electric outlets—two for accessories.
11. Humidifier kettle—provides humidity to the patient.
12. Assist attachment—a selector switch for assisted or controlled ventilation.
13. Deep breathing attachment—a blower that turns on periodically to provide a greatly increased volume.
14. Spirometer—indicates approximate tidal volume.

Procedure for Patient Use

1. Attach power cord to suitable outlet.
2. Fill humidifier with warm water until water level is in the middle of glass gauge.
3. Switch heater to high.
4. Switch on pump, which starts the ventilator.
5. Set tidal volume by turning crank; observe volume scale on lower front of ventilator.
6. Set ceiling pressure by adjusting knurled knob on cap of kettle. To set pressure:
   a. Obstruct ventilator outlet to patient.
   b. Observe pressure monitor for ceiling pressure.
7. Set respiration rate by adjusting inspiratory and expiratory controls on panel.
8. Oxygen may be added through a nipple on the back of the ventilator (refer to preceding formula).
9. Adjust sigh volume and time.
10. Set ventilator in assistor–controller position (if unit is equipped with accessory).
11. Attach spirometer mounting and connect spirometer tee to exhalation port of ventilator.
12. Adjust ventilator alarm (if unit is equipped with accessory).

Cleaning and Sterilization. For cleaning between patients, remove the breathing hoses, **Y**-piece, trap bottles, and other external parts. Cold- or gas-sterilize them. The kettle and metal tube can be disconnected for sterilization also. If they are, the location of all components should be noted carefully. In particular, the valve (between piston and kettle) must be replaced in position to permit proper flow. Tighten joints securely to prevent leakage and loss of intended volume.

Note: For disconnection of humidifier and delivery tubing refer to Figures 5-13 and 5-14.

1. Disconnect clear tygon control tubing from the exhalation valve by loosening the screw clamp.
2. Remove exhalation valve assembly from unit.
3. Disconnect the other end of the clear tygon tubing from the metal outlet from the cylinder by loosening the screw clamp.
4. Disconnect pressure gauge connection tubing from the metal reducing elbow to the inspiratory tubing.
5. Loosen and unscrew the metal fitting on the inside reducing elbow in the cabinet with wrench provided with unit.
6. Loosen and unscrew metal fitting on the outside of the reducing elbow (be careful of rubber washer).
7. Loosen and unscrew metal tee valve, which has pressure gauge connection tubing nipple.
8. Disconnect top metal elbow of large tygon delivery tubing, containing copper wool, by loosening screw clamp.
9. Disconnect the other end of the large delivery tubing by loosening the screw clamp.
10. Loosen and unscrew remaining fitting on top of kettle (be careful of rubber washer).
11. Loosen and unscrew fitting on the clear tygon inlet tubing on top of kettle (be careful of rubber washer).
12. Remove kettle.
13. Disconnect deep breathing tubing from metal tee valve connection.
14. Loosen and unscrew the lower fitting of the metal tee valve (be careful of rubber washer and tee valve: *has check valve*).
15. Loosen and unscrew upper fitting of the metal tee valve (be careful of rubber washer and tee valve: *has check valve*).
16. Loosen and unscrew metal elbow fitting from the outlet of the cylinder (be careful of rubber washer).

Note: An IMV control is available for the Emerson unit.

ENGSTRÖM RESPIRATOR SYSTEM ER 300

I. Introduction

The Engström Respirator (Figure 5-16) is an indirectly acting, increasing force generator consisting of two systems: the primary, or power generating system, and the secondary, or insufflation system. A respiratory bag in an overpressure chamber separates gases of the two systems. The primary system acts pneumatically upon the secondary system.

The system is comprised of three basic units, which when coupled with three patient systems form suitable combinations for prolonged artificial ventilation and for ventilation during anesthesia. One of the units is adapted for treatment of children, but will not be discussed here.

II. Assembly

A. Assemble patient tubing circuit as shown in the diagrams. Be sure that all connections are tight. The CO_2 absorber may be bypassed if the unit is not to be used in anesthesia.

B. Add distilled water to the humidifier so that the float is visible in the middle of the level glass.

C. Fill the water lock with distilled water.

D. Connect high-pressure oxygen hose to inlet of respirator and then to oxygen source.

E. Plug unit into suitable properly grounded receptacle.

III. Checks before connecting to patient

A. Adjustments—Do Not Connect Patient

1. Set pressure limit valve to 50 cm of water.

2. Set multifunction valve lever to *spirometer on* if using Basic Unit ER 311 (other units have spirometer on at all times).

3. Close drain cock on back of spirometer.

4. Turn negative expiratory pressure control knob to minimum setting if it is available on the unit being used.

5. Set switch for rotameter flow to *vaporizer off* position, so that rotameter gas is connected directly to inspiratory line. (On Basic Unit 313, the switch is not included as the rotameter gases are connected directly to the inspiratory line.)

6. Turn end expiratory pressure and expiratory resistance control to neutral position.

7. Turn on main switch.

8. Set respiratory frequency to 20/min.

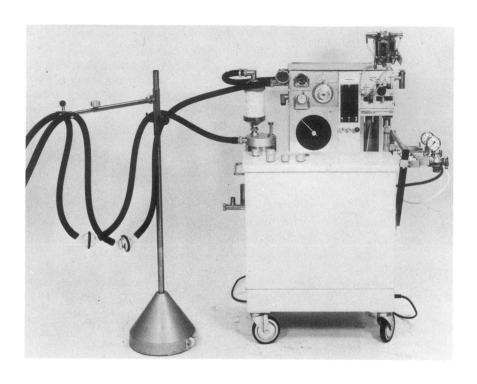

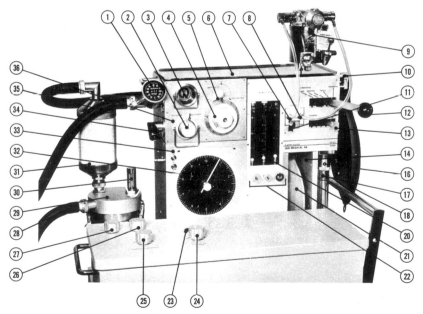

Figure 5-16. Engström Respirator System ER 300. (*Courtesy of LKB Medical, Inc., Rockville, Md.*)

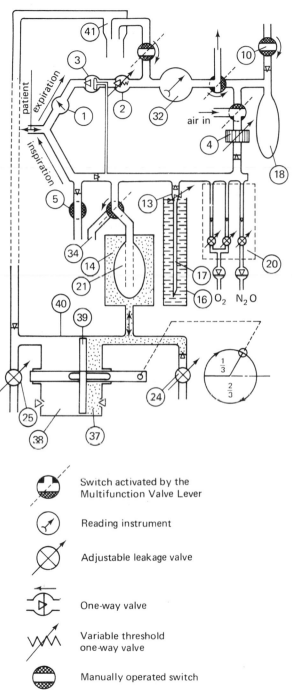

patient

expiration

inspiration

air in

O₂ N₂O

Switch activated by the
Multifunction Valve Lever

Reading instrument

Adjustable leakage valve

One-way valve

Variable threshold
one-way valve

Manually operated switch

Figure 5-16. (*cont.*)

B. Test for tightness of patient system

    1. Attach test lung to patient connection.

    2. Open dosage valve to approximately 10 liters.

    3. Open supplementary air inlet switch.

    4. Turn expiratory resistance control fully clockwise to close expiratory line.

    5. When tubing pressure gauge reads 35 cm of water, turn off respirator.

    6. After 50 sec, the pressure should still be stationary. A decrease would indicate a leak in the patient system.

    7. Return expiratory resistance control to the neutral position and switch on respirator.

C. Test for tightness of respiratory bag

    1. Close air inlet by turning dosage valve fully clockwise; turn off all gas rotameters.

    2. Occlude patient connection with thumb; spirometer and tubing pressure gauge readings should remain stable.

D. Test function of expiratory valve

    1. Attach test lung to patient connection.

    2. You must observe the spirometer and tubing pressure gauge at the same time. On inspiration, as tubing pressure increases, the spirometer should remain absolutely stationary. If movement of the spirometer needle is noted, this indicates a leakage in the expiratory valve; the valve must be removed from its housing and replaced.

E. Test function of dosage valve

    1. Adjust dosage valve to 10 liters.

    2. Adjust emptying pressure to 70 cm of water.

    3. Attach test lung to patient connection and observe the spirometer for 1 min. Frequency must be 20/min; the spirometer should read 10 liters after 20 respirations.

    4. If there is greater than ±5% difference between the dosage valve setting and the return volume on the spirometer, the dosage valve must be recalibrated. (See Engstrom instruction manual for details.)

F. Final adjustment before connecting to patient

    1. Determine minute ventilation required by patient and set according to the ventilation nomogram for the Engstrom Respirator (supplied by the manufacturer; see Figure 5-17). For example, according to the nomogram, for a minute volume of 8 liters/min at 41% oxygen, you would set the oxygen rotameter at 2 liters/min and the

O₂ CONCENTRATION
FOR ENGSTROM RESPIRATOR
O₂ - LPM

L/M	0	1	2	3	4	5	6	7	8	9	10	11	12	13	14	15	16	17	18	19	20	21	22	23	24	25
1	21	100																								
2	21	61	100																							
3	21	47	74	100																						
4	21	41	61	80	100																					
5	21	37	53	68	84	100																				
6	21	34	47	61	74	87	100																			
7	21	32	44	55	66	77	89	100																		
8	21	31	41	51	61	70	80	90	100																	
9	21	30	39	47	56	65	74	82	91	100																
10	21	29	37	45	53	61	68	76	84	92	100															
11	21	28	35	43	50	57	64	71	78	86	93	100														
12	21	28	34	41	47	54	61	67	74	80	87	93	100													
13	21	27	33	39	45	51	57	64	70	76	82	88	94	100												
14	21	27	32	38	44	49	55	61	66	72	77	83	89	94	100											
15	21	26	32	37	42	47	53	58	63	68	74	79	84	89	95	100										
16	21	26	31	36	41	46	51	56	61	65	70	75	80	85	90	95	100									
17	21	26	30	35	40	44	49	54	58	63	67	72	77	81	86	91	95	100								
18	21	25	30	34	39	43	47	52	56	61	65	69	74	78	82	87	91	96	100							
19	21	25	29	33	38	42	46	50	54	58	63	67	71	75	79	83	88	92	96	100						
20	21	25	29	33	37	41	45	49	53	57	61	64	68	72	76	80	84	88	92	96	100					
21	21	25	28	32	36	40	44	47	51	55	59	62	66	70	74	77	81	85	89	92	96	100				
22	21	25	28	32	35	39	43	46	50	53	57	61	64	68	71	75	78	82	86	89	93	96	100			
23	21	24	28	31	35	38	42	45	48	52	55	59	62	66	69	73	76	79	83	86	90	93	97	100		
24	21	24	28	31	34	37	41	44	47	51	54	57	61	64	67	70	74	77	80	84	87	90	93	97	100	
25	21	24	27	30	34	37	40	43	46	49	53	56	59	62	65	68	72	75	78	81	84	87	91	94	97	100

Figure 5-17.

dosage valve at 6 liters/min (room air). The dosage valve setting is derived by subtracting the liter flow of oxygen required from the total desired minute volume.

2. Set the emptying pressure control (if the unit being used is not preset) to regulate the pressure in the overpressure chamber during inspiration. This should be 30 to 50 cm of water above the maximum peak inspiratory pressure indicated on the tubing pressure gauge for 1 min and is read on the scale for emptying pressure control. This may be set at approximately 70 cm of water initially and re-adjusted after connecting patient.

3. Check settings of other controls
   a. Respirator *on*
   b. Frequency
   c. Dosage valve
   d. Rotameter—*vaporizer off*
   e. Multifunction valve lever to *spirometer on*
   f. Pressure limit valve lever (30 to 70 cm of water)
   g. End expiratory pressure and expiratory resistance valve—if desired

      h. Pressure drop alarm—set to about 15 cm of water and switch on alarm

  4. Connect patient

IV. Checks to be made after connecting to patient

  A. Check water lock—if gas bubbles through, it may be due to asynchronous respiration of patient and total ventilation needs adjustment.

  B. Adjust emptying pressure control.

  C. Check for leakage in patient circuit.

V. Cleaning and Sterilization

  A. Disassemble patient system.

    1. Disconnect tubing and remove instrument tray.

    2. Open the door on the right side of the patient system, loosen lock on multifunction valve lever, pull out lever, and remove valve piston.

    3. Remove pressure limit plug-in valve in same manner.

    4. Pull out expiratory valve insert; unscrew butterfly screw on back of expiratory valve.

    5. Remove end expiratory pressure and expiratory resistance control with its valve.

    6. Pull out the tubing pressure gauge.

    7. Unscrew dosage valve (turn counterclockwise) and pull out remaining parts from patient system.

    8. Remove patient system valve box from respirator.

    9. Disassemble humidifier.

    10. Remove Venturi tube and connector for the spirometer.

  B. The following parts may be heat or steam sterilized in an autoclave:

    1. Patient system valve box, after removing parts listed above

    2. End expiratory pressure and expiratory resistance valve

    3. Dosage valve

    4. Expiratory housing after expiratory valve has been removed

    5. Tubing pressure gauge (*not the cable!*)

    6. Multifunction valve piston

    7. Pressure limit plug-in valve

    8. Glass inner water column tube

    9. Metal holder for water lock

    10. Venturi tube

    11. Connector for spirometer

    12. Humidifier

    13. Locks for CO_2 absorber

    14. Respiratory bag (maximum 105°C or cold sterilize)

    15. Patient tubing (maximum 105°C or cold sterilize)

C. The following parts must be cold sterilized:

    1. Spirometer (may also be gas sterilized)

    2. Expiratory valve—do not allow moisture to enter small opening on upper side of valve.

    3. Plexiglass outer water lock container

Note: No alcohol should penetrate into the small holes on the upper side of the valve. The housing of the valve can be autoclaved. Remove the respiratory bag (11) and rinse with a disinfectant or heat sterilize it at 105°C.

D. Disconnect and disassemble the gas humidifier (1); remove, sponge, and rinse in detergent and water; if replacement is necessary, soak the new sponge in detergent and water before use in humidifier to assure maximal humidity output; the rest of the humidifier can be autoclaved.

MONAGHAN 225 VOLUME VENTILATOR

I. Introduction

The Monaghan 225 Volume Ventilator (Figure 5-18) may be operated as an assistor, controller, or assistor/controller. Although it is primarily a volume-cycled unit, it may also be operated on a pressure or time-cycled basis.

    The 225 operates from a 50-psig, 100% oxygen source. The desired oxygen concentration is obtained by the mixture of ambient air and oxygen during exhalation. Thus, the mixture is not affected by inspiratory time, tidal volume, flow rate, or inspiratory pressure. However, use of tidal volumes of less than 100 ml may result in unpredictable and erratic operation and an increase in oxygen concentration.

II. Assembly

A. Screw the support arm into the top of the floor stand.

B. Insert the main line bacteria filter into its bracket, with the flow pointing toward the back of the unit. Tighten the thumb screw.

C. Place the humidifier on the humidifier bracket.

D. Connect a 12-in. corrugated tube from the outlet on the main line bacteria filter to the *inlet* on the humidifier.

E. Connect another 12-in. tube from the *outlet* on the ventilator to the inlet of the bacteria filter.

F. Assemble the patient circuit as shown in the diagrams.

G. Connect the patient supply hose to the humidifier *outlet*.

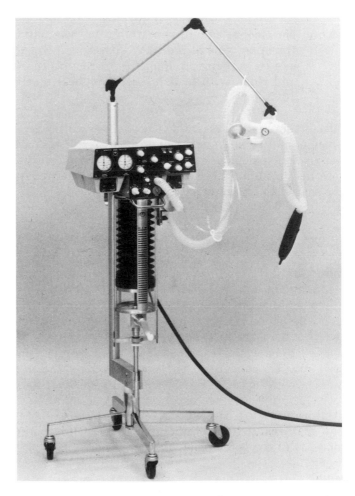

Figure 5-18. Monaghan 225 Volume Ventilator. (*Courtesy of Monaghan, a division of Sandoz-Wander, Inc., Little, Colo.*)

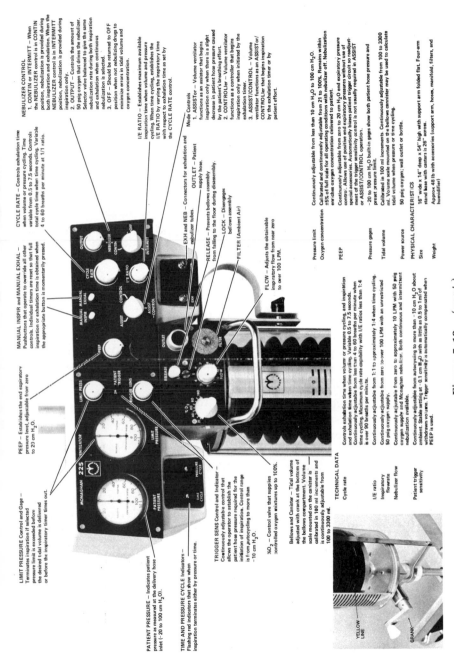

LIMIT PRESSURE Control and Gage — If selected pressure limit is exceeded before the desired tidal volume is delivered or before the inspiratory timer times out.

PATIENT PRESSURE — Indicates patient pressure as measured at the delivery hose inlet (−20 to 100 cm H_2O).

TIME AND PRESSURE CYCLE Indicators — Flashing red indicators that show when inspiration terminates either by pressure or time.

TRIGGER SENS Control and Indicator — Continuously adjustable control that allows the operator to establish the patient hose pressure required for the initiation of inspiration. Control range is from autocycling to more than −10 cm H_2O.

Bellows and Canister — Tidal volume adjusted with crank at the bottom of the bellows compartment. Volume scale mounted on the canister is calibrated in 180 ml increments and is continuously adjustable from 100 to 3300 ml.

%O₂ — Control valve that supplies controlled oxygen mixtures up to 100%.

PEEP — Establishes the end expiratory pressure level, adjustable from zero to 20 cm H_2O.

MANUAL INSPIR and MANUAL EXHAL — Pushbuttons that operate to override all other controls. Individual timers are reset so that full inspiration or exhalation time is obtained when the appropriate button is momentarily pressed.

CYCLE RATE — Controls exhalation time when volume or pressure cycling. Time variable from 0.5 to 7.5 seconds. Controls total cycle time when time cycling. Variable 4 to 60 breaths per minute at 1/1 ratio.

I/E RATIO — Establishes maximum available inspiration time when volume and pressure cycling. When time cycling, establishes the I/E RATIO by varying the inspiratory time with respect to exhalation time as set by the CYCLE RATE control.

NEBULIZER CONTROL
1. CONTIN or INTERMITT — When the NEBULIZER control is in CONTIN position, nebulization is provided during both inspiration and exhalation. When the NEBULIZER control is in INTERMITT position, nebulization is provided during inspiration only.
2. OUTPUT — Controls the amount of 50 psig oxygen that drives the nebulizer. Selector valve balanced to give the same nebulization rate during both inspiration and exhalation when continuous nebulization is selected.
3. OFF — Should be returned to OFF position when not nebulizing drugs to minimize errors in tidal volume and oxygen concentration.

OUTLET — Patient supply hose.

EXH and NEB — Connectors for exhalation and nebulizer tubes.

RELEASE — Prevents bellows assembly from falling to the floor during disassembly.

LOCK — Disengages bellows assembly.

FILTER (Ambient Air)

FLOW — Adjusts the obtainable inspiratory flow from near zero to over 100 LPM.

Mode Controls
1. ASSISTor — Volume ventilator functions as an assistor that begins inspiration only when there is a slight decrease in patient hose pressure caused by the patient's breathing effort.
2. CONTROLer — Volume ventilator functions as a controller that begins inspiration only when initiated by the exhalation timer.
3. ASSIST/CONTROL — Volume ventilator functions as an ASSISTor/CONTROLer that begins inspiration by the exhalation timer or by patient effort.

TECHNICAL DATA

Cycle rate — Controls exhalation time when volume or pressure cycling, and inspiration and exhalation time when time cycling. Variable 0.5 to 7.5 seconds. Continuously adjustable from less than 4 to 60 breaths per minute when time cycling. Maximum cycle rate capability with I/E ratios less than 1:4 is over 90 breaths per minute.

I/E ratio — Continuously adjustable from 1:1 to approximately 1:4 when time cycling. Continuously adjustable from zero to over 50 psig oxygen supply.

Inspiratory flowrate — Continuously adjustable from zero to approximately 10 LPM with 50 psig oxygen supply.

Nebulizer flow — Continuously adjustable from zero to approximately 10 LPM with 50 psig oxygen supply and Mcnaghan nebulizer. Both continuous and intermittent nebulization available.

Patient trigger sensitivity — Continuously adjustable from autocycling to more than −10 cm H_2O about ambient. Stable setting at −0.1 cm H_2O with as little as 0.5 to 1 ml of withdrawn volume. Trigger sensitivity is automatically compensated when PEEP is used.

Pressure limit — Continuously adjustable from less than 10 cm H_2O to 100 cm H_2O.

Oxygen concentration — Calibrated and continuously adjustable from 21 to 100%. Remains within ±5% of full scale for all operating conditions with nebulizer off. Nebulization enriches oxygen concentration delivered to patient.

PEEP — Continuously adjustable from zero to 20 cm H_2O and expiratory pressure control. Allows use of positive end expiratory pressures without use of special accessories. Automatically biases patient trigger circuit so readjustment of the trigger sensitivity control is not usually required in ASSIST or ASSIST/CONTROL operation.

Pressure gages — −20 to 100 cm H_2O built-in gags show both patient hose pressure and preset pressure limit.

Tidal volume — Calibrated in 100 ml increments. Continuously adjustable from 100 to 3300 ml. Volume scale mounted on the bellows canister may be used to calculate tidal volume with pressure or time cycling.

Power source — 50 psig oxygen; wall outlet or bottle.

PHYSICAL CHARACTERISTICS

Size — 16" wide x 14" deep x 54" high with support arm folded flat. Four-arm stand base with casters is 26" across.

Weight — Approx. 48 lb with accessories (support arm, hoses, manifold, filters, and humidifier).

YELLOW LINE

CRANK

Figure 5-18. (cont.)

291

H. Add sterile water to the humidifier.

I. Connect the exhalation and nebulizer tubes to the ports on the unit.

J. Connect a high-pressure hose to the oxygen inlet filter on the unit. Connect the other end to a 40–50 psig oxygen source.

K. Plug the power cord on the humidifier into a 115- or 220-V grounded electrical outlet.

III. Operation
Refer to Figure 5-18 for a complete description of all controls and indicators.

A. Use as a volume instrument
1. Turn the I/E ratio knob fully clockwise.
2. Set the pressure limit control (LIMIT PRESS). Allow for a slightly greater pressure than you expect to need to deliver the desired volume.
3. Set the desired volume by turning the crank located on the bottom of the bellows compartment.
4. Set the flow rate (FLOW) control.
5. Set the frequency (CYCLE RATE).
6. Set the oxygen concentration desired. (With the nebulizer in the *off* position, the percentage of oxygen will be ±5% of the setting.)
7. Select the mode of operation:
   a. Assist
   b. Control
   c. Assist–control
8. Set the sensitivity (TRIGGER SENS) with a test lung or patient attached.
   a. Press and hold the Manual Exhalation button.
   b. At the same time, rotate the sensitivity control clockwise until the indicator (PATIENT TRIGGER) flashes.
   c. Turn sensitivity control counterclockwise just enough to allow indicator to go out.
9. Set PEEP, if desired, using a test lung, or after connecting the ventilator to the patient. The amount of PEEP will be indicated on the PATIENT PRESSURE gauge.
10. Select nebulization—continuous or intermittent, and amount of output.

B. Use as a pressure instrument

All controls are set the same as for volume operation except:

1. Volume—set higher than you expect to be required by the patient.

2. Set pressure limit for desired pressure. It will be indicated on the LIMIT PRESSURE gauge.

C. Use as a time-limited instrument

1. Volume—set higher than expected to be required.

2. Pressure limit—set for greater pressure than you expect to need to deliver the desired volume.

3. Flow rate—set at one (1).

4. Frequency—set CYCLE RATE for an easily determined exhalation time (4 sec, for example).

5. Set I/E ratio.

6. Set desired CYCLE RATE (ratio will remain constant with TIME CYCLE indicator flashing).

7. Adjust flow rate.

8. Set percentage of oxygen.

9. The unit must be adjusted as an assistor–controller or as a controller only. Do not use in the assist mode, as the exhalation timer does not operate.

10. Set PEEP.

11. Select nebulization requirements.

IV. Cleaning and Sterilization

A. Disassemble all parts—tubing, humidifier, etc.

B. Wash in a detergent solution and rinse well.

C. Wipe the outside of the unit with a detergent solution.

D. Unless used in a contaminated atmosphere, the bellows do not require special cleaning or sterilization.

E. The following parts may be sterilized by cold sterilization, autoclaving, or gas sterilization:

1. Nebulizer

2. Patient supply hose and manifold

3. Humidifier

F. The bacteria filters should be *steam autoclaved* only (250° to 300°F (121°–149°C) for 15 min) after each use. Room air dry for 15 to 16 hours minimum.

G. The 225 ventilator may be gas sterilized. All rubber components and filters may be autoclaved at 250°F (121°C) for 15 min.

GILL 1 VOLUME-CONTROLLED RESPIRATOR

I. Introduction

The Gill 1 (Figure 5-19) is a volume-cycled, pressure-limited, electrically powered, positive-pressure ventilator. It may be operated as an assistor, controller, or assistor–controller. It should not be used in an oxygen-enriched atmosphere or in an area where flammable anesthetics are used or stored.

II. Assembly (back panel of Gill 1)

A. Place mainline bacterial filter into its bracket on the rear panel of the unit with the *outlet* end up.

B. Attach outlet tubing coming from rear of the Gill to the tee adapter.

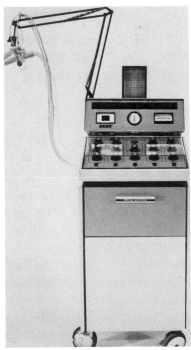

Figure 5-19.   Gill 1 Volume-Controlled Respirator. (*Courtesy of Healthcare Systems, Medical Products Division, Chemetrom Corp., St. Louis, Mo.*)

C. Fit the flexible tee adapter connector over the inlet port of the filter. Insert the tee adapter into the flexible connector.

D. Fit the oxygen sensor over the tee adapter and plug the sensor cord into the oxygen sensor receptacle on the rear panel. *Note:* When the cap of the oxygen sensor is removed, the cell must be installed so that the screened sensing surface is facing out.

E. Fill the humidifier to the correct level (by the outlet port or the access plugs) and clamp into the heating pad.

F. Connect the short humidifier connector hose to the outlet port of the mainline bacterial filter and to the inlet port of the humidifier reservoir.

G. Place the tracking arm into the bracket located on the left or right side of the Gill.

H. Place the spirometer mounting bracket into one of the tracking arm brackets.

I. Attach the assembled spirometer (Bennett model) into the spirometer mounting bracket.

J. Connect one end of the spirometer control tube to the spirometer base and the other end of the spirometer control connector on the rear of the respirator.

K. Attach a collector bottle to the bottom end of the spirometer pole; attach exhalation valve port of the patient manifold to the spirometer by means of corrugated tubing to the port of the collector bottle.

Note: The monitoring spirometer is not recommended for use during intermittent mandatory ventilation (IMV).

III. Assembly of Patient Breathing Circuit

A. Attach manifold assembly to arm as with any other ventilator.

B. Put all small tubing through the retaining clip at the top of the tracking arm.

Note: If the disposable patient breathing circuit you are using does not have a pressure sense line, almost any oxygen connecting tubing may be used for this line.

C. Attach thermometer adapter, thermometer, nebulizer pressure line and filter, pressure sense line, pressure sense line filter, and the pressure sense line adapter to the manifold.

Note: The thermometer, thermometer adapter, pressure sense line filter, pressure sense line adapter, and the nebulizer filter are *not disposable* items. (See cleaning and sterilization.) The nebulizer filter and the pressure sense line filter must be mounted vertically above the patient manifold. If not, condensation will collect in the filter material causing obstruction, and will not drain back into the patient manifold. Proper operation of all pressure sensing controls and alarms also depends on proper installation.

IV. Assembly of Patient Circuit Hoses to the Back Panel of the Gill 1

Note: If oxygen is to be used, attach one end of the O_2 high-pressure line to the O_2 inlet on the back panel of the Gill and the other end to the supply source.

A. Attach the large-bore tubing (inspiratory line) of the patient circuit to the humidifier outlet on the back panel of the Gill.

B. Attach the expiration valve control line, nebulizer pressure line, and the pressure sensor line to their respective ports on the rear panel.

C. Plug power cord into 120-V, 60-cycle, ac *grounded* receptacle.

V. Setup and Test Procedure *Before* Connecting to Patient

A. After assembly as above, push power switch to the *on* position.

Note: After about 40 sec, the breaths per minute display will illuminate.

B. Push test button.

Note: All indicator panel lights should illuminate and all segments of the breaths per minute display should show the numerals 88. The power failure may vary in intensity; if it does not illuminate, change the four AA type batteries in the power failure battery box on the rear panel of the Gill.

C. Check the audible alarm by turning the alarm–reset control to *Loud*. Have the wye open on the patient circuit and push the manual breath switch. The low-pressure alarm should light up at the end of the inspiratory phase, and the audible alarm should sound.

D. Check the inspiration volume indicator; the set control volume and the indicated volume should agree, and the indicator should drop to zero at the end of delivery.

E. Checking for respirator and patient leaks:
   1. Turn the normal breath rate control off.
   2. Turn the nebulizer switch off.
   3. Set normal volume control to 1000 ml.
   4. Set peak flow rate control over 60 liters/min. Occlude the wye connector on the patient circuit. Press and hold the *test* switch. The inspiration volume indicator should drop rapidly to a lesser volume and stop. If the indicator continues to drop toward zero, there is a leak in the system. The leak may be found by occluding the patient tubing at various points of the circuit, while depressing and holding the *test* switch at each point. *Observe the inspiration volume indicator until there is no leak.*

F. Check the *normal* pressure limit.
   1. Set normal volume to 1000 ml.
   2. Set peak flow rate at 40 liters/min.
   3. Set the pressure limit control in turn to 20, 60, and 100 cm of water; at each setting, occlude the airway at the wye connector, and during the inspiratory stroke observe the pressure gauge. The pressure should rise to the set pressure limit, at which point the inspiration cycle should terminate, and the pressure limit alarm should illuminate.

G. Remove the O_2 sensor from the patient breathing circuit and calibrate the O_2 meter to either room air or 100% O_2, whichever is closer to the oxygen concentration to be used.

H. Set O_2 percentage control for desired concentration. Allow approximately 40 sec for O_2 percent meter response.

I. Set normal breath, breath contour, sensitivity, alarm–reset, and sigh controls to desired position.

J. Set temperature control to maintain the desired temperature. Turn control clockwise to increase temperature and consult the airway thermometer for response. Allow 20 minutes for preheating water.

K. If ordered, fill the nebulizer cup at the patient manifold and depress the nebulizer switch on.

L. Connect Gill to patient via patient manifold.

M. Check the system for small air leaks:

1. Set the inflation hold control between 0.6 and 2 sec.

   Note: Continuous use of the inflation hold device may be contraindicated in patients with cardiac problems.

2. Observe the pressure gauge during the next delivery stroke. The needle should rise to peak pressure and then drop suddenly to a point where the breathing circuit pressure and the pressure in the lungs have equalized. The needle will hold at this point for approximately two-thirds of the inflation hold period. If the pressure does not hold at this point, but instead the pressure reading continues to drop, there is an air leak in the system that includes the endotracheal tube and cuff.

3. If there are no significant leaks, turn the inflation hold control off or to the desired setting.

VI. IMV Setup Procedure

A. Connect a straight rubber adapter to the inlet port of the nebulizer on the ventilator circuit.

B. Connect the patient port of a one-way valve (such as Air-Shields E-2) to the straight rubber adapter.

C. Attach the *inspiratory tubing* of the ventilator to the *expiratory port* on the one-way valve.

D. Connect a straight rubber adapter to the *inspiratory port* on the one-way valve.

E. Attach a Venturi-style tee of the desired FIO_2 to the rubber adapter.

   Note: The patient port on the tee must be left open to the atmosphere if accurate FIO_2's are to be maintained.

F. Connect oxygen connecting tubing from the nipple on the Venturi to an oxygen flowmeter and humidifier. Adjust liter flow.

G. Connect large-bore aerosol tubing to humidity adapter on tee; connect other end to all-purpose nebulizer, which is powered by compressed air. Adjust liter flow for adequate humidity.

H. Adjust the IMV interval on the ventilator by turning the thumbwheel to the desired interval between respirator cycles (adjustable from 5 to 199 sec).

I. Depress the IMV *on/off* switch. It will light, and remain illuminated until the IMV mode is canceled. During use of the IMV mode, the normal rate and sigh interval controls do not operate.

VII. Cleaning and Sterilization Procedure

A. Dispose of any disposable items.

B. Dismantle, wash in detergent solution, and rinse well
   1. Humidifier, access caps, and inlet and outlet adapters
   2. Oxygen adapter tee
   3. Humidifier connector hose
   4. Pressure sense adapter
   5. Monitoring spirometer and component parts (except alarm and black valve)
   6. Rubber adapters

C. The above parts may all be gas sterilized.

D. The following should be wiped with 70% isopropyl alcohol and packaged for *steam autoclaving* at 250°F (121°C) for 30 min
   1. Mainline bacteria filter
   2. Nebulizer filter
   3. Pressure sense line filter

E. The following should be wiped with 70% isopropyl alcohol and returned to use
   1. Oxygen sensor probe
   2. Thermometer
   3. Spirometer alarm
   4. Spirometer black valve

F. The exterior of the ventilator should be cleaned with 70% isopropyl alcohol or a mild neutral detergent.

VIII. Alarm Indicators

All alarm indicators are colored red. The following alarms provide the therapist with an indication that a problem has developed.

A. Pressure limit alarm—audiovisual
B. Improper cycle alarm—audiovisual
C. Low pressure alarm—audiovisual
D. Power failure alarm—audiovisual
E. Improper oxygen alarm—audiovisual
F. I/E ratio alarm—visual
G. Fill humidifier alarm—audiovisual

IX. Other Displays and Indicators

A. Inspiration volume indicator displays the exact delivered tidal volume.
B. Pressure gauge displays pressures reached at the patient manifold.
C. Oxygen meter indicates the oxygen concentration in the delivered gas with ±4% accuracy.
D. Breaths per minute display digitally shows patient's respiratory rate per minute averaged over a 30-sec period, in even numbers only. (When the ventilator is first turned on, the display will be blank for approximately 40 sec. When the control panel test switch is pressed, the number 88 should appear to indicate that all segments are functioning.)
E. Circuit breakers and power failure alarms warn the therapist of electrical problems; the two circuit breakers protect the unit from electrical damage.
F. Mode indicators:
    1. Control—green light shows each controlled inspiration.
    2. Assist—amber light shows each patient-initiated inspiration.
    3. Add oxygen—continuous green light shows oxygen is being added to the delivered gas volume.
    4. Sigh—white light shows each sigh volume delivered.
    5. Alarms silent—continuous white light shows that all audible alarms (except power failure) have been silenced. All visual alarms continue to function as normal.

SEARLE ADULT VOLUME VENTILATOR

I. Introduction

The Searle Ventilator (Figure 5-20) is a volume-cycled unit utilizing electronic logic for control and monitoring of the key respiratory parameters. Tidal volume, respiratory rate, and inspiratory flow rate are noninteracting controls that set the basic ventilation pattern.

II. Assembly

A. Attach support arm to handle on ventilator, using handle that provides most mobility, depending on position of unit in relation to patient.

B. Screw IV support pole into remaining handle.

C. Install the spirometer on the right-hand column.

D. Install spirometer liner.

1. Open snap locks on front of spirometer and open door fully.

2. Remove liner from its package.

3. Align liner's connector port with the connector on the 41-in. flexible tubing and snap into place by pressing on rear surface of the liner.

4. After connecting flexible tubing, close door and lock.

5. Attach bracket for humidifier below spirometer.

6. Attach humidifier heating element to bracket.

7. Install humidifier cartridge.

a. Place cartridge (cone down) on heating element.

b. Slide lock ring over cartridge and rotate clockwise. Do not force threaded connection.

8. Suspend suitable solution container from IV support pole and attach tubing set.

9. Connect 12-in. flexible tidal inlet tubing to humidifier cartridge air inlet.

10. Connect 27-in. flexible tidal outlet tube to humidifier cartridge air outlet.

11. Connect other end of 27-in. tube to far left port on manifold.

12. Attach 21-in. flexible patient inhalation tube to far right port on manifold.

13. Attach other end to suitable patient connection (angled or straight wye).

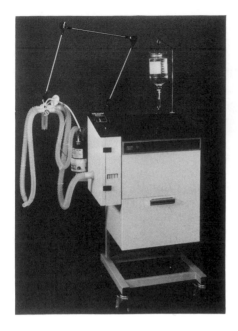

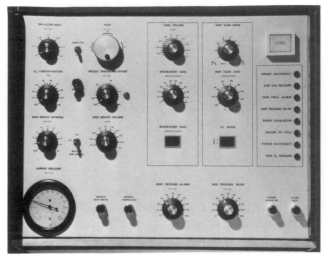

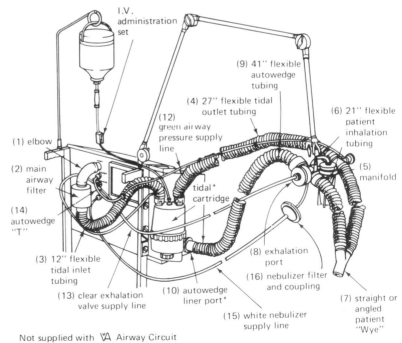

I.V.
administration
set

(9) 41" flexible
autowedge
tubing

(4) 27" flexible tidal
outlet tubing

(6) 21" flexible
patient
inhalation
tubing

(12)
green airway
pressure supply
line

(1) elbow

(5)
manifold

(2) main
airway
filter

tidal*
cartridge

(14)
autowedge
"T"

(8) exhalation
port

(3) 12" flexible
tidal inlet
tubing

(16) nebulizer filter
and coupling

(7) straight or
angled
patient
"Wye"

(13) clear exhalation
valve supply line

(10) autowedge
liner port*

(15) white nebulizer
supply line

Not supplied with VA Airway Circuit

Figure 5-20. Searle Adult Volume Ventilator. (*Courtesy of Searle Cardio-Pulmonary Systems, Inc., a subsidiary of G. D. Searle and Co., Emeryville, Calif.*)

14. Attach another 21-in. tube to the remaining port on the patient connection. Connect the other end to the exhalation port on the near right of the manifold.

15. Connect 41-in. flexible spirometer tubing to the near left exhalation port on the manifold. The other end has already been connected to the spirometer liner port.

16. Attach the pressure supply line (green) to the airway pressure outlet on the rear panel of the unit.

17. Attach the other end to the airway fitting on the manifold.

18. Attach spirometer tee to exhalation valve port on rear of spirometer.

19. Attach clear supply line to tee.

20. Connect other end to exhalation valve port on manifold.

21. Connect 48-in. nebulizer tubing (white) to port on rear of unit.

22. Attach other end to nebulizer bacteria filter and coupling in manifold.

23. Connect spirometer and humidifier power cords to 110-V accessory outlets on back of unit.

24. Plug unit power cord into properly grounded outlet.

25. Press red ventilator and accessory circuit breakers.

26. Attach high-pressure oxygen hose to inlet on unit and then to oxygen source.

III. Operation

A. Turn on power switch.

B. Set desired tidal volume in a range from 0.3 to 2.2 liters.

C. Set the desired respiratory rate from 5 to 60 breaths/min. The average of the last 8 to 10 breaths will be digitally displayed on the rate display.

D. Set the inspiratory flow rate, up to 200 liters/min; this rate will be maintained up to 90 to 100 cm of water airway pressure. The I/E ratio for the average of the last 8 to 10 breaths will be digitally displayed.

E. Set the inspiratory flow taper in the pattern desired, from square to fully tapered wave.

F. Set the inflation flow taper in the pattern desired, from square to fully tapered wave.

G. Set the inflation hold control, if required, from 0 to 3 sec.

H. Select amount of PEEP, if desired, from 0 to 20 cm of water.

I. Set oxygen concentration desired, from 21 to 100%. (100% oxygen can be delivered for a 4-min interval by pushing the 100% oxygen push button; indicator lamp lights during this interval.)

J. Set patient triggering effort to adjust amount of inspiratory effort (from 0 to 20 cm of negative pressure) required for the patient to initiate inspiration. In the *off* position the patient will be unable to initiate inspiration. An indicator lamp shows each breath that is patient triggered.

K. Select interval between each deep breath (1 to 10 min), the number of consecutive deep breaths per cycle (1, 2, or 3), and the volume of each deep breath (0.3 to 2.2 liters). A manual deep breath control allows you to initiate a deep breath (on the next inspiration) at a time other than that set by the above controls.

L. Set inspiratory pressure alarm, which warns of increasing maximum airway pressure during the delivery.

M. Set inspiratory pressure relief for the maximum airway pressure limit. If the limit is exceeded, inspiration automatically ends and any undelivered tidal volume is dumped.

N. If mechanical nebulization is desired, turn on nebulizer switch.

IV. Warning Systems
The unit contains several audiovisual alarms that indicate when preset parameters are not met or when they are exceeded. The indicator lamps are located on the right front panel of the unit. The continuous alarms may be silenced, allowing for a 10-sec "chirp." The reset button resets all activated warning systems.

V. Cleaning and Sterilization
A. The humidifier cartridge and spirometer liner are disposable.
B. Disassemble patient circuit and wash in detergent solution; rinse and dry; cold sterilize or gas sterilize.
C. Autoclave bacteria filters.

BOURNS MODEL LS 104-150 INFANT VENTILATOR WITH MODEL LS 145 OXYGEN BLENDER

I. Classification
A. Assistor, controller, or assistor–controller
B. Volume-, time-, or pressure-cycled

C. Constant flow generator

D. Positive or passive exhalation

E. Pressure limited

II. Features (see Figure 5-21)

A. V_T adjustable from 10 to 150 ml and indicated by meter readout.

B. Respiratory rate adjustable from 5 to 80 and indicated by meter readout.

C. Assist, control, assistor–controller, PEEP, IMV, or CPAP modes of ventilation.

D. Ultrasonic nebulizer provides humidification (0.5 ml/min).

E. Adjustable flow rate from 50 to 200 ml/sec.

F. Adjustable oxygen concentration from 21 to 100% with ±3% accuracy via oxygen blender.

G. Audible alarms for high- and low-pressure (adjustable), apnea and loss of oxygen or air pressure.

H. Audible and visual alarms for high and low pressure.

I. An adjustable pressure relief valve from 25 to 100 cm of water.

J. Pressure capabilities from 0 to 100 cm of water.

K. Patient assist effort from 0.05 to 1.0 cm of water, inspired volume 0.05 ml, 35-ms response.

L. A leak compensator to control sensitivity of the breathing circuit when compensating for minor leaks in the presence of PEEP. Also used to prevent loss of PEEP due to minor leak when in control mode.

III. Operation

A. Preparation

Place the Bourns Model LS 104-150 Infant Ventilator near the infant to reduce tubing length and the Bourns Model LS 145 Oxygen Blender next to the ventilator. Following this step, make the required connections:

1. Electrical supply
   a. Plug the ventilator into a 120-V, ac, 60-Hz grounded electrical source.

2. Gas supply
   a. Connect a 50-psi oxygen source between the 50-psi Oxygen Output (ventilator) and the *To PEEP Valve* (blender).
   b. Connect one end of a high pressure oxygen hose to

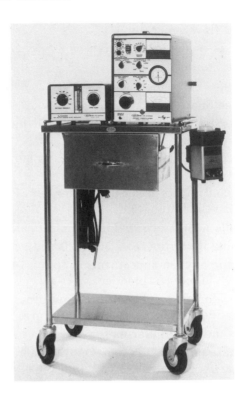

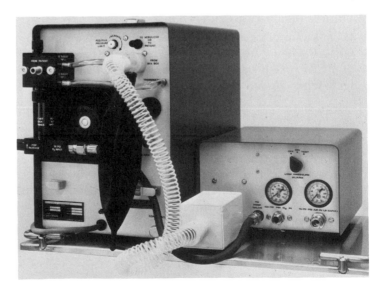

Figure 5-21. Bourns Model LS 1-4-150 Infant Ventilator. (*Courtesy of Bourns Inc., Life Systems Division, Riverdale, Calif.*)

the back of the blender *male DISS Oxygen Fitting*
and the other end to an oxygen cylinder or wall outlet.

   c. Connect one end of a high-pressure air hose to the back
of the blender *male DISS Air Fitting* and the other
end to an air compressor or wall outlet.

3. Blender to ventilator connections

   a. Connect a $\frac{3}{4}$-in. I.D. nonkinkable hose from the *To
Ventilator* port of the blender to the *From Mix Box*
port of the ventilator.

4. Ventilator to Patient connections
Make the following connections:

	Type Hose	From	To
a.	$\frac{3}{8}$-in. I.D. tygon	*To Nebulizer* or to *Patient Fitting* back of ventilator	Nebulizer fitting or the metal fitting, top of humidifier
b.	$\frac{3}{8}$-in. I.D. tygon	Nebulizer fitting or the plastic elbow on the side of humidifier	Black flexible hose adapter
c.	$\frac{3}{8}$-in. I.D. tygon	Black flexible hose tee adapter	*From Patient Fitting* back of ventilator
d.	Black flexible hoses	Each tube connects to an endotracheal tee or corrugated hoses or infant mask (two hoses)	

5. Nebulizer–humidifier

   a. Fill the nebulizer or humidifier to the correct level
with sterile solution. Maintain a constant liquid level
during use.

   b. Place the nebulizer or humidifier on a shelf below the
ventilator and the patient. This will allow water condensate in the tubes to run back to the humidification
source.

6. Setting the ventilator

   a. Perform a system compliance check by using Bourns
compliance calculator.

   b. Set the pressure relief valve on the back of the ventilator to the desired level.

    c. Set the breathing rate.

    d. Adjust the mode selector to assist, control, or assist–control.

    e. Adjust the flow rate to give the I/E ratio desired. The Bourns compliance calculator can be used for this modality.

    f. Set the desired patient effort if in assist mode.

> Note: If PEEP is to be used with assist, it is recommended that the *Patient Effort Control* be placed at mid-range and that the sensitivity be adjusted with the sensitivity control described below. If adjustment of the sensitivity control is not sufficient, then additional range adjustment should be made with the Patient Effort Control.

    g. Set the sigh interval if desired.

    h. Adjust to desired tidal volume. Be sure to correct for compliance loss.

    i. Set the PEEP control to the desired level.

    j. Open the sensitivity control valve all the way (fully counterclockwise).

    k. Set the oxygen concentration to the desired level.

    l. Adjust the high- and low-pressure alarms to the desired levels.

    m. Set the *Low Pressure Alarm Switch* of the blender to the on position.

IV. Cleaning and Sterilization

    A. General maintenance

The Bourns LS 104-150 Infant Ventilator does not contain any "user" serviceable parts. In normal service, lubrication or filter cleaning is not required. It is recommended that the ventilator be returned to the factory every 3000 hours of service for overhaul and relubrication.

    B. External

The external surfaces of the ventilator, mix box, and oxygen controller may be wiped clean after each use with an appropriate germicidal agent. Do not use excessive amounts of liquid cleaning agents. Liquids entering the ventilator or oxygen controller may damage the internal parts. The mix box may be washed internally and externally. Do not allow liquids to enter the bacteria filter.

The bacteria filter may be steam autoclaved 250°F (121°C) for 15 min. Ethylene oxide sterilization of the bacteria filters is not recommended. No known studies have been made of the effectiveness of gaseous sterilization against organisms trapped in loaded filters. The design of the filter is such that normal airing methods and times may not drive off all residual ethylene oxide.

The entire ventilator may be gas sterilized with ethylene oxide at 130°F (54°C) and 8 psig maximum. A 7-day aeration period is required. Shorter aeration periods may be possible with the use of a commercial aerator. Follow the manufacturer's recommendations. Do not aerate at temperatures above 120°F (49°C).

C. Patient circuit

After each patient use or periodically during use, remove and clean the exhalation valve and the tubing system connecting the ventilator to the patient. The tubing and valve may be cleaned by washing in a detergent solution. Rinse thoroughly.

D. Chemical sterilization

Cidex, 2% aqueous activated dialdehyde solution, may be used. Rinse thoroughly after use.

E. Steam autoclaving

The tubing and the exhalation valve may be steam autoclaved (250°F (121°C) for 50 min). Remove plastic knobs before sterilizing. Tygon tubing may change its shape slightly and become cloudy but is still usable. *Do not steam autoclave the entire ventilator.*

F. Ethylene oxide gas sterilization

The tubing and exhalation valve may be gas sterilized. The tubing and exhalation valve diaphragm require an aeration period of 7 days. Shorter aeration periods may be possible by using a commercial aerator. Follow the manufacturer's recommendations. The metal parts of the exhalation valve do not require aeration, but residual gas may be trapped in the internal passages of the valve. Follow the sterilizer manufacturer's recommendations for parts of this nature.

BOURNS BEAR I ADULT VOLUME VENTILATOR

The Bourns Bear I Adult Volume Ventilator (Figure 5-22) is an electronically controlled and pneumatically operated volume-, pressure-, or time-cycled device that delivers accurately controlled air–oxygen

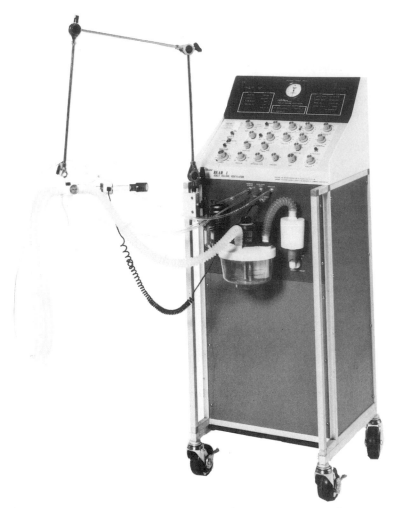

Figure 5-22.   Bear I Adult Volume Ventilator. (*Courtesy of Bourns, Inc.,
Life Systems Division, Riverside, Calif.*)

mixtures. It incorporates constant or decelerating flow and functions
as a controller or an assistor–controller. The ventilator can provide
zero end expiratory pressure (ZEEP), positive end expiratory pressure (PEEP), continuous positive airway pressure (CPAP), a combination of techniques termed synchronous intermittent mandatory
ventilation (SIMV), or an inspiration pause.

Assembly

1. Attach the Bennett cascade humidifier cover to the heater assembly. Turn the two knobs on the humidifier to secure the unit
   in place.

2. Fit the main-flow bacteria filter into the patient output fitting on the front of the ventilator. Observe the flow direction indicated on the filter.

3. Fit the 8-in. flex tube between the bacteria filter outlet and the humidifier inlet.

4. Attach the support arm bracket to either of the handrail supports and tighten. Insert the support arm into the support arm bracket and tighten.

5. Connect the manifold assembly to the support arm with the larger openings facing toward the ventilator.

6. Connect the nebulizer bacteria filter to the white jet connector on the manifold; observe the proper flow direction.

7. Connect the main tube to the humidifier outlet and to the manifold inlet. Connect the $\frac{3}{16}$-in. nebulizer tube to the nebulizer bacteria filter and to the nebulizer connector on the front of the ventilator.

8. Attach the external condenser assembly to the bottom of the support arm bracket by hand tightening the thumbscrew. Cut about 5 to 9 in. of $\frac{1}{4}$-in. tygon tubing and connect one end to the coil assembly and the other end to the fitting marked pressure monitor on the front of the ventilator. The purpose of this assembly is to condense the humidity that may be present in the proximal airway pressure tubing. Should condensation develop, it may be removed by temporarily unscrewing the bowl or the screw under the bowl and emptying it.

9. Connect one end of the two 24-in. circle tubes to the manifold outlet. Connect the other end of the two 24-in. circle tubes to the patient wye. Be sure the proximal airway fitting of the patient wye is on the expiratory side of the patient circuit pointing upward. This will reduce the movement of water up the proximal airway tube.

10. Connect about 4 ft of the $\frac{1}{4}$-in. I.D. tube from the external condenser assembly on the support arm bracket to the proximal airway fitting on the patient wye.

11. Insert the universal adaptor into the large-bore opening of the manifold exhalation valve outlet. Attach the external flow transducer and molded cable assembly to the flow tube. Connect the flow tube into the universal adaptor and the molded cable assembly to the front of the unit marked exhaled flow sensor. Align the connector; gently push it into place and tighten the shell.

12. Attach the $\frac{1}{8}$-in. I.D. exhalation valve tube between the manifold and the front of the machine marked exhalation valve.

13. Attach the air inlet water trap to the air hose assembly. Then

attach the air inlet water trap and the oxygen hose to the rear of the ventilator and to an air/oxygen source. If compressed air is not available, the ventilator will automatically operate from the internal air compressor and only the oxygen hose need be connected.

Operation.   Refer to Figures 5-23 and 5-24 for complete description of all controls and indicators.

1. Following assembly of the patient circuit, but prior to plugging in the ventilator, set the main power switch in the *on* position and verify the audible and visible alarm *vent inoperative*. This tests the power loss alarm batteries.
2. Reset power switch to *off* position; plug electrical cord from ventilator into properly grounded electrical outlet.
3. Attach air and oxygen hoses to air and oxygen source with delivery capability of 30 to 100 psi. If compressed air is not available, the ventilator will automatically operate from the internal air compressor and only the oxygen hose need be connected.
4. Fill the heated humidifier with distilled water to the full mark, setting control at number 6.
5. Adjust the normal rate to desired level.
6. Set the normal pressure limit to maximum (100 cm of water).
7. Set the multiple sigh to the *off* position.
8. Set the sigh volume completely counterclockwise (150 ml).
9. Turn the rate to the minimum position.
10. Adjust the sigh pressure limit to zero.
11. Set the wave form to decelerating flow (tapered), constant flow (square), or a combination in between.
12. Turn the assist sensitivity completely counterclockwise to the position marked less sensitivity.
13. Turn the 1:1 ratio limit to the *on* position.
14. Set the oxygen percentage to the desired level.
15. Set the peak flow to the desired level.
16. Set the inspiratory pause control completely to zero.
17. Set the nebulizer switch to *off*.
18. Turn the PEEP control fully counterclockwise.
19. Set the low inspiratory pressure alarm to zero.
20. Set the minimum exhaled volume alarm to zero.
21. Set the PEEP/CPAP alarm to zero.
22. Set the mode switch to assist–control.

23. Connect a test lung or equivalent to the ventilator.
24. Turn the power switch *on* and observe that the machine is ventilating the test lung. Select mode of operation, control, assist-control, synchronized intermittent mandatory ventilation, or continuous positive airway pressure.

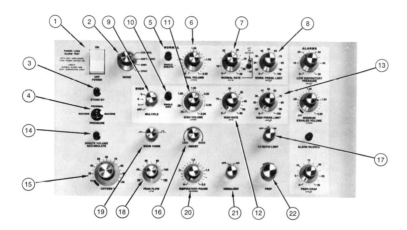

(1) **POWER ON/OFF**—Controls electrical power to the ventilator.

(2) **MODE CONTROL** — Selection of mode of operation.

(3) **STAND-BY** — Controls and alarms disabled except VENT INOPERATIVE and LOW AIR PRESSURE. Ventilator in CPAP mode, audible alarm after 60 seconds. (Display panel shows STAND-BY indicator blinking. Push button to return to normal ventilator operation.)

(4) **PROXIMAL PRESSURE SWITCH** — PROXIMAL position-pressure measured at patient wye; MACHINE position-pressure measured upstream of bacteria filter. (Read on proximal airway pressure gauge.)

(5) **NORMAL SINGLE BREATH** — Manual breath, 100 milliseconds delay prevents double breaths. Operates in all modes.

(6) **TIDAL VOLUME** — 100-2000 ml. When tidal volume is delivered, inspiration ends. (Exhaled tidal volume and minute volume are displayed.)

(7) **NORMAL RATE** — 5-60 BPM; divide by 10-0.5-6 BPM. (Display panel shows RATE ÷ 10 "ON"; breath rate is displayed.)

(8) **NORMAL PRESSURE LIMIT** — 0-100 cmH₂O. When pressure set point is reached, inspiration ends and terminates volume delivery. (Audio-visual alert, PRESS LIMIT on display panel shows pressure reached.)

(9) **MULTIPLE SIGH** — Number of sighs to be delivered in succession at preset intervals. (CONTROL and ASST-CONT modes only.)

(10) **SINGLE SIGH** — Manual sigh, operates in all modes.

(11) **SIGH VOLUME** — 150-3000 ml. When sigh volume is delivered, sigh breath ends.

(12) **SIGH RATE** — 2-60 sighs per hour (CONTROL and ASST-CONT modes only).

(13) **SIGH PRESSURE LIMIT** — 0-100 cmH₂O. When sigh pressure set point is reached, inspiration ends and terminates volume delivery. (Audio-Visual alert, PRESS LIMIT on display panel shows pressure reached.)

(14) **MINUTE VOLUME ACCUMULATE** — Tidal volume accumulates for one minute, displays for second minute, automatically returns to tidal volume. Pushbutton allows immediate return to tidal volume. (MINUTE VOLUME ACCUMULATE indicator blinks during accumulation and remains lit during display.)

(15) **OXYGEN %** — 21-100% oxygen (±3%). Connect to 30-100 psig oxygen source for concentrations higher than 21%. Audio-Visual alert on display panel shows oxygen source pressure less than 30 psig with OXYGEN % control setting higher than 21%.

(16) **ASSIST-SENSITIVITY** — Less (-5 cmH₂O); More (-1 cmH₂O). Senses patient effort, must be adjusted 12-5 o'clock position for ASST-CONT, SIMV, and CPAP to allow proper monitoring and prevent stacked breaths (Display light shows inspiratory source)

(17) **1:1 RATIO LIMIT** — OFF — allows INVERSE I:E RATIO (visual alert only — display panel light shows 1:1 RATIO off). ON — prevents inverse ratio, 1:1 ratio terminates inspiration (Audio-Visual alert).

(18) **PEAK FLOW** — 20-120 LPM. Controls initial flow rate during positive pressure breaths, no affect on spontaneous flow.

(19) **WAVE FORM** — Controls flow patterns delivered during positive pressure breaths.

(20) **INSPIRATORY PAUSE** — 0-2.0 seconds. Delays the beginning of exhalation.

(21) **NEBULIZER** — Allows intermittent administration of medication during positive pressure breaths (10 psig -6 LPM). Does not alter oxygen concentration or tidal volume (display panel light shows NEBULIZER ON).

(22) **PEEP** — 0-30 cmH₂O. Leak make up in all modes except CONTROL (potential spontaneous flow to patient and leak make up is 100 LPM with -1 cmH₂O effort).

CONTROL PANEL

Figure 5-23. Control panel.

DISPLAY PANEL

(1) Indicates by a flashing light that the **EXHALED VOLUME** is being accumulated for one minute. A continuously illuminated indicator signifies that the accumulated **MINUTE VOLUME** is being displayed.

(2) Digital display of **EXHALED VOLUME** on a breath-to-breath basis or **MINUTE VOLUME**.

(3) Digital display of the number of **BREATHS PER MINUTE**. Shows the average of the last twenty seconds and continuously updates itself every second.

(4) Displays level of pressure at the proximal airway from -10 to 100 cmH$_2$O. Machine (system) pressure may also be read on the **PROXIMAL AIRWAY PRESSURE GAUGE** by moving the **PROXIMAL PRESSURE** toggle switch to the left or to the right.

(5) Indicates the **1:1 RATIO LIMIT** switch is in the "OFF" position, permitting inverse **I:E RATIOS** without activating the audible **1:1 RATIO LIMIT** alarm or terminating inspiration.

(6) Digital display of inspiratory time to expiratory time ratio, breath-to-breath. A flashing display indicates greater than a 1:10.0 machine **I:E RATIO**.

(7) **POWER ON** — The machine is plugged into an operating AC power outlet and the POWER switch is "ON".

(8) **STAND-BY** — Controls and alarms disabled, (except VENT INOPERATIVE and LOW AIR PRESS). Ventilator in CPAP mode, STAND-BY indicator blinks, audible alarm after 60 seconds.

(9) **ALARM SILENCE** — Alarms audibly silenced for 60 seconds (exceptions — STAND-BY after 60 seconds elapsed, VENT INOPERATIVE and LOW AIR PRESS).

(10) **NEBULIZER ON** — Nebulizer is on during mechanical inspiration cycle.

(11) **CONTROL** — Ventilator set in CONTROL mode.

(12) **ASST-CONT** — Ventilator set in ASSIST-CONTROL mode.

(13) **SIMV** — Ventilator set in SIMV mode.

(14) **CPAP** — Ventilator set in CPAP mode.

(15) **RATE ÷ 10** — Normal rate is divided by 10 (20 ÷ 10 = 2 BPM)

(16) **SPONTANEOUS** — Patient breath, unassisted (SIMV, CPAP modes).

(17) **CONTROLLED** — Ventilator initiated breath (CONTROL, ASST-CONT, SIMV modes).

(18) **ASSISTED** — Patient initiated breath (ASST-CONT, SIMV modes).

(19) **SIGH** — Sigh breath delivered (Automatic — CONTROL, ASST-CONT; Single — all modes).

(20) **LOW OXYGEN PRESSURE** — Oxygen inlet pressure less than 30 psi and OXYGEN % control set above 21%.

(21) **LOW AIR PRESSURE** — Air pressure less than 9.5 psi.

(22) **PRESSURE LIMIT** — Machine pressure has reached preset level and inspiration terminated (exhaled volume may be less than set tidal volume).

(23) **INVERSE I:E RATIO** — Inspiratory time interval exceeds expiratory time, I:E Ratio less than 1:1. If the 1:1 RATIO LIMIT control is "ON" and the ventilator is in CONTROL mode the 1:1 RATIO LIMIT will terminate inspiration and provide an audible and visual alarm when a 1:1 I:E Ratio is reached.

(24) **LOW PRESSURE** — Inspiratory pressure has not exceeded level set on "LOW INSPIRATORY PRESSURE" alarm.

(25) **LOW PEEP-CPAP** — PEEP/CPAP pressure is less than set on "PEEP/CPAP" control.

(26) **LOW EXHALED VOLUME** — Exhaled volume has not exceeded level set on "MINIMUM EXHALED VOLUME" alarm for three consecutive breaths. Disconnect of clamshell from flow tube will cause alarm on next breath.

(27) **APNEA** — 20 seconds has elapsed since the beginning of the last breath (spontaneous or mechanical).

(28) **VENTILATOR INOPERATIVE** — Total gas, internal electronic or AC power failure. In ASST-CONT, SIMV, or CPAP with PEEP, may be due to patient or circuit disconnect on all models with an "A" following the serial number or units above serial number 1101.

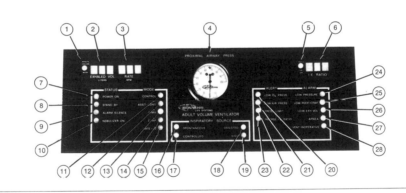

Figure 5-24.   Display panel.

For Patient Ventilation Using the Assist–Control Mode

1. Set the normal rate control to the minimum backup level that is acceptable in the event the patient stops breathing or breathes erratically.

2. Check to see if the peak flow control is set high enough to meet the patient's peak inspiration demands during assisted breaths.

If not, the patient may open the demand valve as necessary to make up the deficit.

3. Readjust the wave form control if necessary.

4. Readjust the tidal volume control to the desired level. For a more accurate delivery of tidal volume, gas lost to total system compliance must be considered.

5. Readjust the normal pressure limit to the desired level. This may be accomplished by temporarily moving the proximal pressure toggle switch to the left or right and reading the proximal airway pressure gauge.

6. Turn the nebulizer control *on* if medication is desired.

7. If sighs are required, set the multiple sigh control, sigh volume control, sigh rate control, and sigh pressure limit control to the desired level.

8. Readjust the oxygen percentage control if necessary.

9. Observe the thermometer; allow 15 min warm-up time for humidifier; if necessary, readjust humidifier temperature.

10. Check to see if the inspiratory pause control is set at zero.

11. Connect patient to ventilator.

12. Observe the patient and display panel.

13. Adjust the assist-sensitivity control to approximately the 2 o'clock position. Be sure the assist indicator on the display panel flashes when the patient takes an assisted breath.

14. If PEEP is used, adjust the PEEP/CPAP alarm about 2 to 3 cm of water below the set PEEP level.

15. Set the low inspiratory pressure alarm by slowly increasing the alarm setting while the ventilator is functioning on the patient. Usually this will be in the range of 5 to 18 cm of water. Then decrease the setting until the alarm ceases.

16. Set the minimum exhaled volume alarm to a level approximately 100 to 200 ml below the exhaled volume digital display.

Cleaning and Sterilization

1. *Ventilator*—except for the display panel, the exterior of the ventilator may be wiped clean with an appropriate bactericidal or germicidal agent. Only alcohol should be used to clean the display panel.

2. *Patient tube system*—The entire patient tube system (except for bacteria filter and thermometer) should be cleaned and sterilized.

3. *Transducer crystals*—These may be wiped clean after each

patient use with an appropriate bactericidal or germicidal agent. The entire molded cable assembly and transducer crystal assembly should not be immersed in liquid or sterilized by ETO gas or steam autoclave.

4. *Bacteria filters*—Under no circumstances should the main flow or nebulizer filters ever be cleaned. They may be sterilized by steam autoclave.

5. *Dust filter*—The air intake filter should be inspected daily. If necessary, it should be removed and vacuum cleaned.

SERVO VENTILATOR 900/900B

The Servo Ventilator 900/900B (Figures 5-25 through 5-27) is an electronically controlled ventilator for intensive care and anesthesia use. It can be set for volume or pressure generated ventilation, controlled or assisted. It is suitable for ventilation of all patients, adults, children, and newborn infants.

Assembly

1. Mount Servo Ventilator on either bedpost, on wall rail, or suitable stand. It may also be placed on the pillar of an anesthesia table or wall stand for anesthesia use.

2. Brief operating and routine cleaning instructions are on the front panel.

3. Make sure that the ventilator is set at the available power supply voltage.

4. Connect the power cable to a wall socket with a protective earth ground.

5. For the U.S. market, the 900B version is provided with a line power switch with a safety catch. Set switch to *on* position by first pulling it out.

6. The green power indicator lamp must light up.

7. Connect the oxygen and compressed air lines to the gas mixer and set the desired oxygen concentration by means of the knob.

8. Set working pressure to 60 cm of water by means of the adjustment screw on the pneumatic unit. The manometer indicates the pressure value.

9. Attach a Bennett cascade humidifier and connect patient tubing to humidifier and ventilator. Insert a thermometer into the inspiratory side of the wye branch with adapter. Autoclavable as well as disposable tubing are available in different lengths

Servo Ventilator 900

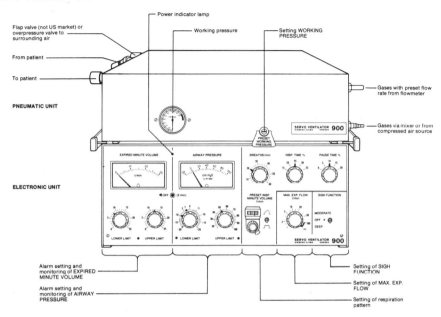

Servo Ventilator 900 B

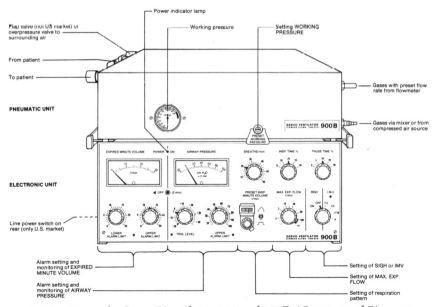

Figure 5-25. Controls, Servo Ventilator 900 and 900B. (*Courtesy of Siemens-Elema AB, Solna Sweden, Siemens Corp., Union, N.J.*)

317

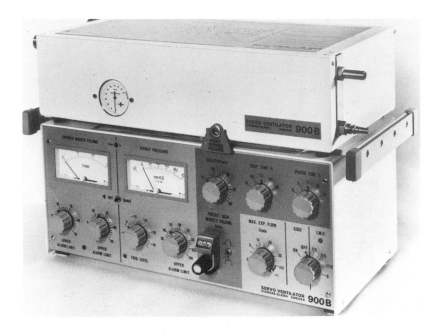

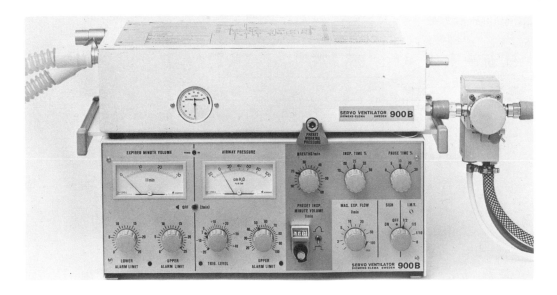

Figure 5-26.   Servo Ventilator 900B. *(Courtesy of Siemens-Elema AB, Solna, Sweden, Siemens Corp., Union, N.J.)*

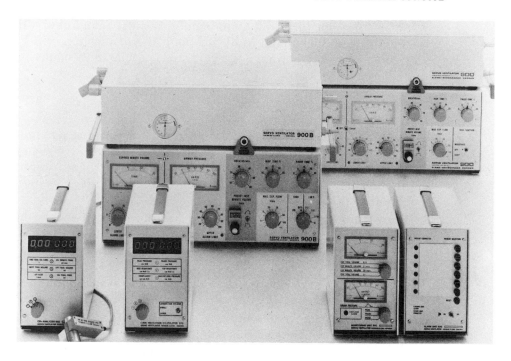

Figure 5-27. Servo Ventilators and Auxiliary Equipment. (*Courtesy of Siemens-Elema AB, Solna, Sweden, Siemens Corp., Union, N.J.*)

and diameters for adults and children. To protect the room air from contamination, an autoclavable bacterial-proof filter can be attached to the expiratory inlet.

10. Set the desired minute volume with the knob *Preset Inspiratory Minute Volume*. Suitable initial values can be calculated from a nomogram (Radford).

11. Set the oxygen flow.

12. The knob Preset Inspiratory Minute Volume may be locked in position by turning the built-in locking button to the right.

13. Set the desired respiration rate knob marked *Breaths/min*.

14. Set the desired values for *Pause Time* and *Inspiratory Time*. The gradations on both dials denote percentage of respiratory cycle.

15. Select a suitable curve shape for the inspiratory flow. Lock the knob *Maximum Expiratory Flow* in the clockwise position.

16. Select the sigh function: using moderate sigh, each hundredth breath; using deep sigh (only SU 900), the inspiration will be trebled in a similar way. For a conscious patient, only moderate sigh should be used.

Operation

1. Connect the ventilator to the patient. Make sure the patient's chest rises and falls in time with the ventilator's frequency and also that the meter *Airway Pressure* indicates the variations in pressure. The meter *Expired Minute Volume* must also indicate the correct value.

2. Make sure that the meter Expired Minute Volume shows the same value as the knob Preset Inspiratory Minute Volume. If these values do not agree, the cause may be leakage in the patient's circuit or extra inspirations triggered by the patient.

3. Set the knob *Expired Minute Volume, Lower Alarm Limit* to a suitable value, usually 10 to 20% below the set minute volume.

4. Set the knob *Expired Minute Volume, Upper Alarm Limit* to 20 to 40% above the meter reading.

5. Adjust the working pressure to approximately 30 cm of water above maximum airway pressure reading.

6. Set *Airway Pressure, Upper Alarm Limit* to a suitable value, usually in mid-position between working pressure and maximum airway pressure reading.

7. Set *Trig Level* to the green marked position T.

8. If auxiliary equipment (such as Monitoring Unit 910, Alarm Unit 920, CO_2 Analyzer 930, and Lung Mechanics Calculator 940) is to be connected to the ventilator, an output junction box must be used.

9. For intermittent mandatory ventilation (IMV) only on Servo Ventilator 900B: if PEEP is to be employed, connect the overpressure (PEEP) valve to the expiratory outlet on the ventilator.

10. Set the Trig Level knob in the T position (above 2 cm of water below atmospheric pressure). If PEEP is employed, set the patient triggering level to 2 cm of water below the desired continuous positive pressure set with the aid of the overpressure (PEEP) valve. If the Trig Level knob is set at a lower value than this, the patient must exert himself more.

11. Change from controlled ventilation to IMV by selecting the desired IMV position. When the IMV function is switched on, the yellow lamp on the IMV dial is illuminated.

12. Check the patient's spontaneous breathing by noting the *Expired Minute Volume* meter, which shows the sum of the controlled minute volume and the spontaneously inspired minute volume.

13. If the magnitude of the Expired Minute Volume meter is too low due to insufficient spontaneous breathing on the part of the patient:

   a. Select a higher IMV frequency so that the number of controlled respirations per minute increases (changing from *f*15 to *f*2).

   b. Consider resumption of controlled ventilation.

14. Special functions

   a. *Restricted expiration flow*—The knob *Maximum Expiratory Flow* should normally be locked in the fully clockwise end position by means of the safety catch and used only when specially indicated. If the knob is set at too low a value, the emptying of the lungs is obstructed.

   b. *Positive end expiration pressure*—If positive end expiration pressure is desired, the external flap not used for the U.S. market at the expiration outlet should be substituted by a springloaded overpressure valve. The overpressure is read on the meter *Airway Pressure* and is regulated by the overpressure valve.

   c. *Negative expiration pressure*—negative phase can be attained by connecting an attachment for negative phase to the expiratory outlet. *Note:* Negative phase cannot be used with IMV.

15. Function check

   a. The apparatus should be disconnected from the patient. To avoid alarm during the check, turn the *Alarm Limit* knobs to end position.

   b. Check that the green power indicator lamp is lit and that the IMV function is in the *off* position.

   c. Check that the manometer shows normal working pressure, also, during the inspiratory phase. A pressure fall to zero during inspiration indicates an insufficient gas supply or leakage in the gas connection or bellows.

   d. Set lowest respiration rate pause time to 20%, and block the opening of the wye branch.

   e. The meter *Airway Pressure* should not show the same value as the manometer *Working Pressure*. The airway pressure must not fall more than a few centimeters of water during the inspiration pause. A large fall indicates leakage in the pneu-

matic unit or in the patient tubing system. During the expiratory phase, airway pressure should fall to zero.

f. Connect a test lung to the patient wye. Set *Preset Inspiratory Minute Volume* to 7.5 liters/min and set respiration rate to 20 breaths/min. The meter *Expired Minute Volume* should now read 7.5 liters/min ±0.5 liters/min.

Cleaning and Maintenance

1. Remove the gas supply lines.

2. Disconnect the power line (cable).

3. Remove the patient tubing system. Clean and sterilize, if they are not disposable.

4. Wipe outside of ventilator with a cloth soaked in disinfectant solution. If solution contains alcohol, the concentration must not exceed 50%.

5. Open the lid on the pneumatic unit and loosen connector from flow transducer in the expiration channel. Grasp metal pipes with one hand and the rubber bend with the other; lift upward.

6. Dismount the different parts and sterilize them in accordance with hospital procedure. Maximum autoclave temperature is 150°C (302°F).

7. The flow transducer is fragile and should be treated with care. Decontaminate the flow transducer by carefully placing it in a normal disinfectant solution for about 1 hour. Then wash the transducer by carefully lowering it into a bowl of distilled water and moving it slowly to and fro. After washing, the transducer is sterilized in an autoclave maximum temperature of 150°C (302°F).

    Note: The flow transducer must not be cleaned by means of ultrasound.

8. Reassemble; make sure that the flow transducer is correctly replaced. The manufacturing number should be visible from above.

9. The inspiration side receives only pure gases, which have passed through a sterile filter. Therefore, a complete cleaning should be carried out when specially indicated, as a rule after every 1000 hours of operating time, indicated on the operating time meter at the rear of the unit, or every 6 months.

10. A routine function test should always be carried out after cleaning the unit.

11. The ventilator should be thoroughly overhauled after each operating period of 1000 hours, and at least every 6 months.

BIO-MED DEVICES IC-2 VENTILATOR

The model IC-2 Ventilator (Figure 5-28) is for respiratory support of adult patients both in hospitals and during transport. It is a pulsatile flow ventilator that may be used in any of the following operating modes: time cycled, either volume or pressure limited, with or without positive end expiratory pressure, intermittent positive pressure ventilation, intermittent mandatory ventilation, synchronized intermittent mandatory ventilation, continuous positive airway pressure, and continuous oxygen administration.

Assembly

1. Connect a 50-psi oxygen source to the power gas supply connector. Only 100% oxygen should be used for proper operation.

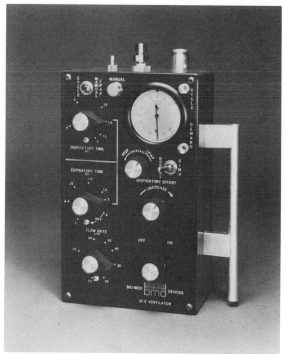

Figure 5-28.   IC-2 Ventilator. (*Courtesy of Bio-Med Devices, Inc., Stamford, Conn.*)

2. Connect the patient gas supply to the *DISS Fitting* labeled patient gas supply. This may be from the output of a blender or any preblended gas mixture of the desired oxygen concentration which delivered to the patient is the same as the oxygen concentration supplied to the ventilator in the patient gas fitting.

3. It is essential that the supplies be regulated to 50-psi sources without flow-restricting devices, such as flowmeters or needle valves. The host fitting should be hand tightened to avoid damage to the fittings. The gas supply should be clean and dry.

4. For patient circuit connection, connect the short piece of corrugated hose to the main patient fitting (output). Connect the other end to the filter with a 6-in. length of hose; connect to the input port of the humidifier.

5. Connect the main patient hose (corrugated) to the output connector of the humidifier.

6. Attach the exhalation valve line to the exhalation valve fitting.

7. Connect the proximal airway pressure line to the pressure guage fitting.

8. Attach patient port of exhalation valve to a test lung. After selecting desired operating parameters, observe proper functioning before attaching to the patient.

Operation

INTERMITTENT POSITIVE PRESSURE VENTILATION (IPPV) OR INTERMITTENT MANDATORY VENTILATION (IMV) WITH OR WITHOUT PEEP. Determine and note patient requirements for respiratory rate, I/E ratio, and tidal volume. Refer to Table 5-4 to find inspiratory time and expiratory time. Obtain the correct flow-rate setting for the desired tidal volume at the set inspiratory time from Table 5-5.

EXAMPLE   Prescribed parameters:

$$\text{Tidal volume} = 500 \text{ ml}$$
$$\text{Respiratory rate} = 20$$
$$\text{I/E ratio} = 1:2$$

From Table 5-4:

$$\text{Inspiratory time} = 1.0 \text{ sec}$$
$$\text{Expiratory time} = 2.0 \text{ sec}$$

From Table 5-5:

$$\text{Flow rate} = 30 \text{ lpm} \ (0.5 \text{ liters/sec})$$

$$\text{Tidal volume (liters)} = \text{flow rate (liters/sec)} \\ \times \text{inspiratory time (sec)}$$

1. Set *on/off* selector to *on.*
2. Set cycle/CPAP-Manual switch to cycle position.
3. Set Normal/SIMV switch in normal position.

TABLE 5-4 Rate and I/E Ratio

Exp. Time (sec)	Insp. Time (sec)					
	0.4	0.5	0.75	1.0	1.5	2
0.5	67 1:1.3	60 1:1	48 1.5:1	40 2:1	30 3:1	24 4:1
0.6	60 1:1.5	55 1:1.2	44 1.3:1	38 1.7:1	29 2.5:1	23 3.3:1
0.75	52 1:1.9	48 1:1.5	40 1:1	34 1.3:1	27 2:1	22 2.7:1
1.0	43 1:2.5	40 1:2	34 1:1.3	30 1:1	24 1.5:1	20 2:1
1.5	32 1:3.8	30 1:3	27 1:2	24 1:1.5	20 1:1	17 1.3:1
2	25 1:5	24 1:4	22 1:2.7	20 1:2	17 1:1.3	15 1:1
4	14 1:10	13 1:8	13 1:5.3	12 1:4	11 1:2.7	10 1:2

$$\text{Respiratory rate} = \frac{60}{\text{insp. time} + \text{exp. time}} \qquad R = \frac{60}{T_I + T_E}$$

TABLE 5-5 Tidal Volume

Flow Rate (lpm)	Insp. Time (sec)					
	0.4	0.5	0.75	1.0	1.5	2
20	130	170	250	330	500	670
30	200	250	375	500	750	1000
40	270	330	500	670	1000	1330
50	330	420	630	830	1250	1670
60	400	500	750	1000	1500	2000
70	470	580	875	1170	1750	2330
75	500	630	940	1250	1880	2500

Tidal volume (ml) = insp. time (sec) × flow rate (ml/sec) $V_T = T_I \times \dot{V}_I$

4. Set maximum pressure control fully counterclockwise, and PEEP/CPAP control fully clockwise to zero.

5. Adjust inspiratory time and expiratory time controls to required settings.

6. Set flow-rate control to proper position to give desired tidal volume according to Table 5-5.

7. Set desired oxygen concentration with blender control.

8. Attach test lung to patient port and observe proper cycling.

9. Connect to patient.

10. Set inspiratory effort control for proper patient triggering.

11. If PEEP is to be used, set the desired level using the PEEP/CPAP control. Adjust control until the pressure gauge indicates the desired level during the expiratory time. Note that the PEEP level is somewhat sensitive to flow rate. The PEEP control should be set with the flow rate used. When using PEEP, the inspiratory effort control should be reset to compensate for each PEEP level used.

12. For intermittent mandatory ventilation (IMV), the inspiratory effort control should be locked out by turning clockwise, and a constant flow source with one-way valve should be connected to the patient circuit. Determine prescribed tidal volume, inspiratory time, and rate. IMV is set simply by increasing expiratory time in the IMV range from 4 to 4.5 sec.

SYNCHRONIZED INTERMITTENT MANDATORY VENTILATION (SIMV).   The procedure is similar to IMV as noted above, with the following differences:

1. Normal/SIMV selector is set to SIMV position.

2. Set inspiratory effort control for proper patient triggering.

3. Set PEEP level, making certain to readjust the inspiratory effort to compensate for PEEP.

4. Observe assist breath following termination of expiratory time. Adjust tidal valve equal to inspiratory time times flow rate to proper level.

Note: In the SIMV mode, the IC-2 functions as an assistor; therefore, it is necessary that an apnea alarm be used at all times to signal the cessation of spontaneous breathing. In SIMV the demand indicator alone will show spontaneous breaths, while both demand and cycle indicators together indicate an assist breath.

CONTINUOUS POSITIVE AIRWAY PRESSURE (CPAP)

1. Set the PEEP/CPAP control fully clockwise (zero).
2. Cycle/CPAP-Manual switch to CPAP-Manual position.
3. Turn expiratory time control fully clockwise to maximum.
4. Set Normal/SIMV switch to SIMV.
5. Adjust inspiratory time and flow rate to give administered gas volume sufficient to meet patient demand.
6. Connect the test lung.
7. Set desired CPAP level using the PEEP/CPAP control.
8. Adjust inspiratory effort for preset CPAP level for proper patient triggering; *note* that it is essential with the triggered demand flow of the IC-2 that the inspiratory effort be properly adjusted to assure that the patient can obtain gas. As in the SIMV mode, no external constant flow source is necessary.
9. Connect to patient and observe pressure gauge. Adjust inspiratory time and/or flow rate to assure that sufficient gas is provided and that the CPAP level is maintained. In CPAP only, the demand indicator will be activated.

MANUAL CYCLING

1. Set Cycle/CPAP-Manual to CPAP-Manual position.
2. Set Normal/SIMV selector to SIMV (optional). Set expiratory time to maximum.
3. Set desired inspiratory flow rate.
4. Set maximum pressure level (rear panel control) by occluding patient port, depressing manual control, and adjusting maximum pressure.
5. Adjust PEEP level in manner similar to maximum pressure, if it is desired to have PEEP during manual cycles.
6. Ventilate test lung by depressing manual button and observing pressure gauge for proper operation.
7. Connect to patient and ventilate by depressing manual button for the desired inspiratory time. Observe chest excursion and pressure gauge for proper operation.

Maintenance

1. The IC-2 Ventilator should be protected from abusive mechanical shock and kept in a clean condition.

2. The instrument should be returned to Bio-Med Devices, Inc., for repair.

3. The supplied patient circuit is disposable and should be replaced for every patient or during extended periods for a single patient. It is recommended that the patient circuit be changed at least every 24 hours.

4. Care should be taken in connecting supply hoses to the power oxygen and air fittings. Hand tightening of these fittings is sufficient. Do not overtighten with a wrench, as the fittings could be damaged.

5. The accuracy of the instrument's indicators and controls should be retained over its life as long as it has not been subjected to abuse. The calibration of the pressure gauge, flow control, and timing controls may be checked with relative ease.

6. Annual preventive maintenance must be performed at the end of the first year or the second year of the guarantee will be voided.

BOURNS BP 200 INFANT PRESSURE VENTILATOR

The Bourns BP 200 Infant Pressure Ventilator (Figure 5-29) is a pneumatically operated, electronically controlled, time-cycled device. It is a constant or continuous flow generator that functions as a controller. The ventilator can provide zero end expiratory pressure (ZEEP), positive end expiratory pressure (PEEP), continuous positive airway pressure (CPAP), a combination of techniques timed, intermittent mandatory ventilation (IMV), or an inspiratory plateau.

Assembly

1. Attach the oxygen hose to the oxygen inlet port on rear of ventilator; oxygen source of 30 to 75 psi of pressure at flow rates of up to 30 liters/min is required.

2. Attach the air hose to the air inlet port on the rear of the ventilator; air source of 15 to 75 psi of pressure at flow rates of up to 22 liters/min is required.

3. Connect assembly hose between the ventilator and the PEEP jet fitting.

4. Connect $\frac{3}{8}$-in. tygon tubing between ventilator and heated humidifier inflow connection port. Approximately 1 ft of tubing will be necessary.

5. Connect $\frac{3}{8}$-in. tygon tubing on both the inflow and outflow connection ports of the heated humidifier. On the outflow port

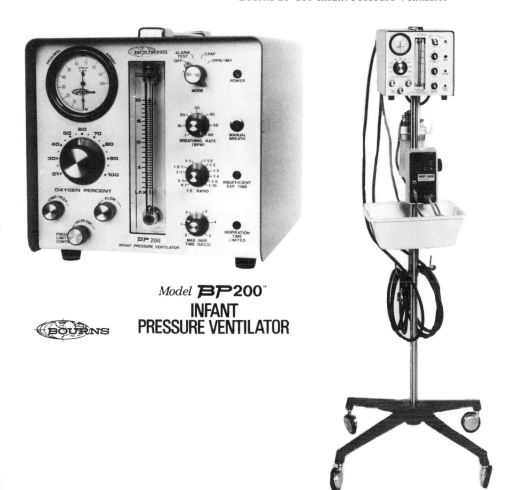

Model **BP 200**
INFANT
PRESSURE VENTILATOR

Figure 5-29.   Bourns BP 200 Infant Pressure Ventilator. (*Courtesy of Bourns, Inc., Life Systems Division, Riverside, Calif.*)

approximately 3 ft of tubing is used to attach to either the infant bed arm or to the adaptor.

6. Adaptor is used to connect $\frac{3}{8}$-in. tygon tubing to flexible hose.

7. Flexible hose connects between endotracheal tee adaptor and adaptor.

8. Endotracheal tee adaptor attaches to both ends of flexible hose and provides a means of connection to the patient.

9. Attach $\frac{3}{8}$-in. tygon tubing from patient fitting on back of ventilator to adaptor on the flexible hose. Approximately 4 ft of tubing is usually necessary.

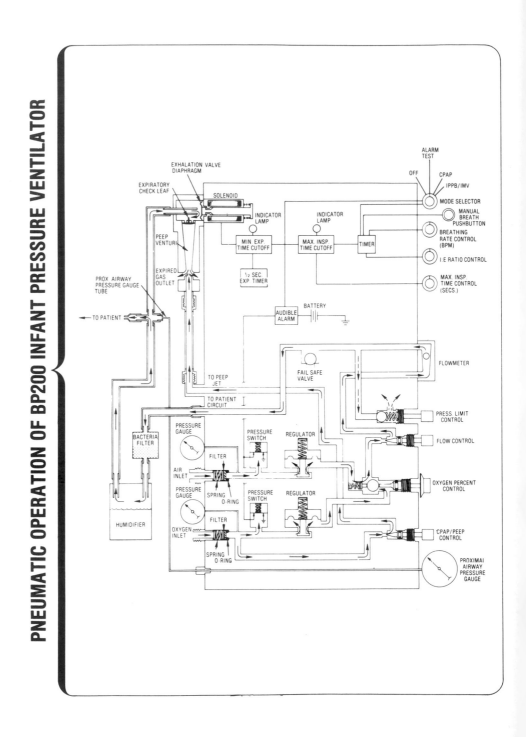

PNEUMATIC OPERATION OF BP200 INFANT PRESSURE VENTILATOR

ALARMS
(CONTINUOUS AUDIBLE AND VISUAL)

CONDITION	CORRECTIVE ACTION
Loss of air and/or oxygen pressure (below 15 psig (1 Kg/cm²)—air, 30 psig (2 Kg/cm²)—oxygen)	Check inlet pressure gauges and correct gas supply problem.
Electrical power failure or electrical power disconnect (Ventilator)	Check electrical power cord and reestablish electrical power.
Overtemperature	Check temperature at proximal airway. a. If greater than 104°F (40°C), check temperature at humidifier. If excessive temperature is indicated: 1) empty water from humidifier; 2) replace with room temperature, sterile distilled water; 3) reduce temperature setting on immersion heater; 4) observe temperature on probe thermometer during warm-up period to assure it does not overshoot safe range (98-108°F). If immersion heater is already set at minimum, replace with properly functioning heater. b. If less than 104°F (40°C) refer overtemperature alarm to a qualified service technician.

INDICATORS
(VISUAL)

CONDITION	CORRECTIVE ACTION
INSPIRATION TIME LIMITED	a. In IPPB mode, review BREATHING RATE and I:E RATIO control settings for desired level. If controls are set as clinically desired, increase the MAXIMUM INSPIRATION TIME control until the INSPIRATION TIME LIMITED indicator stops blinking. b. In IMV Mode — normal. Indicates inspiratory time is being limited according to setting of MAXIMUM INSPIRATION TIME control.
INSUFFICIENT EXPIRATORY TIME	Review BREATHING RATE and I:E RATIO control settings.

WARNING: When the ventilator is connected to the patient, it is recommended that someone be in attendance at all times in order to detect an alarm or other indication of a problem.

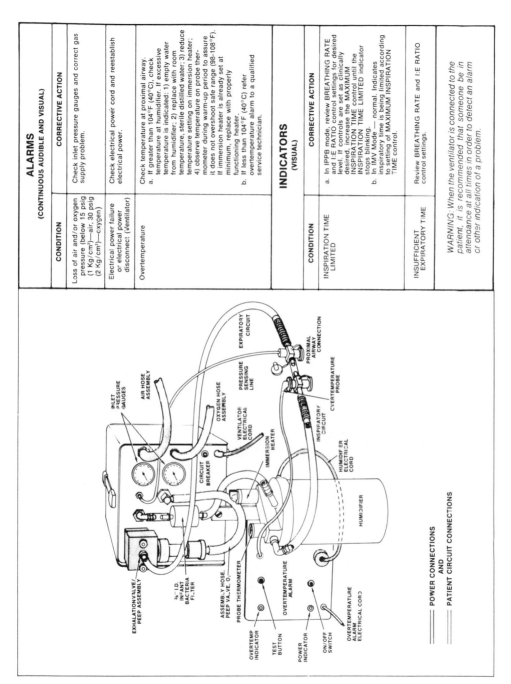

Figure 5-30. Pneumatic Operation of BP 200 Infant Pressure Ventilator.

331

10. Connect the airway pressure gauge tube from the back of venti-
    lator to the 11-mm infant endotracheal connector at the proximal
    airway. Approximately 5 ft of $\frac{1}{8}$-in. tygon tubing is necessary.

Operation.   Refer to Figure 5-31 for complete description of all controls and indicators.

*FOR INTERMITTENT POSITIVE PRESSURE VENTILATION
(IPPV)*

1. Check out complete infant ventilator system.
2. Fill heated humidifier with sterile water to full mark. Select
   the desired setting of warm, tepid, or cold on the humidifier.
3. Plug the electrical cord of the ventilator and humidifier into a
   properly grounded outlet.
4. Attach the air and oxygen hose assemblies to an appropriate
   gas source.
5. Switch mode control from *off* position to *Alarm Test*, and then
   to IPPB mode.
6. Turn the pressure limit control to 80 cm of water.
7. Set the respiratory rate control to the desired level.

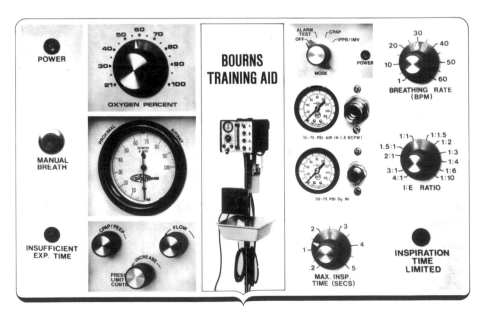

Figure 5-31.

DESCRIPTION OF CONTROLS AND INDICATORS

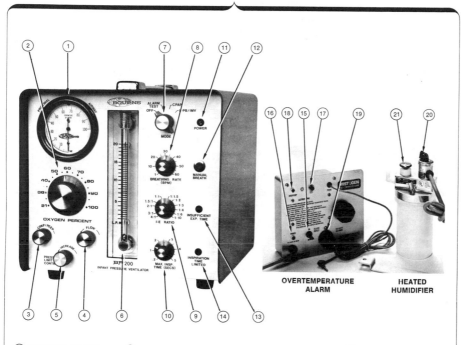

OVERTEMPERATURE
ALARM

HEATED
HUMIDIFIER

(1) **PROXIMAL AIRWAY PRESSURE GAUGE**

Displays level of pressure at the proximal airway from 0–100 cmH₂O.

(2) **OXYGEN PERCENT**

Continuously adjustable to any level from 21–100% oxygen.

(3) **CPAP/PEEP**

Continuously adjustable level of end expiratory pressure between 0–20 cmH₂O (with 42 psig or more O₂ inlet pressure). If O₂ inlet pressure is less than 42 psig, the inlet pressure must be constant to insure constant CPAP/PEEP level.

(4) **FLOW**

Continuously adjustable over the range of 0–20 LPM as read on the flowmeter.

(5) **PRESSURE LIMIT**

A pop-off valve prevents excessive inspiratory pressures. Continuously adjustable from 10–80 cmH₂O. Also used to establish an inspiratory plateau.

(6) **FLOWMETER**

Displays gas flowrate to the patient circuit from 0–20 LPM.

Note: The gas flow to the patient may be reduced during the pop-off period by the action of the PRESSURE LIMIT control.

(7) **MODE**

Off —All electronic controls are off.

Alarm —Closes the alarm circuit to
Test   test the 1.5 volt "D" size alkaline battery and audible alarm buzzer.

Note: The alarm battery is accessible by removing the cover plate under the infant ventilator.

CPAP —Activates the pneumatic and electrical power alarm circuits. If a loss of air and/or oxygen inlet pressures occur, the audible battery operated alarm will sound. Also allows use of the MANUAL BREATH pushbutton control.

IPPB/ —Time cycles the ventilator and
IMV   activates both the pneumatic and electrical power loss alarm circuits. If a loss of air and/or oxygen inlet pressures occur, or if a power failure or disconnect occurs, the battery operated audible alarm will sound.

(8) **BREATHING RATE**

Adjustable control of respiratory rate from 1–60 breaths per minute (BPM).

(9) **I:E RATIO**

Calibrated selection of I:E RATIO from 4:1 to 1:10.

(10) **MAXIMUM INSPIRATION TIME**

Adjustable from 0.2–5.0 seconds. This control limits the inspiration time independently of the BREATHING RATE and I:E RATIO controls. It may be used as an override to prevent excessive inspiratory time periods or as a primary control of inspiratory time at lower breathing rates.

During the normal IPPB mode of operation, this control should be set at a level above the inspiratory time period the patient is actually receiving. This will prevent the MAXIMUM INSPIRATION TIME control from overriding the I:E RATIO control. During the IMV mode of operation this control should be set at whatever length of inspiration the clinician wants the patient to receive.

(11) **POWER**

Indicates electrical power to the ventilator has been turned on.

(12) **MANUAL BREATH**

Operational in CPAP mode only. Allows one manual breath on each actuation. Inspiratory time is controlled by ventilator settings of BREATHING RATE, I:E RATIO, and MAXIMUM INSPIRATION TIME controls.

(13) **INSUFFICIENT EXHALATION TIME**

Indicates an internal timer is preventing exhalation periods shorter than 0.45–0.55 seconds.

NOTE· Review the BREATHING RATE and I:E RATIO control settings to be sure sufficient exhalation times are being provided to prevent gas trapping in the lung.

(14) **INSPIRATION TIME LIMITED**

Indicates MAXIMUM INSPIRATION TIME control is overriding the BREATHING RATE and I:E RATIO controls and terminating inspiration. During normal IPPB mode of operation the MAXIMUM INSPIRATION TIME control should be set to a level where the INSPIRATION TIME LIMITED indicator does not blink. During low breathing rate IMV, the MAXIMUM INSPIRATION TIME control should be set at the prescribed limit. The limiting action will be indicated by a blink of the INSPIRATION TIME LIMITED indicator at the end of each controlled inspiration.

(15) **ON/OFF**

Turns on electrical power to the over-temperature alarm.

(16) **POWER**

Indicates electrical power to the over-temperature alarm has been turned on.

(17) **TEST**

Press to test audible and visual OVER-TEMP alarm. Cancel by moving ON/OFF switch to "OFF".

(18) **OVERTEMP**

Indicates via an audible and visual alarm that inspired gas temperature at the probe is 104°F (40°C).

(19) **HEATER OUTLET**

Immersion heater electrical plug connects here. Electrical power discontinued to heater during overtemperature condition.

(20) **TEMPERATURE CONTROL**

The temperature of the inspired gas going to the patient is regulated by an adjustable thermostat which controls the water temperature. The adjustable thermostat has three areas of temperature settings as a guide — warm, tepid and cold.

(21) **PROBE THERMOMETER**

Indicates the temperature of the inspired gas leaving the heated humidifier.

Figure 5-31. *(cont.)*

8. Set the I:E ratio control to the desired level.
9. Set the maximum inspiration time control to the desired level. In the IPPB mode of operation this is when the inspiration time limited indicator stops blinking.
10. Adjust the flow rate so that the desired pressure level, as indicated on the pressure manometer, is approximately 5 cm of water higher than desired.
11. Use the pressure limit control to reduce the pressure as indicated on the proximal airway gauge to the desired level.
12. Adjust for desired PEEP level by turning the CPAP/PEEP control and observing the proximal airway pressure gauge.
13. Select the desired oxygen concentration.
14. Connect ventilator to patient.

OPERATION FOR INTERMITTENT MANDATORY VENTILATION (IMV)

1. Follow all steps outlined for IPPV operation.
2. Turn the respiratory rate control to the desired level.
3. Adjust the maximum inspiration time control to the level of inspiratory time desired.

Note: During low breathing rate IMV the primary control of inspiratory time is the maximum inspiration time control and not the I:E ratio control.

OPERATION FOR CONTINUOUS POSITIVE AIRWAY PRESSURE (CPAP)

1. Check out complete infant ventilator system.
2. Fill heated humidifier with sterile water to full mark. Select the desired setting of warm, tepid, or cold on the humidifier.
3. Plug the electrical cord of the ventilator and humidifier into a properly grounded outlet.
4. Attach the air and oxygen hose assemblies to an appropriate gas source.
5. Switch mode control from *off* position to *Alarm Test*, and then to CPAP mode.
6. Adjust flow rate to desired level as indicated on the flowmeter.
7. Adjust for desired CPAP level by turning the CPAP control and observing the proximal airway gauge.
8. Select desired oxygen concentration.

9. Set the pressure limit control.
10. Connect the ventilator to the patient.

   Note: The manual breath push button is operational in the
   CPAP mode only. Inspiratory time is controlled by the
   ventilator settings of breathing rate, I:E ratio, and maximum inspiration time controls.

Cleaning and Sterilization

1. *Ventilator*—The exterior of the ventilator may be wiped clean
   with an appropriate bactericidal or germicidal agent.
2. *Patient tube system*—The entire patient tube system (except
   for bacteria filter) should be cleaned and sterilized.
3. *Heated humidifier*—Remove and clean humidifier, and then
   sterilize; do not wash, rinse, or immerse the probe thermometer
   or heating element in a solution.
4. *Bacteria filter*—Under no circumstances should the bacteria
   filter ever be cleaned. It may be sterilized by steam autoclave.
5. *Exhalation valve/PEEP assembly*—Remove and clean the entire
   exhalation valve/PEEP assembly. Make sure the various components are properly reassembled.

TECHNIQUE FOR WEANING A PATIENT FROM THE VENTILATOR

Four criteria should be met before consideration is given to weaning
a patient from a ventilator:

1. Clinically stable status with normal blood pressure and pulse.
2. Forced vital capacity of at least 15 cc per kg of body weight.
3. Normal or stable arterial blood gases.
4. An inspiratory force of at least 20 cm of water pressure.

   The technique should be as follows:

1. The physician must order the length of time the patient will be
   off the ventilator.
2. When the patient is off the ventilator, the nurse should monitor
   vital signs every 15 min or more or less frequently as indicated
   by the patient's condition.

3. Observe for poor tolerance of the patient while off the ventilator, such as shallow respirations, increase or decrease in pulse rate, increase or decrease in blood pressure, perspiration, and a low tidal volume.

4. The respiratory therapist should check the patient's vital capacity with a meter such as the Wright Respirometer when the patient is taken off the ventilator, and check whether increased breathing difficulty is noted during the weaning time.

5. The respiratory therapist should see that adequately humidified oxygen is provided when the patient is off the ventilator; preferably the FIO_2 should be at least the same concentration as it was for breathing on the ventilator.

6. The endotracheal or tracheostomy cuff must be deflated when the patient is off the ventilator; it should be reinflated when the patient has something to eat or drink unless specified otherwise; deflation should be preceded by suction.

7. Preparation should be made for blood gases to be drawn before and at the end of the initial weaning; further blood gases will be ordered at the physician's discretion.

8. The therapist should work with the patient, encouraging breathing control exercises during the weaning period.

9. The initial period off the ventilator and the subsequent intervals are somewhat arbitrary and are determined by the clinical condition of the patient and the periodic assessment of the criteria listed above.

INTERMITTENT MANDATORY VENTILATION (IMV)

I. Introduction

IMV is a relatively new concept that enables the patient to breathe spontaneously at his own rate while receiving a hyperinflation from the ventilator at regular preset intervals. The rate of the ventilator is gradually decreased until the patient is breathing entirely on his own.

Although IMV may be used when the patient is initially placed on the ventilator, its primary use has been to make the weaning process less traumatic for the patient and more successful than conventional methods.

If IMV is used for weaning, the patient must meet certain parameters, that is, adequate arterial blood gases, spontaneous breathing, adequate tidal volume, and stable vital signs.

There are two types of IMV setups—ambient and pressure.

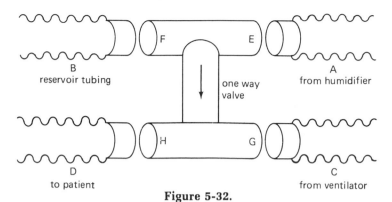

B
reservoir tubing

F

E

one way
valve

A
from humidifier

H

G

D
to patient

C
from ventilator

Figure 5-32.

II. Ambient Setup
  A. Equipment
     1. Puritan jar with immersion heater
     2. Aerosol tubing
     3. One-way valve
     4. Rubber adapter
     5. Flow regulator
  B. Procedure (see Figure 5-32)
     1. Set up the aerosol unit as for an aerosol tee.
     2. Attach the aerosol tubing (A) to the one-way valve as
         shown to port (E). Observe arrow on diagram that indi-
         cates flow.
     3. Attach a length of aerosol tubing (approximately 18 in.)
         to port (F) opposite aerosol setup.
     4. Attach the inspiratory line from the ventilator (C) to port
         (G) on one-way valve.
     5. Add extension (D) from port (H) to patient.
     6. Adjust FIO_2 for nebulizer the same as that on ventilator.

III. Pressure Setup (see Figure 5-33)
  A. Equipment
     1. One-way valve with hose connector
     2. Two-liter reservoir bag
     3. Oxygen supply tubing
     4. Flow regulator or oxygen blender
  B. Procedure
     1. Attach one-way valve (A) to outlet on ventilator humidi-
         fier. Note arrow indicating flow.

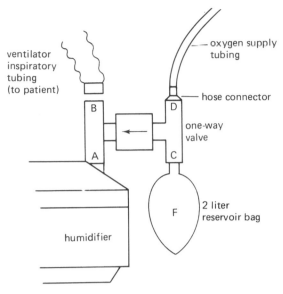

Figure 5-33.

2. Attach ventilator inspiratory tubing (E) to port (B) of valve.
3. Attach 2-liter bag to port (C) of valve.
4. Attach oxygen supply tubing (G) to port (D) of valve and then to regulator or oxygen blender. Adjust FIO_2 so that it is the same as that delivered by the ventilator.

PROCEDURE FOR USE OF THE HEALTHDYNE IMV CONTROLLER (INTERMITTENT MANDATORY VENTILATION)

I. Introduction
The Healthdyne IMV Controller (Figure 5-34) allows the use of IMV on the MA-1 ventilator without modification of the ventilator itself. This allows you to control the rate of the ventilator below six breaths per minute.

II. Installation
The IMV Controller must be connected to the internal circuitry of the ventilator. This procedure is best carried out by a service representative or other individual with thorough knowledge of both the ventilator and controller. Once in place, the ventilator may be used with or without the controller in operation. The IMV Controller is electrically powered independently of the ventilator.

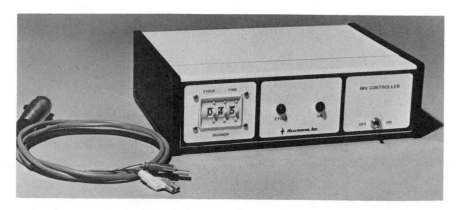

Figure 5-34. Healthdyne IMV Controller. (*Courtesy of Healthdyne, Inc., Atlanta, Ga.*)

III. Procedure
   A. Assemble the IMV setup as described previously.
   B. For use with MA-1 ventilator:
      1. Plug output cable into rear of controller.
      2. Plug the ac power cord for the controller and the Ma-1 into suitable electrical outlets and turn both units *on*.
      3. Set the MA-1 rate control in the *off* position.
      4. Set the desired rate for IMV by setting *Cycle Time* on the controller.

      Note: The IMV Controller is calibrated in seconds and allows the ventilator to cycle through a range from 5 to 199 sec.

      a. If the physician orders IMV, for example, every 30 sec, simply set the controller to read 030 for a rate of 2 breaths/min. (Divide the number of seconds in a minute by the frequency to determine rate.)
      b. If the physician orders IMV at a specific number of cycles per minute, for example, 4, set the controller at 015. (Divide number of cycles per minute into 60.)
      5. It is not necessary to use the *Sigh* controls or sensitivity on the MA-1.
      6. Peak flow, normal volume, pressure limit and FIO_2 (of the ventilator) may be set as desired.
      7. The IMV Controller has an *on/off* switch. Two lights are found in the middle panel of the unit. One indicates that

the controller is in operation; the other indicates each cycle that is initiated by the ventilator–controller unit.

C. *Note:* Do not set the IMV Controller's respiratory cycle below 5 sec as the ventilator will not cycle.

IV. Cleaning and Sterilization
The IMV Controller does not require sterilization as it is not in the patient circuit. It may be wiped down externally with alcohol if necessary, but do not allow moisture to enter controller.

EXERCISES

1. How would you determine the presence of a partial obstruction in the tracheostomy tube of a patient on an MA-1?
2. How would you determine the presence of a leak in the tubing system of a PR-2?
3. Describe the physical and emotional support necessary to the patient being weaned from a ventilator.
4. Classify the following mechanical ventilators: (a) Bennett PR-2, (b) Bennett MA-1, (c) Bourns, (d) Searles.
5. What aspects of ventilator function do you feel should be monitored most frequently?
6. Describe what you feel is a good system for weaning a patient from mechanical ventilation.
7. Compare the advantages and disadvantages of the two types of IMV setups—ambient and pressure.

UNIT 6

ACCESSORY DEVICES FOR RESPIRATORY THERAPY

This unit surveys some of the most commonly used accessories and their procedures. The procedures we present are guidelines, which you may modify to fit your present department.

LT 60 BUNN ALARM SYSTEM

The LT 60 Bunn Alarm System (Figure 6-1) is used with either pressure or volume ventilators. Its intent is to guard against failure of the ventilator to cycle, pressure drop, or pressure increase. It also indicates patient inspiratory effort.

Table of Controls

1. Low-pressure control—set from 10 to 60 cm of water pressure; if pressure falls below preset pressure setting, the alarm will go off and the red light will glow.
2. High-pressure control—set from 20 to 60 cm of water pressure; when pressure exceeds preset pressure, the alarm will go off and the yellow light will glow.
3. Reset button—resets the low-pressure alarm.
4. Time delay adjustment—sets the length of time before the low-pressure alarm will go off.
5. Inspiratory effort indicator—tells you when the patient is creating any inspiratory effort.

341

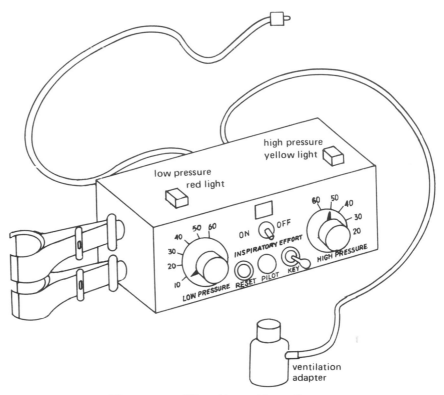

Figure 6-1.   LT 60 Bunn Alarm System.

6. Key switch—turns the unit on and off.
7. Test batteries button—checks if batteries are good; batteries' power is used for operation of the power failure alarm only.

Operation

1. Connect clamps of alarm on a stable structure or pedestal mount.
2. Connect ventilator adapter of alarm to outlet of ventilator before connecting the humidifier.
3. Set desired low- and high-pressure setting; set delay and inspiration effort on or off.
4. Plug unit into proper electrical outlet, grounded.
5. Turn unit on by switching the key to *on* position; you may remove the key if you wish and attach it to the magnetized key keeper on side of unit.
6. Reset low- and high-pressure setting when the ventilator is in operation.

TIMETER LOW/HIGH PRESSURE ALERT

The Timeter Pressure Alarm System is a solid-state, battery-operated unit designed to be used with any neonatal and adult volume or pressure cycled ventilator for the purpose of monitoring changes in airway pressure. The unit automatically turns on when attached to the patient circuit and is designed to be used where circuit pressure is 10 to 70 cm of water on CMV or IMV.

Table of Controls (refer to Figure 6-2)

1. Mode switch—CMV, continuous mandatory ventilation; IMV, intermittent mandatory ventilation.
2. Pressure cycle light-emitting diode (LED) (yellow)—flashes when proper pressure setting is achieved. Operating normally when the LED only is flashing during the mandatory breaths.
3. Manual—manually sets alarming circuit in order to check circuit and batteries.
4. Inhibit—manually silences alarm after low-pressure condition exists for delay time period.
5. Manual override sequence—to silence alarm before delay time period, push manual, then inhibit. Unit will now stay silenced. Inhibit will not silence low-battery alarm condition.
6. Pressure adjust—two-in-one pressure adjust control knob for simultaneously setting low- and high-pressure limits.

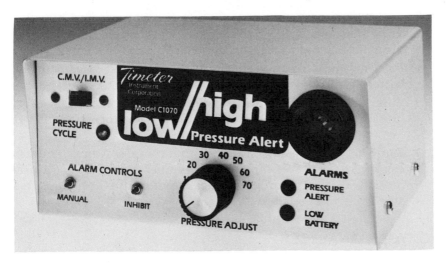

Figure 6-2. Timeter Low/High Pressure Alert. (*Courtesy of Timeter Instrument Corp., Lancaster, Pa.*)

7. Low-battery LED (red)—this LED will be very dimly lit during normal operation. When brightly lit, it indicates batteries are to be changed.

8. Pressure alert LED (red)—lights continuously when low-pressure condition exists and intermittently when mandatory breath pressure exceeds pressure adjust setting.

9. Audible alarm—sounds continuously when low-pressure adjust low limit is not obtained. Also sounds continuously when low battery level is reached. Sounds intermittently when high-pressure limit occurs.

10. Pressure connector cap—must be removed to attach pressure sensing tube. To remove, pull out; this turns power on. Attach pressure connector cap to back of alarm by placing flat magnetic side of cap against rear panel.

Operation.   After ventilator is attached to the patient and ventilator settings are selected, the following instruction should be used.

Note: Do not use near flammable anesthetics.

1. Select CMV or IMV.
2. Set Pressure Adjust to 40.
3. Remove pressure connector cap from back of alarm.
4. Attach one end of pressure sensing tube to pressure connector on rear panel of alarm unit. Leave other end disconnected.
5. If alarm sounds, push *Inhibit.*
6. Test unit.
7. Turn Pressure Adjust clockwise to approximately 10 above pressure reading on ventilator airway pressure gauge.
8. Push Manual; alarm will sound (no sound indicates complete battery failure). Push Inhibit to silence.
9. With all final adjustments completed on ventilator, attach pressure setting tee to patient circuit. Alarm will sound indicating automatic turn on.
10. For final adjustment, slowly turn Pressure Adjust counter-clockwise until Pressure Adjust number correlates with peak pressure on ventilator pressure gauge, and only the yellow pressure cycle LED flashes.

IMI PORTABLE OXYGEN ANALYZER

The IMI Portable Oxygen Analyzer (Figure 6-3) is designed to monitor oxygen concentration in controlled environments such as tents, incubators, and oxygen hoods, and may also be adapted for ventilator

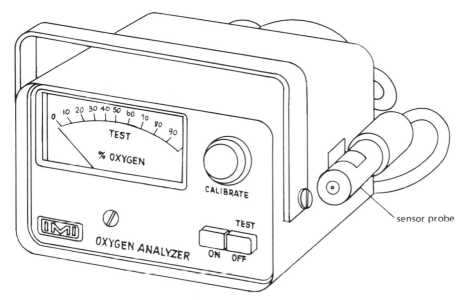

Figure 6-3. IMI Portable Oxygen Analyzer.

use. It comes with a portable sensor probe that is exposed to the environment to be monitored, and immediate readout is obtained. The unit is powered by two transistor radio batteries and its accuracy is ±2% of the full scale. It is lightweight and may be easily carried from place to place.

Operation

1. Place unit on flat surface.
2. Test unit by pressing the button marked test; if the batteries are good, the needle will go to the green area between the 40% and 60% marks; if the needle falls below the 40% mark, change batteries.
3. Replace batteries by tipping the unit upside down and removing the two thumbscrews holding the batteries in place.
4. Pull the plate out carefully and the batteries will be exposed.
5. Remove the two terminal connections, replace with new batteries, and reconnect the terminal connection.
6. Place battery plate back into unit carefully and replace two thumbscrews.
7. Repress test button to check new batteries.
8. Press button marked *on*.
9. Expose sensor to room air and wait 20 to 30 sec to stabilize unit.

10. Adjust unit with calibrate knob until needle is located on 20.9%.

11. If batteries are good and calibration cannot be adjusted to 20.9%, the sensor will have to be replaced.

12. Replacement of sensor is by means of an oxygen sensor change kit that is supplied by the IMI Corporation.

13. Expose sensor to the environment to be analyzed.

14. Push test button to turn unit *off*.

HARRIS 330A OXYGEN ANALYZER

The Harris 330A Oxygen Analyzer (Figure 6-4) is designed for continuous monitoring of environmental oxygen concentration. The unit operates on a Teledyne microfuel cell, which has a life cycle of approximately 18 months of continuous operation. The cell, when no longer functioning, can be easily replaced. The oxygen analyzer is unaffected by relative humidity and may be sterilized with ethylene oxide.

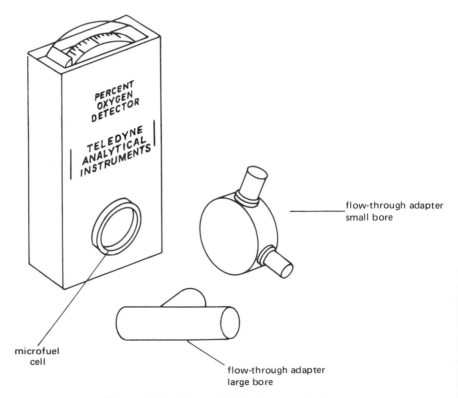

Figure 6-4.   Harris 330A Oxygen Analyzer.

For operation of the unit, select a proper flow-through adapter —either small bore or large bore. Place the adapter into the cell unit of the analyzer and connect tubing to the inlet of the unit. Attach the other end of the adapter to the outlet tubing; then attach tubing and adapters to patient. The analyzer will respond 90% in 30 sec and is accurate within 2% of the full scale.

BECKMAN D2 OXYGEN ANALYZER

The measurement of oxygen has far-reaching importance in science and medicine. Applications include safeguarding newborn premature infants by measuring oxygen concentration in incubator air and also measuring the oxygen in inspiratory air produced by respirators.

The Beckman D2 Oxygen Analyzer (Figure 6-5) is portable, simple to operate, and provides reliable oxygen measurements almost anywhere with safety. The instrument is powered by two flashlight batteries. The scale of each instrument is calibrated for partial pressure of oxygen in millimeters of mercury; the percentage of oxygen at a barometric pressure of 760 mm Hg also is indicated on each scale.

Principle of Operation

The Beckman D2 Oxygen Analyzer is based on a simple phenomenon —the magnetic susceptibility of oxygen. Oxygen is strongly para-

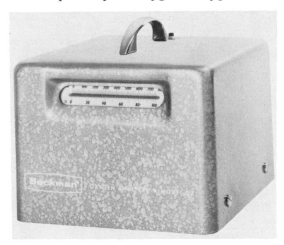

Figure 6-5.   Beckman D2 Oxygen Analyzer. (*Courtesy of Beckman Instruments, Inc.*)

magnetic (attracted by a magnetic field), while other common gases, with a few exceptions, are slightly diamagnetic (repelled by a magnetic field). The susceptibility of oxygen can be thought of as a measure of the propensity of an oxygen molecule to become a temporary magnet when placed in a magnetic field; this is analogous to the effects of a magnetic field on soft iron. Diamagnetic gases are comparable to nonmagnetic materials.

The heart of the oxygen-measuring system is a small glass dumbbell suspended on a taut, durable, quartz fiber in a nonuniform magnetic field. At equilibrium the magnetic force on the dumbbell is balanced by the torque of the quartz fiber. When a gas sample containing oxygen is drawn into the test chamber surrounding the dumbbell, the magnetic force is altered. This change in force allows the dumbbell to rotate. The degree of rotation is proportional to the change in force; the change in force is proportional to the partial pressure of oxygen in the sample. A small mirror attached to, and rotating with, the dumbbell throws a focus of light on the instru-

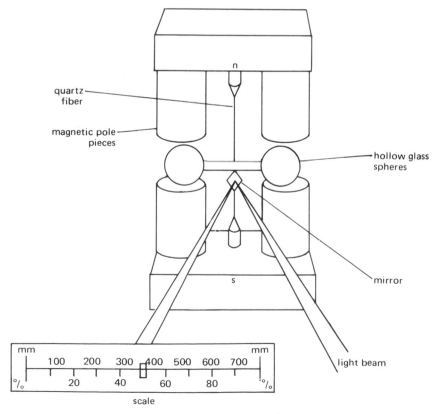

Figure 6-6.   Schematic view of oxygen analyzer measuring system.

ment's translucent scale. The position of the light beam on the scale indicates the partial pressure of the oxygen (see Figure 6-6).

Operating Instructions

1. Remove protective rubber bulb from the sampling tube and place the end of the sampling tube at the point from which sample is desired.
2. Squeeze and release the aspirator bulb slowly ten to twelve times to make certain that new sample fills the analyzer.
3. Press light switch on top of instrument.
4. Read oxygen concentration in gas sample from position of light beam on graduated scale.

   Note: The sampling tube is provided with an adapter to fit standard Luer-type needles. These needles, which may be inserted through rubber walls without damage, are convenient for obtaining samples from respirators, masks, and rubber bladders.

The Instrument

Scale Graduation.   The scale is graduated for 0 to 100% oxygen and 0 to 760 mm Hg oxygen partial pressure. For oxygen partial pressure measurement, the scale readings are correct regardless of ambient barometric pressure and altitudes. However, the oxygen percentage readings are affected by the barometric pressure and should be corrected whenever the instrument is used at high altitudes. Values to be added to the percentage reading to correct for lower barometric pressure at higher altitudes are listed in Table 6-1.

Moisture.   Moisture should not be permitted to condense within the instrument. It is advisable, therefore, to dry the gas sample by passing it through the silica gel drying tube included with the instrument. Water vapor, as such, is not harmful and measurements may be made on either a dry or wet basis; however, readings must be corrected to compensate for moisture. A lower oxygen content will be observed if a wet gas is analyzed than if the gas sample is dried before analysis. The magnitude of this difference is directly related to the water vapor content of the sample gas. For example, dry air contains 20.9% oxygen. At a barometric pressure of 760 mm Hg, the oxygen partial pressure of dry air is 159 mm Hg (760 $\times$ 0.209). In air saturated with moisture at body temperature (98.6°F), the water

TABLE 6-1   Corrections for Changes in Altitudes and Barometric Pressure

Altitude (ft)	Barometric Pressure (mm Hg)	Scale Readings (%)										
		0	10	20	30	40	50	60	70	80	90	100
0	760	0	0	0	0	0	0	0	0	0	0	0
350	750	0	0	0	0	1	1	1	1	1	1	—
700	740	0	0	1	1	1	1	2	2	2	2	—
1050	730	0	0	1	1	2	2	2	2	3	4	—
1400	720	0	1	1	2	2	3	3	4	4	5	—
1750	710	0	1	1	2	3	4	4	5	6	6	—
2100	700	0	1	2	3	3	4	5	6	7	8	—
2450	690	0	1	2	3	4	5	6	7	8	9	—
2800	680	0	1	2	4	5	6	7	8	9	10	—
3200	670	0	1	3	4	5	7	8	9	11	—	—
3600	660	0	2	3	5	6	8	9	11	12	—	—
4000	650	0	2	3	5	7	8	10	12	14	—	—
4400	640	0	2	4	6	8	9	11	13	15	—	—
4800	630	0	2	4	6	8	10	12	14	17	—	—
5200	620	0	2	5	7	9	11	14	16	18	—	—
5600	610	0	2	5	7	10	12	15	17	20	—	—
6050	600	0	3	5	8	11	13	16	19	—	—	—
6500	590	0	3	6	9	11	14	17	20	—	—	—
6920	580	0	3	6	9	12	16	19	22	—	—	—
7410	570	0	3	7	10	13	17	20	23	—	—	—
7900	560	0	4	7	11	14	18	21	25	—	—	—

Actual oxygen percentage equals reading in percent plus number shown in table.

vapor partial pressure is 47 mm Hg, so that the oxygen partial pressure in air saturated with moisture at 98.6°F is

$$159 \times \frac{760 - 47}{760} = 149 \text{ mm Hg}$$

As a further example, if air saturated at 98.6°F is cooled to 32°F (by an ice pack), water will condense until the water vapor partial pressure is only 4.6 mm Hg. The oxygen partial pressure of the cooled gas will be

$$159 \times \frac{760 - 4.6}{760} = 158 \text{ mm Hg}$$

Temperature. The readings of the analyzer are affected by temperature. The instrument has been calibrated at 72°F. The accuracy at that temperature is ±2% of the full scale. The influence of the ambient temperature is at minimum near the center point of the scale and increases proportionally to a maximum at the high and the lower ends of the range.

For each degree Fahrenheit decrease from 72°F, the indicated oxygen concentration at the upper end of the scale is approximately 0.25% of full scale less than the true oxygen concentration, while the indicator valve at the lower (zero) end of the scale is higher than the true oxygen concentration by the same amount. A decrease of the ambient temperature has the opposite effect; that is, for each degree Fahrenheit decrease from 72°F, the indicated oxygen concentration at the upper end of the scale is 0.25% of the full scale more than the true oxygen concentration.

Drying Tube.   The drying tube contains indicating-type silica gel desiccant, normally blue in color. When the color changes to pink, the silica gel has lost its drying power and should be replaced. Exhausted tubes may be refilled from bottles of fresh bulk (mesh size 6-16) silica gel or the silica gel may be regenerated by heating to about 300°F.

Important: Fresh cotton packing (commercial grade) should be used each time the silica gel is replaced.

Aspirator Bulb.   Aspirator bulbs used with the model D2 draw the sample gas through the analyzer. When the bulb is squeezed, the air inside the bulb is expelled through the check valve. As the bulb returns to its normal state, it draws a gas sample from its source through the sampling hose, the drying tube, and then the analyzer.

Aspirator bulbs not obtained from Beckman Instruments probably operate backward. When this occurs, room air will be pushed into the analyzer each time the bulb is squeezed, and the analyzer will read above 21% oxygen.

An easy test of bulb operation is as follows: Make sure that the bulb is connected to the analyzer, the analyzer to the drying tube, and that all sample lines are clear. Squeeze the bulb while holding one hand an inch or so from the check valve end of the bulb. Air should be felt being expelled from the valve each time the bulb is squeezed. If not, reverse the check valve in the end of the bulb and repeat the test.

Maintenance.   For maintenance check the manual, *Beckman Instructions, D2 Oxygen Analyzer.*

BIO MARINE OXYGEN ANALYZER WITH DIGITAL DISPLAY

I. Introduction

The Bio Marine Oxygen Analyzer (Figure 6-7) is a portable unit that provides a continuous digital display of oxygen concentra-

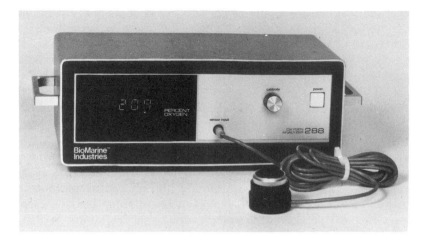

Figure 6-7.   Bio Marine Oxygen Analyzer. (*Courtesy of Bio Marine Industries, Inc., Malvern, Pa.*)

tions from 0 to 100%. It is temperature controlled (32° to 104°F (0°C–40°C) automatically and performs accurately in high humidity.

II. Operation
   A. Plug the Bio Marine Analyzer into a properly grounded 110-V ac receptacle.
   B. Attach the sensor to the analyzer.
   C. Depress the *on* switch; the button should light.
   D. Check calibration:
      1. If the Bio Marine is to be used for measuring oxygen levels below 50%, use ambient air. Rotate the calibration knob until the meter reads 20.9%.
      2. If the Bio Marine is to be used for measuring oxygen levels above 50%, calibrate to 100% (or known gas mixture):
         a. Attach in-line adapter; expose sensor to flow of gas for 2 min, or
         b. Place sensor in small polyethylene bag; direct flow of gas into bag at 5 liters/min for 5 min.
   E. For *direct exposure* analysis, such as in a tent, place the sensor in the atmosphere to be analyzed for 1 min. The percentage of oxygen concentration will be digitally displayed.
   F. For *sample* analysis, such as a ventilator, attach a suitable adapter so that the gas flow is directed over the sensor face.

G. If the remote sensor is to be used in high-humidity atmospheres, attach the high-humidity adapter so that moisture does not collect on the sensor face.

BECKMAN OM-15 OXYGEN MONITOR

The Beckman OM-15 Oxygen Monitor (Figure 6-8) is an instrument that measures the partial pressure of oxygen. The oxygen level displayed may be calibrated in concentration units for convenience. The detection and measurement of oxygen are accomplished using a polarographic oxygen sensor. Sensor output current developed in the presence of oxygen is amplified and temperature compensated. The amplified signal is then used to drive a digital panel meter, selectable to display either partial pressure of oxygen in kilopascals

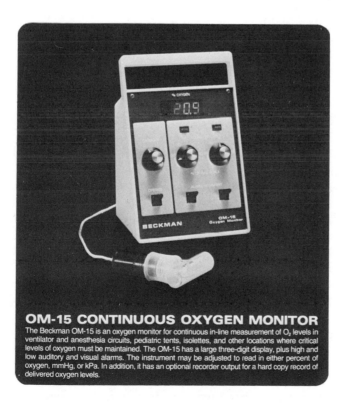

OM-15 CONTINUOUS OXYGEN MONITOR

The Beckman OM-15 is an oxygen monitor for continuous in-line measurement of O_2 levels in ventilator and anesthesia circuits, pediatric tents, isolettes, and other locations where critical levels of oxygen must be maintained. The OM-15 has a large three-digit display, plus high and low auditory and visual alarms. The instrument may be adjusted to read in either percent of oxygen, mmHg, or kPa. In addition, it has an optional recorder output for a hard copy record of delivered oxygen levels.

Figure 6-8. Beckman OM-15 Continuous Oxygen Monitor. (*Courtesy of Beckman Instruments, Inc., Schiller Park, Ill.*)

or in millimeters of mercury or oxygen concentration in percentage. Visual and audible alarms may be set for both high and low oxygen levels.

Assembly

1. Connect oxygen sensor cable to sensor connector on console rear panel.
2. Screw oxygen sensor into cable receptacle.
3. If desired mount the OM-15 to a pole or other vertical or horizontal support.
4. Connect power cord to a properly grounded electrical outlet.
5. Place operate switch in *up* position.
6. After allowing instrument to warm up approximately 5 min, perform calibration as indicated. *Two-point calibration* procedure is recommended for maximum accuracy and performance verification.
   a. Allow the instrument and sensor to warm up a minimum of 5 minutes.
   b. Place sensor in 100% oxygen and allow to stabilize for at least 1 min. Adjust the calibrate control if necessary so that the display reads 100% oxygen or the correct oxygen partial pressure.
   c. Place the sensor in room air and allow to stabilize for 1 min. Verify that the meter reads 20.9% oxygen or the correct partial pressure within 1% of the reading obtained in (b) above.
7. *Single-point calibration* on air may be used for rapid instrument setup but does not necessarily ensure the accuracy at high levels provided by the *two-point calibration* method.
   a. Allow the instrument and sensor to warm up a minimum of 5 min.
   b. Place the sensor in room air and allow to stabilize for at least 1 min. Adjust the calibrate control if necessary so that the meter reads 20.9% oxygen or the correct oxygen partial pressure.

Operation

1. Place the oxygen sensor in gas to be monitored. The sensor tee fitting and adapter may be used to connect two 22-mm tubings. Position tee so that face of sensor is facing down.
2. Set the low alarm to the desired level by rotating the low alarm

set/inhibit switch. The alarm level will be shown on the digital display. Set the high alarm in the same way, using the Hi alarm level control and Hi alarm set/inhibit switch. Alarm levels may be approximately set by rotating the control to the level indicated by the knob pointer. The exact level set may then be verified by pressing down the corresponding alarm set/inhibit switch.

3. Read the monitored oxygen level from the digital display.

4. If the oxygen monitor is not to be used for several hours, it is recommended that the instrument be shut down to prevent unnecessary operation of the oxygen sensor.

   a. Place the operate switch in down position.

   b. Remove the sensor from the monitored atmosphere and shake out any accumulated moisture.

   Note: It is good practice to mount or position the sensor so the membrane faces downward, causing condensation to drain away from the membrane.

Cleaning and Disinfecting

1. *Console*—Before attempting to clean the console, disconnect the power cord from the electrical outlet. To clean, a mild detergent such as alconox may be used. Isopropyl alcohol or ethyl alcohol may be used to clean and disinfect.

Note: Do not apply alcohol to the console front panel. Cleaning cloths should only be moistened and must not allow cleaning solution to flow into the console.

2. *Oxygen sensor*—It may be necessary to clean and disinfect the oxygen sensor, the sensor receptacle, and the connecting sensor cable. When the sensor becomes contaminated with foreign matter, remove it from its receptacle and soak it in distilled water. Shake the sensor gently to remove any solids, and resoak with gentle wiping until the sensor is thoroughly clean. Dry the sensor thoroughly before screwing it back into its receptacle. To disinfect the sensor, place it in a container with the receptacle, cable, tee, and adapter, and use ethylene oxide at room temperature.

Note: Do not place sensor in an autoclave to sterilize it.

VENTRONICS POLAROGRAPHIC OXYGEN MONITOR AND ANALYZER

The Polarographic Oxygen Monitor and Analyzer (Figure 6-9) are digital display units with a disposable polarographic sensor cell and temperature compensation that takes place directly in the sensing environment. They have a response time that gives 97% of any change in oxygen concentration in less than 12 sec. They provide accuracy of ±2%, and a total analytical range of 5% to 100% oxygen.

Operation

1. *On/Off Procedure*—Activate the unit by plugging the connector of the oxygen sensor into the connector socket on the rear of the monitor or analyzer. The connector must be in proper position, with the cord on the right side of the connector.

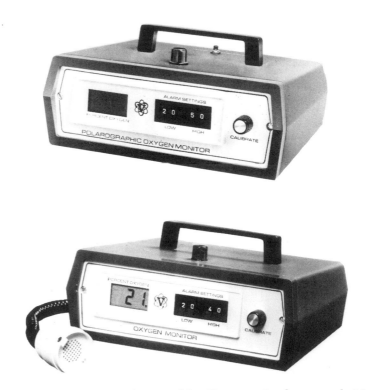

Figure 6-9. Ventronics Polarographic Oxygen Analyzer and Monitor. (*Courtesy of Ventronics Division of Hudson, Temecula, Calif.*)

Note: The unit requires approximately 5 min to polarize, during which time numbers will flash rapidly on the digital readout. The unit is ready for use (polarized) when the display *ceases* blinking. To turn the unit *off,* simply unplug the connector.

2. *Calibration*—When the sensor is polarized, calibrate the unit in room air to 21% oxygen. Turn the calibration knob until 20 appears; then turn the knob clockwise until 21 appears with a decimal point after it (21.).

Note: Decimal point must be present to achieve full stated accuracy. To calibrate at 100%, expose the sensor for about 1 min to 100% oxygen. Then adjust the calibration knob until 100 appears.

3. Place sensor into medium to be analyzed.
4. Set high and low alarm on monitor only.
5. Alarm silence button on monitor only will silence the alarm for 30 sec.
6. *Battery life*—a minus sign will appear at the *left* of the digital display when the batteries are 90% expended. The batteries should be replaced with two 9-V batteries.
7. *Sensor life*—When the sensor is near the end of its useful life, its output will gradually become nonlinear (reading farthest from the calibration point will lose accuracy). To assure the accuracy of the unit, the sensor condition should be checked daily. Calibrate the units to 21%; then check the reading in 100% oxygen. If the reading is below 98% or above 102%, the sensor cell should be replaced. To replace sensor cell, pull on the exposed rim at the end of the sensor assembly unit. The cell separates from its holder. To install the new sensor cell, line up the three prongs on the cell with the holes at the bottom of the holder. Then slide the cell into its holder; when you feel the prongs line up with their holes, press the sensor cell in until it is completely flush with the holder.

Cleaning and Sterilization

1. Wipe off case with damp cloth or alcohol.
2. The polarographic sensor may be cleaned with alcohol or sterilized in buffered glutaraldehyde.

IL 406 OXYGEN ANALYZER

The IL 406 oxygen analyzer is designed to spot check or to continuously monitor oxygen tension in a gaseous atmosphere. It comes with a single scale meter: 0 to 100% O_2. It is *not* equipped with an audio or visual alarm. It is powered by two mercury batteries; *use only 4.05-V mercury batteries.*

Battery Installation

1. Remove the back panel screw in the center of the back cover, and then slide out battery holder board.
2. Insert one battery at a time, noting the polarity labels in the battery holder. The polarity of mercury batteries is reversed from other types of batteries; the positive end (+) end is the flat end.
3. Take the sensor from its package and remove yellow protective cap. (Save this cap.) Check the condition of the membrane cap; look for cracks, pinholes, or moisture on the sensing end.
4. Place the sensor connector into the receptacle under the left side of the circuit board. Be sure that the large-diameter pin is inserted into the corresponding large-diameter socket. *Be careful not to force this connection.*
5. Rotate the twist lock ring on the connector until it is fully engaged.
6. To have maximum precision, the sensor should be allowed to warm up for a period of 1 to 2 hours on *initial* installation. If the sensor is kept plugged into the unit during this time, no waiting period is necessary before calibration.
7. Remove the manifold from the instrument; attach both male ends of the manifold to the patient breathing circuit. Be certain you have a tight fit.
8. The sensor is inserted into the manifold up to the "stop" in the 15-mm port. The sensor should be placed vertically with membrane down and cable end up.

Daily Checklist of Calibration and Operation

1. With the unit upright and the function switch in the standby position, check to see that the meter reads zero. If not, adjust the meter zero (screw head in center of the front panel) to obtain a reading of 0% O_2.
2. Press the battery check button. The meter reading should be

above 82 and below 94. If not, replace with new 4.05-V mercury batteries.

3. Turn the function switch to the *on* position. Expose the sensor to dry 100% O_2 and adjust the calibrate control so that the meter reads 100% O_2. Expose the sensor to room air. The meter reading should return to 21% O_2 (±2% O_2 within 30 sec).

4. Check that sensor and manifold are secured in the patient breathing circuit.

5. Readjust flowmeter as required.

Storage and Return to Service

1. For *storage up to 30 days*, the temperature of the storage area must be maintained between 0° to 40°C (32° to 104°F).

2. The batteries and the O_2 sensor should remain in place with the instrument function switch in the standby position. The membrane end of the sensor should remain plugged into the manifold or be reinstalled into the yellow protective cap originally supplied with the sensor.

3. Daily checklist must be performed before the instrument is returned to service.

4. *Storage over 30 days*, or when the temperature limits in the storage area exceed 0° to 40°C. The following must be performed:
   a. Turn function switch to standby.
   b. Disconnect O_2 sensor and replace yellow protective cap originally supplied.
   c. Remove both batteries from unit.
   d. Store in an area where temperatures are maintained between −40° to +65°C (−40° to +149°F).

5. When returning to service:
   a. Replace membrane with a new one or *recharge the sensor.*
   b. Reassemble unit as per battery installation.
   c. Perform daily checklist.

Changing the Electrolyte and/or the Membrane (recharging)

1. With the function switch set to standby, disconnect the sensor cord from the unit. The O-ring on the sensor provides a snug fit on the manifold. Grasp the sensor firmly and pull it out of the manifold with a clockwise motion to overcome the snugness of the O-ring.

2. At a sink, carefully unscrew the membrane cap from the sensor body. Hold sensor in a vertical position with the cable end up.

3. Flush the sensor body and inside of the membrane cap with tap water. Shake off the excess water and rub the cathode end (the silver tip at the end of black stem) with a rough paper towel. Tap the open end of the membrane cap down on the towel to remove excess water droplets.

4. Invert the rinsed membrane cap and slowly fill it with electrolyte gel to within $\frac{1}{4}$ in. of the top of the cap. *Do not touch the membrane itself.*

5. Insert the sensor body at an angle into the membrane cap so that trapped air bubbles can escape through the vent groove.

6. Straignten the sensor body and slowly screw it into the membrane cap. Use a paper towel to keep excess electrolyte gel off the fingers and away from the outer membrane surface at the end of the membrane cap.

7. Using a paper towel, tighten the assembly securely.

8. Rinse off the sensor with tap water and blot dry with a paper towel.

9. Replace the sensor in the manifold and connect the sensor cord to the instrument.

10. Proceed with daily checklist.

Cleaning and Sterilizing. The surface of the instrument can be cleaned periodically by wiping with a cloth moistened with 70% isopropyl alcohol. It is recommended that the batteries be removed before clɔaning.

To clean the sensor, turn the function switch to standby and unlock and disconnect sensor connector from the instrument. The sensor then may be placed in a sterilizing solution such as Cidex, following the manufacturer's instructions.

Ethylene oxide sterilization (low-temperature method) requires that the batteries be removed from the instrument and that the membrane cap be loosened one full turn on the sensor to allow pressure relief during the sterilization process. After sterilization, the electrolyte gel must be changed.

Preventive Maintenance

1. *Every 3 months*—Change electrolyte gel in the sensor.

2. *Every year*—Attach new membrane cap with electrolyte. Install new batteries.

These schedules may have to be changed or altered if instrument is subject to heavy usage.

BENNETT MONITORING SPIROMETER AND SPIROMETER ALARM

The Bennett Monitoring Spirometer (Figure 6-10) is designed for use with ventilators to give a visual indication of expired tidal volumes. It should be used in conjunction with the Bennett Monitoring Spirometer Alarm or other alarm systems.

I. Bennett Monitoring Spirometer
   A. Assembly (see Figure 6-11)
      1. Turn the spirometer base over.

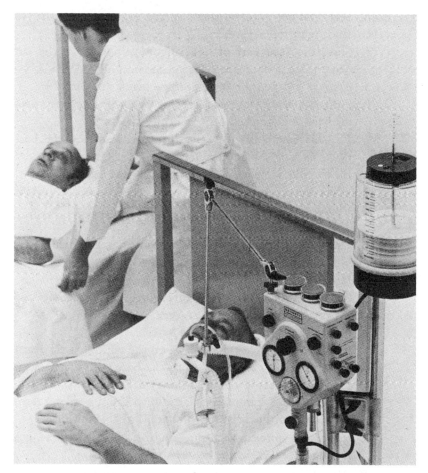

Figure 6-10.   Bennett Monitoring Spirometer and Alarm mounted on Bennett Respiration Unit Model PR-2. (*Courtesy of Puritan-Bennett Corp., Kansas City, Mo.*)

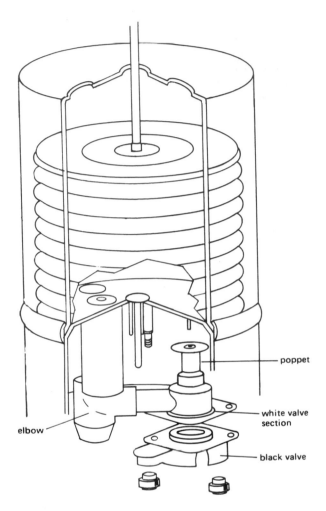

Figure 6-11.   Assembly of the Bennett Monitoring Spirometer.

2. Assemble the poppet by placing silicone disc between metal poppet and plastic screw; tighten, but do not bend disc.

3. Slide poppet onto its guide on the base (between the two studs with metal threads).

4. Slide the oval end of the silicone elbow onto the corresponding port on the white valve section.

5. Slightly dampen the O-ring on the black valve.

6. Push the black valve section into the white section, making sure to align the holes on both sides.

7. Fit this assembly over the threaded studs on the base, thus covering the poppet.

8. Fit the silicone elbow over the outlet on the base.

9. When the assembly is properly seated, secure it, using two thumbscrews.

10. Turn the base over.

11. Place the silicone leaf over the inlet stud, which resembles a wheel with spokes.

12. Place the pushrod into its hole in the center of the base.

13. Place the small silicone diaphragm over the center stud, making sure that it is well seated.

14. Place the ring seal around the base.

15. Fit the bellows over the groove on the white plastic disc.

16. Set the bellows assembly onto the base with the flange of the bellows evenly arranged onto the base.

17. Assemble the spirometer alarm onto the spirometer dome according to the directions in Part II of this outline.

18. Place the spirometer dome on the base, with the post through the hole in the center top of the dome.

19. Seal with the ring.

20. Check the spirometer for leaks:
    a. Turn the spirometer over to fill the bellows.
    b. Return the spirometer to an upright position.
    c. If the bellows falls more than 300 cc in a minute, check all connections.

21. Mount the spirometer according to the procedure for the specific ventilator.

II. Bennett Monitoring Spirometer Alarm

   A. Assembly (see Figure 6-12)

      1. Fit the alarm over the spirometer dome, with the feet of the alarm in the holes on the top of the dome.

      2. Secure the alarm by engaging all four of its feet with the clamp.

      3. Assemble the spirometer as directed in Part I of this outline.

      4. Place the meter stick into the center post.

   B. To set alarm (Figure 6-13)

      1. Observe tidal volume on the spirometer.

      2. Remove the collecting tube from the manifold.

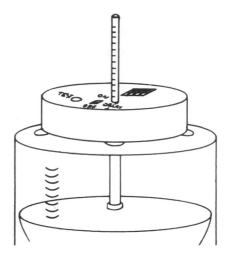

Figure 6-12.   Assembly of the Bennett Monitoring Spirometer Alarm.

3. Set the meter stick slightly below the desired tidal volume, so that if the tidal volume does not reach the desired volume, the alarm will sound.
4. Turn switch to *on.*
5. Push the test button and release; the alarm should sound.
6. Lift the bellows until the alarm stops.
7. Maintain this position; the alarm should sound again in approximately 20 sec.

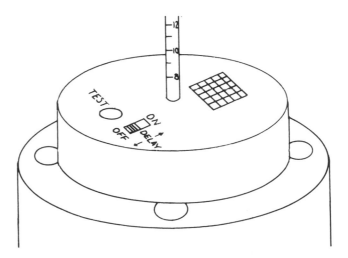

Figure 6-13.   Setting the Bennett Monitoring Spirometer Alarm.

8. Lift the bellows again to stop the alarm.

9. Release the post; turn the switch off and then on; the alarm should sound in approximately 1 min; turn the switch off and on (see Figure 6-11).

10. Replace the collecting tube.

11. If the tidal volume is readjusted, the alarm must be readjusted.

III. Cleaning

   A. Disassemble all parts of the spirometer as completely as possible.

   B. Set aside the black valve section of the spirometer, and also the alarm; these may not be submerged in fluids, but can be gas sterilized.

   C. After processing, all parts of the spirometer except those mentioned above may be cold sterilized in Cidex or gas sterilized; however, gas sterilization tends to glaze the plastic dome.

BENNETT MONITORING SPIROMETER ALARM: NEW STYLE

The Bennett Spirometer Alarm is an independently battery operated monitor designed to give an audible signal when a set tidal volume is not reached. A flag switch turns the alarm on and off. The alarm may be installed or removed from the spirometer by turning and lifting. It is not necessary to remove the dome to do so.

To Set the Alarm

1. Remove the collecting tube from the manifold.

2. Set the metering stick for approximately 10% less than the desired volume.

3. Set warning time, usually 15 to 20 sec. This ensures that if the desired volume is not reached, a warning will sound within that time.

4. Lower the flag to activate the alarm.

5. Press and hold the *test* button. The alarm should sound and the light activate.

6. Release the *test* button. Within the set warning time the alarm should sound and light.

7. Press the *Silence* button. The audible warning should cease, but reactivate in 60 sec.

8. Lift the bellows slowly above the desired volume. The alarm should cease. Hold the bellows in this position; the alarm should activate. Lift the bellows to a greater volume and then allow the spirometer to dump. The alarm should cease.

9. Reconnect the collecting tube.

Special Notes

1. Do not use the alarm unless it is functioning properly.

2. If the normal volume is readjusted, the alarm metering stick must be also.

3. Do not turn alarm *off* unless the patient will be disconnected from the ventilator for an extended period of time.

Cleaning and Sterilization. Since the alarm is not in the patient system, it need not be sterilized. After each use, wipe the alarm with alcohol to clean.

BENNETT TEMPERATURE ALARM

The Bennett Temperature Alarm (Figure 6-14) is designed for use with heated humidifiers or nebulizers, and warns visually and audibly if the temperature in the patient circuit exceeds the settings of 104°F (40°C) or 115°F (46°C).

Assembly

1. Install the adapter with connector downstream of any sidearm nebulizer to avoid the cooling effect of such a nebulizer. The adapter may be attached at the outlet of the nebulizer manifold if an extension or circle tube is used.

2. Connect the cord to the alarm, using a push–twist motion.

3. Attach the alarm to the support arm, allowing for mobility of the cord.

4. Connect the sensor to the cord with a push–twist motion.

5. Push sensor into adapter.

Operation

1. To test the alarm, press the *Test/Reset* button. The alarm should be loud and undistorted and the light should be bright. Do not use if either alarm does not function properly.

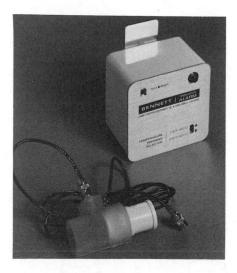

Figure 6-14. Bennett Temperature Alarm. (*Courtesy of Bennett Respiration Products, Santa Monica, Calif.*)

2. Set temperature warning selector.
   a. 104°F if sensor is close to patient.
   b. 115°F if sensor is separated from patient by extension or circle tube.
3. If the alarm sounds during operation, rearrange tubing system to bypass the humidifier.
4. Press *Test/Reset* button to silence alarm, once sensor has cooled below warning temperature.
5. Correct condition causing warning; change humidifier as necessary. Monitor patient, humidifier, and thermometer.

Cleaning and Sterilization.   When removing the sensor from the adapter, first disconnect the cord. The alarm proper and the cord are not in the patient circuit; dry and wipe clean. Do not allow liquid to enter the alarm case or the cord connections. The adapter, connector, and the removable sensor may be cold sterilized, gas sterilized or autoclaved (250°F for 15 min). Wrap the parts in muslin.

WRIGHT RESPIROMETER

The Wright Respirometer, which is supplied complete with adapters in a zippered case, has a watch-face-type dial protected by a clear plastic cover plate. See Figure 6-15. The dial is marked in 100 divisions and numbered at every tenth division. One complete revolu-

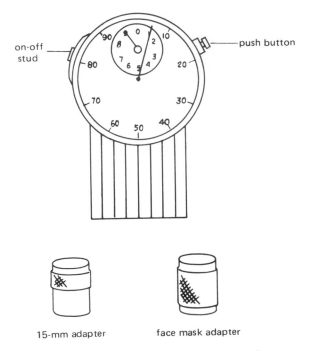

Figure 6-15. Wright Respirometer and adapters.

tion of the large hand indicates a volume of 100 liters. A smaller scale on the upper part of the main dial is marked in 100 divisions with the numerals 0.1, 0.2, and so on, at appropriate intervals. One complete revolution of the hand of this small dial indicates a volume of 1 liter. A spring-loaded button for resetting the hands to zero positions and an *on/off* control in the form of a sliding stud are mounted on the outside of the instrument.

Operating Instructions

1. The respirometer has an inspiratory port and an expiratory port. The flow of gas through the instrument is in one direction only; on reversal of the flow, the hands remain stationary. For most of our purposes, the expiratory port is used.
2. The *on/off* stud may be used to stop the flow at the end of any respiration.
3. The respirometer may be inserted into any part of a gas circuit to measure flow, using a suitable adapter. Tidal volume and minute volume may be measured in this manner.
4. Expiratory tidal volume, minute volume, and vital capacity may be measured directly from a patient by attaching a flex

tube with a mouthpiece, mask, or tracheotomy adapter to the expiratory port of the instrument and having the patient exhale. (For TV and MV, patient breathes as normally as possible. For VC have the patient inhale deeply and exhale as much as possible.)

5. The respirometer can be used to ensure that a ventilator is delivering the volume for which it is set.

6. Reading the dials:
   a. Reset dials to zero.
   b. Take the measurement.
   c. Move *on/off* stud to *off*.
   d. Reading volume less than 1 liter entails using only the small dial. Each graduation represents 0.01 liter or 10 ml. Slightly longer graduations indicate 0.1 liter (100 ml), 0.2 liter (200 ml), and so on.
   e. Use the small dial as a guide, reading first the fraction of a liter that is recorded. Then refer to the large dial to determine the number of full liters recorded. Care must be taken not to read a greater number of liters than is actually recorded. Hold the respirometer so that you look directly down on it.

Cleaning and Sterilization

1. The outside of the instrument may be wiped with alcohol.
2. The respirometer may be gas sterilized. Tape it securely in its case. Leave the case open when packaging. Mark package *Fragile*.

VERIFLO MR-1 RESPIRATOR OXYGEN CONTROLLER

The need for the ability to deliver a variety of oxygen and air mixtures in an adjustable ratio for ventilators, incubators, masks, and various other respiratory therapy equipment has led to the designing of the Veriflo MR-1 Respirator Oxygen Controller (Figure 6-16). This device has a self-regulating feature that maintains the desired percentage of oxygen regardless of wide variations in flow that result from fluctuations in the patient's respiration rate, tidal volume, or back pressure from the ventilator or other equipment.

I. Installation
   A. Mounting
      1. The MR-1 may be wall mounted using the wall-mounting plate accessory; the handle at the rear of the MR-1 may then be easily slid into the slot on the wall plate.

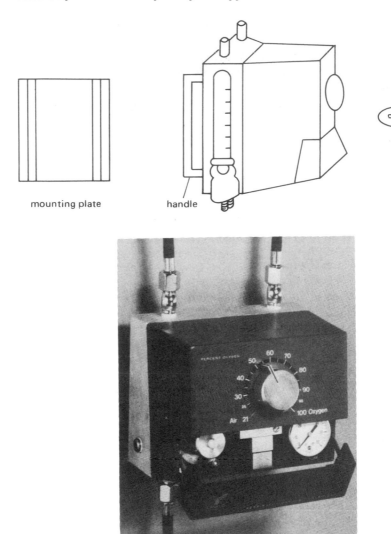

mounting plate   handle   pole bracket

Figure 6-16. Veriflo MR-1 Centilator Oxygen Controller. (*Courtesy of Veriflo Corp.*)

    2. The MR-1 may be mounted on a portable pole and base by attaching a universal clamp and bracket to the pole and then fitting the handle on the unit into the bracket.

B. Oxygen and air supplies

    1. The line pressure for both air and oxygen should fall between 50 and 60 psi pressure and the supply pressure should never exceed 70 psi; for the best results, the two supply pressures should fall within ±5 psi of each other.

2. Attach one end of the oxygen hose to the MR-1 oxygen inlet fitting (it is marked *oxy*), and then attach the other end to a high-pressure regulator (for use with cylinders) or to the proper adapter for pipeline use; to prevent leakage, make sure that all fittings are properly tightened.

3. Attach one end of the air inlet hose to the inlet fitting on the unit (marked *air*), and then attach the other end to a high-pressure regulator or the proper adapter for pipeline use; tighten all connections.

C. Installation for use with the Bennett PR-1 and PR-2 ventilators

1. Attach oxygen and air inlet hoses as described.

2. Attach one end of the outlet hose to the outlet on the bottom of the unit; make sure the connection is tight.

3. Attach the other end of the outlet hose to the oxygen inlet fitting on the ventilator.

4. Set the ventilator for 100% oxygen.

5. Set the desired oxygen concentration on the MR-1 unit.

6. Operate the ventilator as usual.

D. Installation for use with Bird ventilators

1. An adapter kit is required for use of the MR-1 oxygen controller; after installation according to the factory specifications, the kit remains in place.

2. The ventilator may be run in either the air-mix position or the 100% oxygen position.

3. Set the desired oxygen concentration on the MR-1 unit.

4. Operate the ventilator in the usual manner.

II. Operation

A. Starting procedure

1. Attach air and oxygen supplies.

2. Check both inlet and outlet pressures.

a. The lower hinged panel swngs down to expose the pressure gauge.

b. The pressure indicator selector is directly beneath the pressure gauge; set the indicator at each of the three positions: left for air, center for mixture outlet, and right for oxygen (see Figure 6-17). The air and oxygen readings should fall between 50 and 60 psi and should be within ±5 psi of one another. The mixture outlet should read 40 psi or at least 10 psi below the oxygen and air inlet readings.

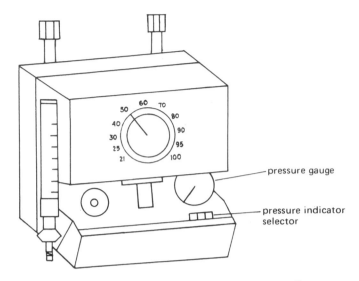

Figure 6-17. Veriflo MR-1 Oxygen Controller.

    c. This procedure should be repeated each time the audible alarm sounds and each time the unit is activated.

   3. To set the desired oxygen percentage, rotate the percent oxygen knob to the proper setting.

B. Operation of the audible alarm

   1. Alarm will sound for the following reasons:

    a. Inlet oxygen pressure falls below 40 psi.

    b. Inlet air pressure falls below 40 psi.

    c. Outlet pressure falls below 20 psi.

   2. If alarm sounds, all pressure must be monitored to determine the cause.

   3. If the air supply fails, the unit will continue to operate with pure oxygen; however, the flow capacity will be reduced proportionately to the setting. For example, at 100% the flow would be normal, while at 21% oxygen it would be zero.

C. Outlet pressure adjustment

   1. The outlet pressure is factory set at 40 psi, nominal.

   2. It is screwdriver-adjustable to vary pressure from 5 to 45 psi; the outlet pressure should be at least 10 psi below the inlet pressure.

   3. To increase pressure, turn the control clockwise, and to reduce pressure, turn the control counterclockwise.

Caution: Although the MR-1 unit is accurate within ±2% of the settings, periodic oxygen analysis should be done.

III. Maintenance

A. The two inlet filters should be replaced at no greater than 6-month intervals; to do so, remove the inlet fittings, remove the used filters, and replace inlet fittings.

B. If necessary, the MR-1 unit may be gas sterilized with ethylene oxide.

BIRD OXYGEN BLENDER

The Bird Oxygen Blender (Figure 6-18) is designed to regulate the concentration of oxygen being delivered by mechanical ventilation to the patient. Utilizing the mixture of oxygen and air, a wide variety of oxygen concentrations may be delivered.

Mounting.   The Bird Oxygen Blender may be mounted on a portable pedestal or in line. Make sure that the blender comes before the ventilator source inlet.

Oxygen and Air Supply

1. Attach one end of the oxygen supply tubing to the oxygen blender and the other end to a 50-psi oxygen source.

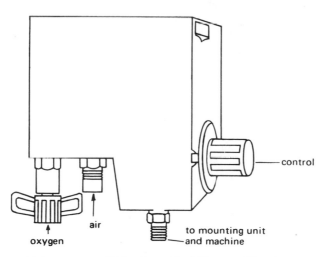

Figure 6-18.   Side view, Bird Oxygen Blender.

2. Attach one end of the compressed-air supply tubing to the blender and the other end to a 50-psi compressed-air source.
3. Attach blender to mounting unit of Bird ventilator to be used.
4. Attach Bird ventilator to be used.
5. Set ventilator on 100% setting so there is no air dilution.
6. Set desired oxygen percentage.
7. Check percentage of oxygen with an oxygen analyzer.

BENDIX RESPIRATORY SUPPORT SYSTEM

I. Introduction

The Bendix Respiratory Support System (RSS) (Figure 6-19) was designed to provide oxygen concentrations of 48 to 90%, utilizing flow rates from 10 to 20 liters/min. It is also capable of supplying 0 to 30 cm of water pressure for IPPB treatments or medicated aerosol therapy.

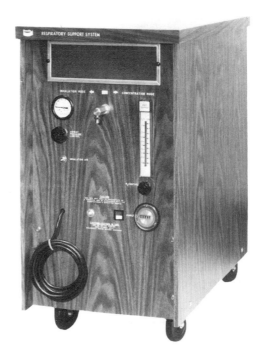

Figure 6-19.   Bendix Respiratory Support System. (*Courtesy of the Bendix Corp., Instruments and Life Support Division, Davenport, Iowa.*)

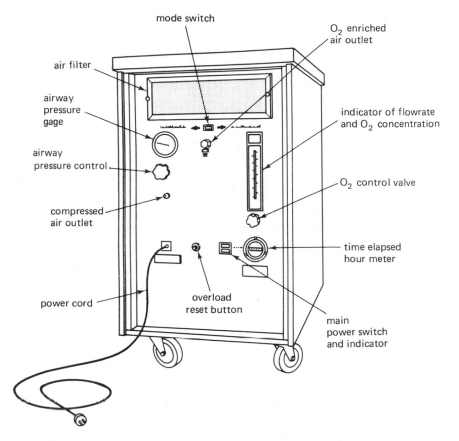

mode switch

O_2 enriched air outlet

air filter

airway pressure gage

indicator of flowrate and O_2 concentration

airway pressure control

O_2 control valve

compressed air outlet

time elapsed hour meter

power cord

overload reset button

main power switch and indicator

Figure 6-19. (cont.) Bendix Respiratory Support System—rear view.

II. Procedure

A. Place RSS unit with long dimension against wall.

B. Plug power cord into a properly grounded 115-V electrical outlet.

C. Press *Power* switch; amber light should go on. If it does not, press reset button.

D. For use with nasal cannula or face mask (concentration mode)

    1. Attach humidifier to threaded outlet in center of console. Do not use nebulizer or dual-purpose device as they will not operate properly.

    2. Attach delivery device desired (cannula or mask).

    3. Push switch at top of console to *Concentration Mode.*

4. Turn O_2 *Control* counterclockwise until desired flow rate is shown on indicator.

5. When using a Venturi-type mask, set the flow rate for 1 liter more than is indicated on the mask. Allow to stabilize for 30 min, analyze, and readjust flow rate as necessary.

E. For use with Bennett TA-1 handpiece:

1. Assemble handpiece and instill medication prescribed.

2. Attach handpiece supply tubing to compressed air outlet.

3. Push switch at top of console to *Inhalation Mode*.

4. Rotate *Airway Pressure Control* clockwise until gauge indicates prescribed pressure.

F. For use with hand-held nebulizer

1. Attach nebulizer supply tubing to compressed air outlet.

2. Push switch at top of console to *Inhalation Mode*.

3. To set mist desired, rotate *Airway Pressure Control* clockwise.

III. Guidelines for Respiratory Support System Use with Nasal Cannula

In calculating the following guideline graph for cannula therapy with the RSS, an I/E ratio of 1/1.5 is assumed.

Liter Flow Rate from RSS

6	48%	43%	39%	36%	34%	32%	31%
5	46%	41%	38%	35%	33%	32%	31%
4	44%	39%	36%	34%	32%	31%	30%
3	40%	36%	33%	31%	30%	29%	28%
2	34%	31%	30%	28%	27%	26%	26%
Patient Minute Volume (liters)	4	5	6	7	8	9	10

Approximate Inspired Oxygen Concentration (FIO_2)

IV. Routine Maintenance

A. *Each 24 hours of operation:* Remove, clean, and replace the air inlet filter. Clean by brushing, vacuuming, or washing in a detergent solution.

B. *Each 750 hours of operation:* Replace the felt inlet filter.

C. *As required:* Clean outside of the cabinet by wiping with any household cleaning solution. Clean any accessories used with the RSS according to the manufacturer's instructions.

Note: All filters should be in place when operating the RSS. Occluded filters will cause the unit performance to degrade.

Important: Additional maintenance at 750, 3000 and 6000 hours is required to assure proper operation.

DeVILBISS DeVo$_2$ OXYGEN CONCENTRATOR

The DeVilbiss DeVo$_2$ Oxygen Concentrator (Figure 6-20) is designed with the capability of providing an oxygen concentration of 94% at a flow of 2 liters/min. To accomplish this, a process similar to filtration is used.

Room air, which is composed basically of 21% oxygen and 78% nitrogen, is drawn into the DeVo$_2$ by a compressor. Before reaching the compressor, the air passes through a dust filter, a felt prefilter, and a high-efficiency bacteria filter. From the bacteria filter the room air enters a diaphragm-type compressor, which produces clean oil- and graphite-free air. The compressed air temperature is lowered with the aid of a heat exchanger and air flow from a cooling fan (Figure 6-21).

After passing through the heat exchanger, the compressed air is directed into one of two cylinders containing a complex inorganic silicate called *molecular sieve*. It is a unique property of the material that it selectively absorbs nitrogen from the room air, thereby producing oxygen-concentrated gas.

Because there are two cylinders of molecular sieve material available, one cylinder is alternately pressurized to produce oxygen while the other cylinder is being depressurized and flushed of the nitrogen it has collected. This process is called a *pressure swing cycle*, and it occurs automatically every 30 sec, assuring the patient of a continuous, uninterrupted supply of oxygen.

The gas is then directed through a check valve to an accumulator tank, a pressure regulator, and a second high-efficiency bacteria filter. An adjustable flowmeter on the DeVo$_2$ control panel permits control overflow of oxygen-rich gas to the patient at the level prescribed by the physician.

Installation

Locate the oxygen concentrator such that the operating controls are convenient to the patient. It must be accessible to a 115-V, 60-cycle, 15-A grounded electrical receptacle that is independent of other appliances.

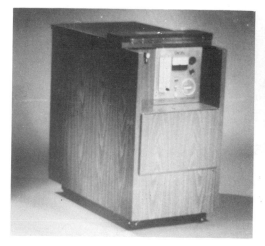

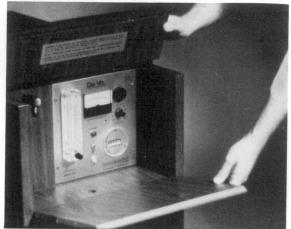

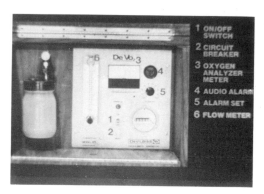

1 ON/OFF SWITCH
2 CIRCUIT BREAKER
3 OXYGEN ANALYZER METER
4 AUDIO ALARM
5 ALARM SET
6 FLOW METER

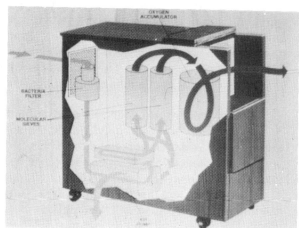

Figure 6-20.   DeVilbiss DeVO$_2$ Oxygen Concentrator. (*Courtesy of the DeVilbiss Co., Somerset, Pa.*)

The oxygen concentrator should not be located adjacent to radiators, heaters, or hot-air registers. Do not position the back of the unit closer than 3 in. from a wall, draperies, or other surfaces that could interfere with the air.

Note: Always observe the warning imprint on the oxygen concentrator.

Procedure

1. With the power switch in the *off* position, plug the power cord into a 115-V, 60-cycle, 15-A grounded electrical outlet. The use

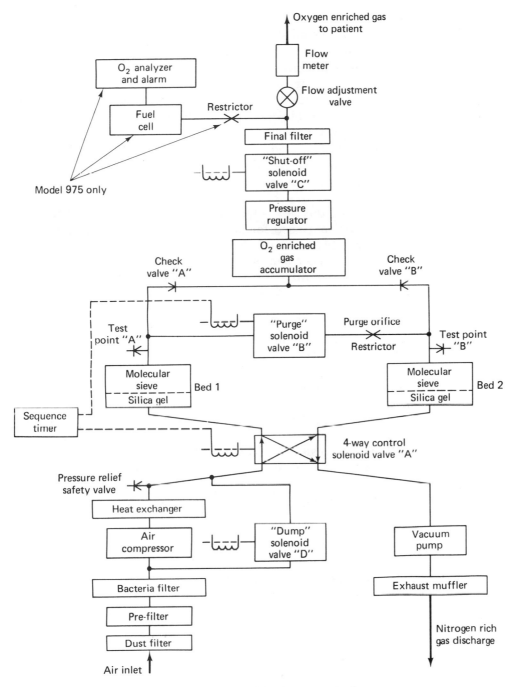

Figure 6-21.   Schematic of DeVo$_2$ Oxygen Concentrator.

of a three-wire adapter is not recommended, but if used, the adapter pigtail must be adequately grounded.

2. Turn power switch on. If the pilot light does not illuminate, press the white circuit breaker reset button on the front panel. If the pilot light still fails to illuminate, do not reset the circuit breaker, but check power cord for proper insertion; check to see if receptacle is powered. If oxygen concentrator still fails to operate, call for service.

3. With the DeVo$_2$ operating, slowly turn the flow-rate control until the center of the ball in the flow-rate indicator corresponds to the number of liters per minute prescribed by the physician.

> *Note:* When the DeVo$_2$ Oxygen Concentrator is first turned on (or if not used for an extended period of time, approximately 30 min to 1 hour will be required for the flow rate and oxygen concentration to stabilize. The flow rate may drift slightly during this period of time and should be monitored and readjusted if necessary.

4. If a humidifier has not been prescribed by the physician, a 9-16/18 nut and tapered hose fitting will be needed to accept the $\frac{3}{16}$-in. I.D. delivery tubing.

5. If a humidifier has been prescribed, attach a bubble-type humidifier to the threaded oxygen outlet.

> *Note:* Only bubble-type humidifiers should be used.

6. Attach the desired length of $\frac{3}{16}$-in. I.D. oxygen tubing to the unit or humidifier and attach either a cannula or a mask.

Routine Maintenance

1. The humidifiers should be cleaned daily. The patient should remove, empty, and clean the bubble-type humidifier, cannula, or mask prescribed by the physician and refill the humidifier in accordance with his recommendations.

2. The gross particle filter should be removed and cleaned by the patient weekly.

> *Note:* To remove and wash the dust filter located on the rear panel of the DeVo$_2$:
> a. Remove the two-wing screw that holds the filter and frame to the back panel.
> b. Wash the entire assembly in warm, soapy water and rinse. Shake excess water from the filter.

    c. Use a lint-free paper towel or absorbent cloth to re-
move excess water from the filter, and permit the filter
to dry before replacement.

Note: The gross particle filter should be monitored more closely
in environments with abnormal amounts of particulate
matter in the air. Operation of the DeVo$_2$ without the filter will prematurely occlude the felt prefilter and cause
a decrease in performance.

3. To test the audible oxygen alarm system on the model 965, remove the line cord from the 115-V ac outlet and turn the power
switch to the *on* position. If the alarm is not heard or sounds
weak, replace the batteries located in the inside rear of the cabinet. Check the audible alarm on model 975 by turning the power
switch on and rotating the oxygen alarm adjustment to the test
position (clockwise); the alarm should sound.

4. Additional maintenance at 2000, 9000, and 27,000 hours is required to assure proper operation.

BOURNS MODEL LS 160 VENTILATOR MONITOR

I. Introduction

The Bourns Model LS 160 Ventilator Monitor (Figure 6-22) utilizes a solid-state pressure transducer to sense pressure levels
in the patient circuit of a ventilator. It has no moving parts; it
should not be used in the presence of flammable anesthetics.

II. Operation

    A. Place the monitor on top of the ventilator or connect directly
to the ventilator by attaching a bracket.

    B. Connect the sampling adapter to the inspiratory line of the
patient circuit.

    C. Attach oxygen tubing from the sampling adapter and the
Monitor Input in front of unit.

    D. Plug power cord into 115-V ac, grounded outlet.

    E. Set desired parameters

        1. Low rate

        2. High rate

        3. PEEP

        4. Low pressure

        5. High pressure

    F. Set *Infant* or *Adult* mode

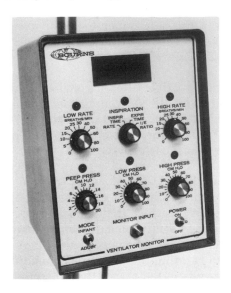

Figure 6-22. Bourns Model LS 160 Ventilator Monitor. (*Courtesy of Bourns, Inc., Life Support Division, Riverside, Calif.*)

G. Turn on power switch

H. I/E ratio, expiratory time, inspiratory time, inspiration, and rate may be dialed, and are displayed digitally.

I. All alarms are audible and visual, except the power failure alarm, which sounds if line power is lost when the power switch is in the *on* position.

BOURNS MODEL LS 75 VENTILATION MONITOR

I. Introduction

The Bourns Model LS 75 Ventilation Monitor (Figure 6-23) may be used for those patients having normal respiratory function (spontaneous mode) or may be connected to any ventilator or anesthesia circuit. The monitor has no moving parts and is battery operated.

II. Operation

A. Spontaneous Mode

1. Attach mouthpiece or mask to flow tube.

2. Press the *Spontaneous Mode* button.

3. Cumulative tidal volume will be displayed for 1 min; thereafter, the monitor will show minute volume and respiratory rate alternately for an additional minute.

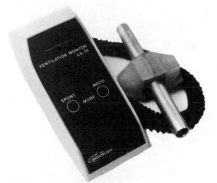

Figure 6-23. Bourns Model LS 75 Ventilation Monitor. (*Courtesy of Bourns, Inc., Life Support Division, Riverside, Calif.*)

    4. The unit will automatically turn itself off to conserve battery power.

    5. The sensor flow tube may be sterilized with ethylene oxide.

B. Mechanical Mode

    1. Attach sensor flow tube to the exhalation valve of the ventilator or anesthesia circuit.

    2. Press the *Mechanical Mode* button.

    3. Cumulative tidal volumes will be displayed for 1 min; thereafter, the monitor will show minute volume and respiratory rate alternately for an additional minute.

    4. The unit will automatically turn itself off to conserve battery power.

INCENTIVE SPIROMETRY

Studies have shown that the incidence of postoperative atelectasis may account for 90% or more of postoperative pulmonary complications. This is due to shallow, monotonous breathing as a result of pain, long-term anesthesia, narcotics, immobility, and many other factors. The result is gradual, progressive alveolar collapse, leading to reductions in total lung capacity, tidal volume, vital capacity, and functional residual capacity. Ventilation–perfusion abnormalities follow, leading to an increased alveolar–arterial oxygen gradient and decreased arterial oxygen tension. Work of breathing is greatly increased.

    Periodic, sustained, maximal inflations, because they interrupt the pattern of shallow, monotonous breathing, should prevent or minimize atelectasis. It is with this goal in mind that several manu-

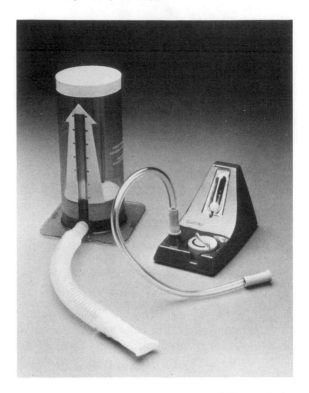

Figure 6-24.   Incentive Spirometer. (*Courtesy of Cutter Laboratories, Inc., Covina, Calif.*)

facturers have designed *incentive spirometers* (see Figure 6-24). These devices are intended to encourage the patient to take a deep breath and, very importantly, to *hold it* before exhaling. Depending on the unit, the incentive will be to light a clown's nose, raise a ball in a column, or raise a bellows to a prescribed volume. As the patient's ability to take a deep breath increases, so also can the goal be advanced.

For the purpose of this discussion, we will review three incentive spirometers that are representative of the basic types available.

Spirocare Incentive Breathing Exerciser: Marion Laboratories

This is an electronic device that utilizes a feedback system. It contains two volume scales, one of which sets the patient's goal while the other approximates the patient's actual performance. The goal scale can be set in either of two ranges: 500 to 2750 ml in volume increments of about 250 ml, or 1000 to 5500 ml in volume increments of about 500 ml. When the patient inhales, he illuminates a light panel equal to the cumulative volume of air he has inspired. When he reaches the preset goal volume, a light marked *hold* will illuminate (this sign may be replaced by a clown's face, the object being to make the clown's nose light up; adults as well as children enjoy this). The light will remain illuminated for approximately 2.5 sec after inspiration ceases. The patient should be encouraged to hold inspiration until the light goes out.

The Spirocare also has controls that allow the therapist to set the number of times the patient should achieve his goal volume in a prescribed period of time. A digital display then records each breath that reaches this volume.

The Spirocare may be used by more than one patient simply by changing the disposable flow tube through which the patient breathes.

U-Mid/Volume Plus Respiratory Exerciser: Bard Parker

This is a disposable, single-patient device that utilizes a bellows to record the patient's inspired volume. Ideally, the patient's goal volume should be determined preoperatively and recorded on the side of the exerciser. To reach this goal postoperatively represents his incentive. If such a procedure is not possible, the therapist can set a reasonable goal volume initially and gradually increase this as the patient improves.

When the patient has reached his peak inspiration, he should be encouraged to hold inspiration with the glottis open for 2 to 5 sec. The Volume Plus unit can be adapted for use with the intubated or tracheostomized patient. Since the Volume Plus unit records volume rather than flow, patients will still register a reading on the bellows even if unable to produce a preset minimum flow rate, as required by some devices.

Uniflo and Triflo Respiratory Exercisers: Chesebrough-Ponds, Inc.

These disposable, single-patient devices depend on air flow to raise a ball in a cylinder, and thus have the patient reach his goal.

Uniflo. When the patient inhales, air flow through a cylinder raises the ball. The goal is to have the patient continue to inhale to keep the ball suspended at the top of the cylinder for approximately 5 sec.

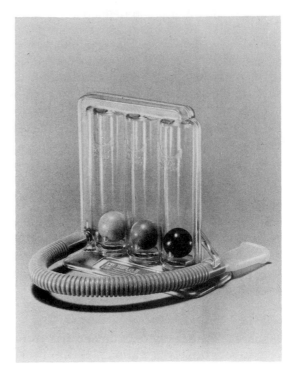

Figure 6-25.   Triflo Respiratory Exerciser. (*Courtesy of Chesebrough Ponds, Inc., Greenwich, Conn.*)

Triflo.   This is a three-chambered device (see Figure 6-25); each chamber contains a ball. The object of the exerciser is to have the patient continue to inhale until the balls in the first two chambers have risen to the tops of their columns, but to have the third ball remain stationary.

BLOW BOTTLES

Blow bottles, although not a new concept, have recently gained popularity as a method to encourage maximal ventilatory effort and forced expiration "exercise." Resistance is provided by blowing water from one bottle to another. The unit described below is disposable.

Procedure

1. Fill one chamber with 900 cc of H_2O.
2. Remove blue coloring tablet from packet, drop in water, and allow to dissolve.

3. Remove covers from both patient mouthpieces.

4. Position patient in upright position.

5. Have patient inspire deeply and blow into mouthpiece on tubing connected to the water-filled chamber, thus transferring the water to the second bottle.

6. This procedure can be repeated, blowing the water alternately from one bottle to the other as often as is desired or directed by the physician.

7. Replace covers on the mouthpieces when the treatment is completed.

PROCEDURE FOR USE OF POSITIVE END-EXPIRATORY PRESSURE

Positive End-Expiratory Pressure (PEEP) (Figure 6-26) is defined as mechanical ventilation against a threshold resistance. Many of the newer ventilators have controls or accessories for the application of PEEP. A similar therapy may be accomplished by having a patient on a ventilator exhale through a tube placed under water.

The objective of treatment with PEEP is to enhance oxygen transport using as low inspired oxygen fractions as possible. The mechanism involved is to increase functional residual capacity and to prevent or resolve diffuse microatelectasis, thus improving ventilation.

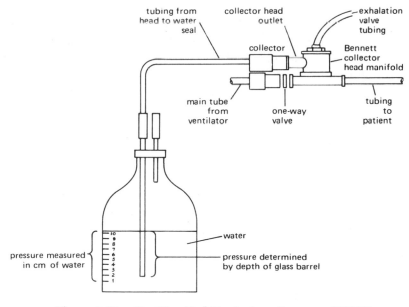

Figure 6-26. Positive End-Expiratory Pressure (PEEP).

When first used, PEEP necessitated using the ventilator in the control mode, sedating the patient if necessary. Now, however, it has been found that by setting the ventilator in the assist mode and adjusting the sensitivity to maximum (minimum patient effort required to begin inspiration) PEEP can still be maintained with less trauma to the patient. This is particularly effective when using the Bennett MA-1.

I. Equipment (all equipment should be sterile)
   A. Ventilator
   B. A 2600-ml chest bottle with rubber stopper and two pieces of glass tubing, one approximately 5 in. long and one approximately 12 in. long
      1. The 12-in. tube should be marked with an electric engraver from 0 to 10 cm, using the end of the tubing as the zero point.
      2. Mark the chest bottle in the same manner, using, for example, the 800-ml line as the zero point.
   C. Disposable tubing such as that used with humidity collars
   D. Two 15-mm adapters
   E. Two tapered flex tubes
   F. Tape
   G. Sterile water

II. Assembly
   A. Insert stopper into bottle; the zero marking on the glass tubing should be even with the 800-ml marking on the bottle; if it is not, adjust the tubing, being careful not to contaminate the part of the tubing below the stopper.
   B. Add sterile water to the bottle until it reaches the marking on the tubing equal to the centimeters of water pressure ordered by the physician.
   C. Tape the stopper so that there is no air leak around it.
   D. Connect the tapered flex tube to the top end of the longer piece of glass tubing.
   E. Connect one end cf the expiratory tubing from the ventilator to the tapered flex tube, using a 15-mm adapter.
   F. Connect the other end of the tubing to the exhalation port on the ventilator manifold.
   G. Connect the other tapered flex tube to the short piece of glass tubing, and, using a 15-mm adapter, connect the disposable tubing to the collector jar of the spirometer.

H. Bubbling should be observed in the bottle with each exhalation.

I. When using Bennett Respiration Units PR-1 or PR-2, a one-way valve should be used in line between the main tube from the ventilator and the manifold.

III. Monitoring

A. Water level in chest bottle—never drain condensation from the tubing system back into the chest bottle, as this increases the pressure; add or drain water as necessary to maintain the desired level.

B. Blood gases—particularly observe for increased $PaCO_2$; if this occurs, therapy may be discontinued; PaO_2 will indicate effectiveness of therapy.

C. Vital signs—notify physician of any changes.

D. Cardiac output—notify physician if this decreases.

IV. Cleaning

A. The entire setup should be changed daily.

B. Equipment that is not disposable may be cold or gas sterilized.

PROCEDURE FOR USE OF CONTINUOUS POSITIVE PRESSURE BREATHING

The terms continuous positive pressure breathing (CPPB) and continuous positive airway pressure (CPAP) are used interchangeably when referring to nonventilator breathing against a threshold resistance. It is useful in the treatment of those patients who are unable to maintain an adequate PaO_2 even when inhaling high FIO_2's, but who do not require mechanical ventilation.

I. Equipment

A. A 2600-ml chest bottle, marked as described under Part II of this outline

B. Two lengths (60 in. each) of large-bore disposable tubing

C. One tapered flex tube

D. One standard flex tube

E. One 15-mm adapter

F. Bennett Seal with strap or adapter for tracheostomy or endotracheal tube

G. One-way valve such as Air-Shields E-2
H. Nebulizer with dilution control such as Puritan All-Purpose Jar
I. Nose clips
J. Sterile water
K. Rubber adapter
L. Five-liter anesthesia bag
M. Aerosol
N. Tape

II. Assembly (Figure 6-27)
  A. All equipment should be sterilized before use.
  B. The chest bottle should be marked form 0 to 10 cms, using the 800-ml line on the bottle as the zero point; an electric engraver gives permanent markings.
  C. The rubber stopper for the chest bottle is fitted with two lengths of plastic tubing, one approximately 12 in. long and

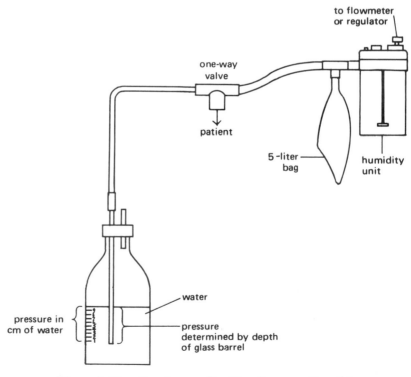

Figure 6-27. Continuous Positive Pressure Breathing.

one approximately 5 inch. long; the longer tube is also marked from 0 to 10 cm, using the lower tip as the zero point. The two zero points must be lined up; it is best to do this before adding water to the bottle, as there is less distortion.

D. Add sterile water to the bottle until the water reaches the level of pressure ordered by the physician; the actual expiratory pressure is determined by the distance the tube is under water.

E. Insert the rubber stopper and plastic tubes; tape firmly in place to prevent any air leaks, and also to discourage tampering.

F. Connect a tapered flex tube to the top end of the 12-in. plastic tube and insert 15-mm adapter into the flex tube.

G. Connect one end of a length of disposable tubing to the adapter.

H. The Puritan All-Purpose Jar is used to humidify the inspired air; the dilution control on the nebulizer head allows for the delivery of 40%, 70%, or 100% oxygen.

I. Fill the jar with sterile water to the fill line; a heating element may be used; however, such use will result in more condensation in the tubing system and therefore will require close observation.

J. To ensure that the patient always has an adequate flow of gas available, an anesthesia bag is inserted next to the outlet port on the nebulizer, using a rubber adapter and an aerosol tee; the bag acts as a reservoir and is especially important for patients having a large minute volume.

K. Attach one end of the second length of disposable tubing to the aerosol tee on the Puritan All-Purpose Jar.

L. The one-way valve has three ports: inspiratory port, expiratory port, and patient port. It is essential that the tubings be connected correctly or the patient could be asphyxiated.

M. Connect the free end of the disposable tubing coming from the Puritan All-Purpose Jar to the inspiratory port on the one-way valve; this is the inspiratory line.

N. Connect the free end of the disposable tubing coming from the long plastic tube on the chest bottle to the expiratory port on the one-way valve; this is the expiratory line.

O. If the patient has a tracheostomy or endotracheal tube in place, the patient port on the valve will most likely fit directly onto the tube; for the patient who does not have a tube, we add a flex tube and Bennett Seal with strap.

P. Connect a low-pressure oxygen hose to the top of the Puritan All-Purpose Jar, and connect the other end to the bottom of a flowmeter; turn on the cylinder valve and adjust to approximately 8 liters/min of oxygen; adjustment of flows may be needed to obtain a specific FIO_2.

III. Procedure

A. You are now ready to adjust the Bennett Seal to the patient; it must fit securely so that there are no air leaks; apply the nose clips; it is essential that the patient keep both the seal and clips in place during the therapy, if it is to be effective.

B. Notice the bubbling of the water in the chest bottle as the patient exhales; if there is no bubbling, it indicates that either there is a leak in the system, or the patient is apneic. If the patient experiences any difficulty, it may indicate that the valve needs cleaning, as moisture and medication tend to freeze the one-way valve.

IV. Monitoring

A. Blood pressure and pulse should be monitored hourly.

B. Tidal volume should be monitored hourly.

C. Blood gases should be drawn within an hour of starting the therapy, as they give the best indication of the effectiveness of the CPPB.

D. Condensation from the tubing system should never be emptied into the chest bottle, as this will increase the pressure; if excess water does collect, the level should be adjusted; conversely, water may be added to maintain the desired level.

E. Water should be added, as needed, to the nebulizer.

F. Check FIO_2 with oxygen analyzer and positive pressure by means of a pressure or water manometer.

V. Cleaning

A. The entire setup should be changed daily.

B. Dispose of the tubing system.

C. Disassemble the one-way valve.

D. Remaining equipment may be cold or gas sterilized.

CONTINUOUS POSITIVE AIRWAY PRESSURE

Continuous Positive Airway Pressure (CPAP) may be defined as a pressure above atmospheric maintained at the airway opening throughout the respiratory cycle during spontaneous breathing. This procedure is now being used more and more in the care of the newborn with respiratory distress syndrome.

Treatment with CPAP involves attaching an infant who is breathing spontaneously to a system that applies a constant pressure to the airway. Examples of CPAP delivery system are nasal prongs, head hood, face mask, and endotracheal tube.

CPAP is most effective in the treatment of respiratory distress syndrome; it also may be used in the resuscitation of the newborn at birth, to treat intractable apnea in premature infants, and in the postoperative care of infants. It is useful in the care of infants suffering from heart failure associated with pulmonary edema and in the treatment of respiratory failure due to meconium aspiration or pneumonia.

In using CPAP, complications that might develop are reduction in cardiac output, pressure necrosis, pulmonary air leak, and airway drying and probable obstruction. Intensive monitoring should be done on infants using CPAP; observation of vital signs, for airway obstruction, and for gastrointestinal tract distention are some of the most critical.

BIRD NEONATAL CPAP GENERATOR

The Bird Neonatal CPAP Generator (Figure 6-28) is a pneumatically driven device with controls for an accurate selection of continuous positive airway pressure (CPAP), FIO_2, and nebulizer output to the neonate.

Assembly

1. Install post in base.
2. Place collar hanger on post and tighten 13 in. from top of base.
3. Place utility tray on post and slide down to collar hanger.
4. Install dovetail mount bracket near top of post.
5. Slide blender into bracket.
6. Connect CPAP generator to blender (use only low-flow blender).
7. Attach mounting bracket to post and tighten in position 10 in. below CPAP generator.

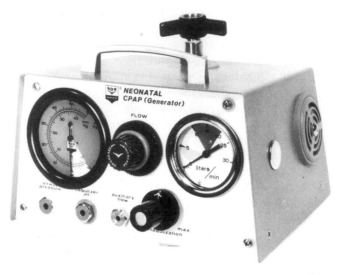

Figure 6-28. Bird Neonatal CPAP Generator. (*Courtesy of Bird Corp., Palm Springs, Calif.*)

8. Connect oxygen and air gas lines to bottom of blender.
9. Connect large-diameter green tube to a female side of nebulizer tee.
10. Connect small green tube to nebulizer jet outlet on face of CPAP generator and tall socket of 500-ml nebulizer.
11. Connect long small-diameter tubing from tubing bifurcation to airway pressure monitor outlet on face of CPAP generator.
12. Connect small clear tube to auxiliary flow socket on CPAP generator and either short socket of the 500-ml nebulizer.

Patient Breathing Circuit Assembly

1. Insert the keyed adapter of the master tee assembly into the mount bracket until spring-loaded pin engages hole in adapter, securing master tee assembly in proper position.
2. Check to ensure that expiratory flow gradient port on side of shuttle valve is blocked with a tapered plug.
3. Into the tee fitting atop the shuttle valve, insert the relief valve into the rear port and the 500-ml micronebulizer into the front port.
4. Install tee into the outlet of the 500-ml nebulizer.
5. Place small therapy micronebulizer in the backside of the tee with its stopper in place.

6. Install the Airbird valve assembly on the Airbird bag and place into the open end of the master tee.
7. Mount the outflow valve atop the Airbird valve with the red PEEP control lever in front.
8. Mount extension arm bracket on post and install extension arm.

Operation

1. Breathing circuit—assemble and attach to generator.
   a. Connect large-bore green tube to 500-ml nebulizer and to water trap.
   b. Connect large-bore red tubing to bottom of shuttle valve and to water trap.
   c. Connect small-bore green tubing with double-ended patient wye connector to water trap.
   d. Connect small-bore red tubing attached to other side of wye connector to water trap with large-bore red tubing.
   e. Place breathing circuit in extension arm clamp and position water traps so that reservoirs are down.
2. Power source—connected and on (generator operates from a source pressure of 50 psi).
3. Adjust gas flow to patient need; flow between 2 and 15 liters/min should be selected by rotating the flow control clockwise.
4. End expiratory pressure—adjust to desired level. The amount of CPAP is selected by rotating a red control lever located on the bottom of the Bird outflow valve housing.
5. Adjust nebulizer output. Desired nebulizer output can be selected by rotating the nebulization control full clockwise for maximum aerosol production.
6. Check operation of pressure relief circuit. Occlude gas flow from the patient wye at the end of the breathing circuit and note pressure rise on the pressure manometer. This pressure should not exceed 88 cm of water (65 mm Hg).
7. Check all alarms for function:
   a. Oxygen blender alarm.
   b. The overpressure governor should release at approximately 88 cm of water and sound an alarm.
8. Connecting the patient—prior to attaching a patient to the CPAP system, the patient's airway should be cleared of obstruction and the patient should be ventilating on his own at a rate and depth sufficient to maintain desired $PaCO_2$ and pH levels. Determine patient minute volume requirement and adjust

CPAP flow to ensure elimination of CO_2 from the breathing circuit during exhalation.

9. Using the Airbird Resuscitator—when it becomes desirable to assist or control the patient's ventilatory efforts, the Airbird Manual Resuscitator can be used by squeezing the bulb at a preselected rate and volume.

CARDIOPULMONARY RESUSCITATION

Cardiac arrest occurs when there is no electrical activity of the heart (asystole) or when an irregular heart rhythm (arrhythmia) develops that cannot sustain adequate blood pressure. Examples of arrhythmias are *ventricular fibrillation*, where the ventricles beat in a bizarre pattern without effective ventricular contraction and cardiac output, and *ventricular tachycardia*, which is characterized by rapid regular or only slightly irregular beats of 150 to 200/min.

Respiratory arrest may occur as a result of airway obstruction, depression of the respiratory center (as from drug overdose), asphyxiation or trauma, or as a direct result of cardiac arrest. The latter occurs due to the resultant hypoxemia and hypercapnia associated with a cardiac arrest.

Cardiopulmonary resuscitation (CPR) is the action taken to restore spontaneous respiration and/or heartbeat following their cessation either individually or in combination. A cardiopulmonary arrest constitutes a true medical emergency and requires prompt action of all members of the health team.

I. Signs of an Arrest
   A. Respiratory Arrest
      1. Apnea
      2. Dilatation of pupils
      3. Cyanosis (except with carbon monoxide poisoning)
      4. Unconsciousness
   B. Cardiac Arrest
      1. Apnea
      2. Dilatation of pupils
      3. Absence of pulse and heartbeat (check pulse at carotid and femoral sites)

II. Equipment
   A. Cardiac arrest cart—should contain all equipment and medications required for intubation, emergency, and definitive treatment.

    B. Tracheal suction machine

    C. Defibrillator (a battery-operated model that can be stored and charged on the arrest cart is convenient)

    D. Manual resuscitator and airways

    E. Cardiac arrest board

    F. EKG machine—some defibrillators have this built in.

III.   Procedure

    A. When a state of true arrest is determined, start resuscitation immediately and summon help. *Do not leave the patient.*

    B. Position patient flat in bed to facilitate venous return.

    C. Establish patency of airway (Figure 6-29)

        1. Clear oral cavity, but *do not* place fingers in patient's mouth, as a severe bite could result; use gauze pads, and the like.

        2. Suction, if necessary

    D. Hyperextend the neck to prevent occlusion of the posterior pharynx by the base of the tongue.

        1. Support back of head with one hand.

        2. Press downward on the patient's forehead with the other hand, thus tilting the chin upward and backward.

OR

        3. Stand behind the patient's head, placing one hand on either side of the chin, with the fingers at the mandibular notch.

        4. Push the lower jaw forward and at the same time extend the head backward.

    E. Insert airway, using the size most appropriate to the size of the patient. An airway that is too large or too small can interfere with proper ventilation.

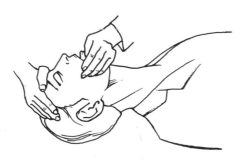

Figure 6-29.

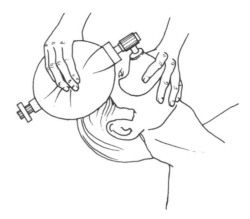

Figure 6-30.

F. Aerate the patient's lungs (Figure 6-30)
1. Use bag/mask unit with bag attached to oxygen (flow-meter should be set on *Flush*).
2. Place mask over patient's nose and mouth; squeeze bag five times. It is necessary to ventilate the patient before beginning external cardiac compression since there is no value in circulating nonoxygenated blood.

G. Begin external cardiac massage (Figure 6-31)
1. Place arrest board under patient's back, still maintaining hyperextension of the neck. The board provides a firm surface to aid in compression of the heart.
2. Unless you are extremely tall, it is advisable to stand on a stool. Otherwise, you are more likely to exert pressure on the patient's chest at an angle, thus increasing

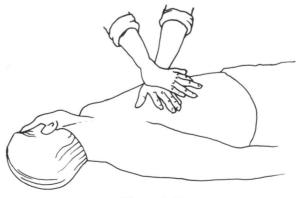

Figure 6-31.

the possibility of rib fractures and their resultant complications.

3. Place the heel of your left hand on the lower third of the patient's sternum. Keep fingers extended.

4. Place the heel of your right hand over the heel of your left hand. Keep fingers extended.

5. With your elbows straight, depress the sternum $1\frac{1}{2}$ to 2 in. and release.

6. The heart is thus compressed between the sternum and the spinal column (supported by the arrest board).

7. If you are alone:
   a. Ventilate three times.
   b. Apply compression 15 times.
   c. Maintain this pattern until help arrives.

8. If you have help:
   a. Ventilate one time.
   b. Apply compression five times.
   c. Maintain this pattern; it is necessary to intersperse the ventilations between compressions, while maintaining rhythmic compressions.

9. Another individual should determine the effectiveness of the procedure by monitoring:
   a. Femoral and carotid pulses
   b. Pupil reaction and size
   c. Spontaneous respirations

10. Defibrillation may be necessary.

11. *Precordial thump* (Figure 6-32). The use of the precordial thump may be effective on adult patients who have no pulse as a result of a witnessed cardiac arrest or who are being monitored or paced for known atrioventricular block. It is not recommended, however, for children, nor has its effectiveness been determined in cases of myocardial anoxia, such as may occur in the unmonitored or unwitnessed cardiac arrest.
   a. The thump should be delivered within the first minute after cardiac arrest from a height of 8 to 12 in. over the chest.
   b. Deliver a sharp, quick single blow over the midportion of the sternum using the bottom, fleshy portion of the fist.
   c. If there is no *immediate* response, begin other CPR measures at once.
   d. The precordial thump may be integrated into basic

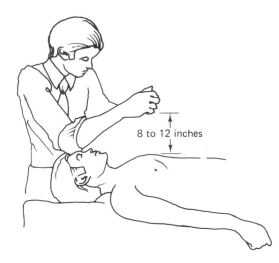

8 to 12 inches

Figure 6-32.

CPR procedures; however, the thump should not interfere with the administration of external cardiac compression.

IV. Definitive Treatment
   A. Medications commonly administered during an arrest
      1. Adrenalin—to stimulate weak or absent cardiac contractions.
      2. Calcium chloride—increases the force of ventricular contractions.
      3. Pronestyl—reduces heart irritability; treatment of ventricular tachycardia.
      4. Xylocaine—treatment of ventricular tachycardia.
      5. NaHCO$_3$—counteracts acidosis.
      6. Aramine—raises blood pressure.
      7. Levophed—raises blood pressure.
   B. Intubation
      1. The insertion of an endotracheal tube may be necessary to facilitate removal of secretions and attaching a ventilator.
      2. This procedure should be carried out by the individual with the greatest expertise—an anesthetist or specially trained respiratory therapist. The procedure must be done as quickly and atraumatically as possible.
   C. Defibrillation
      1. Consists of electrical shock administered to the heart in an effort to stop ventricular fibrillation and establish

a coordinated cardiac rhythm. It is not effective when asystole is the cause of cardiac arrest.

2. Defibrillation should be done only by individuals who have been well versed in the technique and complications of the procedure.

D. Mechanical ventilation

1. When the patient has been resuscitated from a cardiac standpoint, if he is still unable to ventilate adequately, a mechanical ventilator may be needed.

2. The choice of ventilator will depend on the primary disease condition that the patient has.

E. Other measures

1. Oxygen administration by cannula or mask may be indicated to relieve hypoxia in those patients not requiring mechanical ventilation.

2. After the crisis is over, diagnostic procedures must be initiated to determine the exact cause of the arrest.

3. Blood gases will be drawn periodically during the arrest procedure and until the patient's condition is stabilized.

V. Mouth-to-Mouth Resuscitation (Figure 6-33)

In the absence of resuscitating equipment such as a bag/mask unit, it may be necessary to begin artificial ventilation by other methods. This procedure, as well as external cardiac compression, should also be taught to the lay public for emergency use outside a hospital situation.

A. Establish a patent airway as for use with a bag/mask unit. This may be enough to establish spontaneous ventilation.

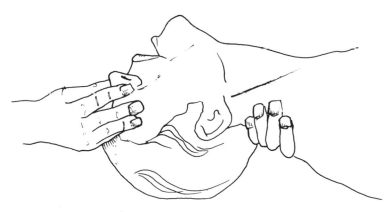

Figure 6-33.

B. Position yourself at the patient's side. Use the hand behind the patient's neck to maintain maximal backward tilt of the head.

C. With the thumb and index finger of the other hand, pinch the patient's nose, at the same time exerting pressure on the forehead to maintain the backward tilt of the head.

D. Open your mouth widely and take a deep breath.

E. Make a tight seal around the patient's mouth and blow into his mouth. Remove your mouth.

F. Initially give four quick full breaths without allowing for full lung deflations between breaths.

G. Thereafter repeat the cycle once every 5 sec, allowing the patient to exhale passively.

H. If mouth-to-mouth ventilation is performed adequately, you will be able to see the patient's chest rise and fall as well as hear and feel the air escape during exhalation. You should also feel the resistance and compliance of the patient's lungs as they expand in your own airways.

VI. Resuscitation of Infants and Children

A. Open airway as for adult; however, avoid an exaggerated head tilt position, as this may obstruct airways.

B. Cover both the mouth and nose of the child with your mouth; use smaller breaths, delivered once every 3 sec.

C. Infants—use only the tips of the index and middle fingers for external cardiac compression, depressing the mid-sternum $\frac{1}{2}$ to $\frac{3}{4}$ in. at a rate of 80 to 100/min with breaths after each five compressions.

D. Young children—use only the heel of one hand, depressing the mid-sternum $\frac{3}{4}$ to $1\frac{1}{2}$ in. at a rate of 80 to 100/min with breaths after each five compressions.

VII. The Role of the Respiratory Therapist

The duties of the respiratory therapist during an arrest will vary according to the institution in which he works. Generally, however, he will be involved in operating the manual resuscitator, setting up and operating the ventilator, and, possibly, intubation.

AIR-SHIELDS AMBU MANUAL RESUSCITATOR

I. Assembly

A. Always keep the unit completely assembled and ready for use.

B. Insert inspiratory port of one-way valve into bag.

C. Squeeze bag and observe movement of the disc inside valve; if it does not move freely, the valve has been inserted into the bag incorrectly.

D. If the patient to be resuscitated has an endotracheal tube or tracheostomy tube with a standard adapter, no mask is needed; merely fit the remaining port on the one-way valve directly over the tube adapter.

E. If a mask is to be used, fit the mask adapter over the remaining port on the one-way valve; when the bag is squeezed, you should feel a flow of air through the mask.

F. Connect one end of a length of small-bore tubing to the oxygen input nipple on the bag.

G. Connect the other end of the small-bore tubing to a flowmeter.

H. Turn oxygen flow to 15 liters/min.

II. Operation

A. Use with mask

1. Position patient's head so that jaw is forward, head tilted back.

2. Place the mask firmly on patient's face, with narrowed portion over bridge of nose and rounded portion of cushion between chin and lower lip.

3. Squeeze the bag firmly, observing the rise of the chest.

4. Release the bag for exhalation.

5. Repeat, allowing 1 sec for inspiration and 2 sec for expiration.

6. If manually resuscitating a patient who is also receiving closed cardiac massage, a rhythm must be set up; for example, five chest compressions to one lung inflation.

B. Use without mask (for endotracheal or tracheostomy tube)

1. Position patient's head so that you have free access to tube.

2. Connect the patient port on the one-way valve to the patient's tube.

3. Continue as for use with mask (explained above).

C. Resuscitator for high oxygen administration

1. Pull out valve device on bottom of bag about $\frac{3}{4}$ in.

2. Attach oxygen supply tubing, 6 to 8 ft in length, to valve nipple.

3. Thread oxygen supply tubing through a 3-ft-long large-bore tubing and connect over valve.

III. Cleaning
A. Disassemble bag, valve, and mask.
B. Clean the outside of the bag with a chemical germicide.
C. Although the company recommends gas sterilization with ethylene oxide for the bag, it has been our experience that complete aeration is a problem unless an aeration cabinet is used.
D. The mask and valve may be gas or cold sterilized; if gas is used, remove plug from mask before packaging.

PURITAN MANUAL RESUSCITATOR

I. Assembly
A. Always keep the unit assembled and ready for use.
B. Place plastic elbow over bushing on the bag; the elbow will only fit in one position.
C. Attach the valve to the elbow.
D. If a mask is to be used, attach the mask to the valve.
E. Attach one end of a length of small-bore tubing to an oxygen regulator with flowmeter.
F. Attach the other end to the hose nipple located on the valve.
G. Set liter flow for 15 liters/min.

II. Operation
A. Position the patient
B. Use of mask
1. Place mask on face with narrow part of mask over bridge of nose and rounded portion of cushion between lower lip and chin.
2. Squeeze the bag firmly, then release; the slower the bag is released, the higher the concentration of oxygen delivered with the next inspiration will be.
3. Continue as above.
C. Use without mask
1. Place connection on valve over tube adapter.
2. Squeeze bag firmly, then release; the slower the bag is released, the higher the concentration of oxygen delivered with the next inspiration will be.
3. Continue as above.

III. Cleaning
  A. Disassemble bag, mask, elbow, and valve.
  B. All the above parts may be steam autoclaved, gas sterilized, or chemically cold sterilized.

HOPE RESUSCITATOR

I. Assembly
  A. The entire unit should be assembled and stored as such for emergency use.
  B. Attach mask, if necessary, to valve.
  C. Attach one end of a length of small-bore tubing to the oxygen inlet on the valve housing.
  D. Connect the other end of the tubing to a regulator with flowmeter.
  E. Set oxygen flow for 15 liters/min (an adapter for high oxygen administration is commercially available).

II. Operation
  A. Position patient.
  B. If mask is to be used, place narrow portion over bridge of nose and rounded part of cushion between chin and lower lip.
  C. If mask is not used, place connector on valve housing over adapter on endotracheal tube.
  D. Squeeze bag firmly and release; allow more time for exhalation than for inhalation.

III. Cleaning
  A. Disassemble all parts as completely as possible.
  B. All components may be sterilized with gas- or cold-sterilizing agents.

EXERCISES

1. Describe the indications and contraindications for PEEP.
2. What is the effect of increasing the liter flow of gas to a manual resuscitating bag?
3. Compare the advantages and disadvantages of weaning using an aerosol tee.

4. What is the purpose of silica gel in a Beckman D-2 Analyzer? In a Mira?

5. What parameters would you check to determine the accuracy of an oxygen analyzer?

6. List two methods of providing CPAP to premature infants.

7. List some of the possible complications of the use of CPAP.

RESPIRATORY THERAPY DEPARTMENT RECORDS

The Joint Commission for Accreditation of Hospitals has determined that documentation of a patient's entire course of respiratory therapy is a necessity. With this in mind, we have designed the protocol for the initiation of such therapies in our department. Although they will of necessity have to be modified for use by others, it is our hope that they will serve as a guide to improved patient care.

PROTOCOL FOR INITIATION OF RESPIRATORY THERAPEUTIC PROCEDURES

I. A written order, signed by the requesting physician, must be submitted to the Respiratory Therapy Department before initiation of the therapy. One copy of the order will be retained in the patient's chart.

II. Upon receiving the written order, the therapist will review the patient's chart and perform an initial assessment (see attached guide) of the patient to determine the indication for therapy and its objectives. The patient should meet at least one of the following criteria.

A. Difficulty mobilizing secretions due to poor cough or tenacious secretions.

B. Strong clinical indication or x-ray evidence of atelectasis.

C. Conditions conducive to atelectasis or retention of secretions that are not preventable by simpler means.

    D. Evidence of bronchospasm.

    E. Decreased alveolar ventilation as evidenced by arterial blood gases, tidal volume measurement, auscultation, respiratory rate, depth of breathing, x-ray, and/or pulmonary function studies.

III. The initial assessment, form _____, upon completion, will be placed in the patient's permanent record.

IV. In the event there is no clear justification for the procedure, or there is a question of contraindication or a question regarding the appropriateness of the therapy, the following procedure will be enacted.

    A. The therapist will include a SOAP note on the progress sheet indicating reason for the decision, and that the physician will be consulted.

    B. All such inclusions in the chart must be signed by the therapist, giving full name and title.

    C. The therapist will follow-up by consulting with the requesting physician to determine if reassessment is necessary.

    D. If a mutually agreed upon decision cannot be reached, the matter will be referred to the medical director of the Respiratory Therapy Department for final determination.

V. If the therapist determines that the patient is a candidate for respiratory therapy, he will so note on the assessment form and take necessary steps to initiate the treatments.

VI. Each treatment administered shall be assessed in terms of the patient's cooperation, the immediate results, and any side effects, and such information noted on the Respiratory Therapy Flow Sheet in the patient's chart. If at any time during the course of the patient's therapy there is a significant change in the patient's condition or an adverse reaction occurs, the therapist will so note on the patient flow sheet, SOAP a progress note, and indicate on the chart "Physician, please see respiratory therapy progress note and advise." The therapist will also report the specific problem to the nursing staff.

VII. Upon completion of the five-day course of therapy (as per the original order), the therapist will include a final assessment of the effects of the therapy in the progress notes. At that time, he will also place a sticker in the progress note requesting an evaluation by the physician.

Respiratory Therapy Department
Respiratory Therapy Requisition

Room Number _____
Date Ordered _____
Date Discontinued _____

Respiratory Diagnosis _____

Objectives of Therapy: Please Check
- ☐ Mobilize and liquefy secretions
- ☐ Relieve and/or prevent atelectasis
- ☐ Relieve bronchospasm
- ☐ Improve or promote cough

- ☐ Improve alveolar ventilation
- ☐ Sputum collection
- ☐ Other (specify)

Precautions (specify) _____

☐ IPPB
☐ IPPB with PEPB

Frequency _____
Treatment at night (11 to 7)
☐ Yes   ☐ No
☐ Compressed air
☐ Oxygen enrichment
Peak inspiratory pressure _____ cm of H_2O
  (usual 10 to 20 cm of H_2O)
Expiratory pressure (if desired) _____ cm of H_2O

Medication:
Isoproterenol 0.25% _____ ml
Normal saline _____ ml
Sterile water _____ ml
Acetylcysteine 10% _____ ml
Isoetharine HCl 1% _____ ml
Other _____

☐ Heated Aerosol
  Frequency _____
  Solution _____
  Duration _____

☐ Ultrasonic Neb.
  (with sterile water)
  Frequency _____
  Duration _____

Chest Physiotherapy
  ☐ Bronchial drainage
Lobes involved:

Percussion:
  ☐ Yes   ☐ No
Breathing exercises

☐ Incentive Spirometer
  Frequency _____

☐ Self
☐ Follow-up

☐ Other Respiratory
  Therapy Procedures
  (specify)

_____
House Physician's Signature

This order will automatically be discontinued after five (5) days. If the patient requires additional treatment, a new written order will be necessary, as well as a progress note by the physician in the patient's chart indicating necessity for continuation.

PROTOCOL FOR INITIATION OF OXYGEN–HUMIDITY THERAPY

I. A written order, signed by the requesting physician, must be submitted to the Respiratory Therapy Department before initiation of the therapy. One copy of the order will be retained in the patient's chart.

Note: If, in an emergency situation, it is necessary for the nursing staff to initiate the therapy, the signed order must be forwarded to Respiratory Therapy immediately upon completion of such action.

II. The patient requiring oxygen therapy should meet at least one of the following criteria:
A. Emergency occurrence: no ABG's (Arterial Blood Gases)
1. Shock
2. Myocardial infarction
3. Pulmonary edema
4. Pulmonary embolism
5. Sudden onset of dyspnea
B. Hypoxemia of cardiac or pulmonary nature as evidenced by arterial blood gas: P_aO_2 less than 70 mm Hg on room air.
C. Severe anemia
D. Carbon monoxide poisoning and/or smoke inhalation
E. Sleep hypoxemia

III. Upon receiving the written order, the therapist will take the necessary steps to initiate the therapy.

IV. The therapist will then perform an initial assessment (see attached guide) of the patient to determine the indication for therapy and its objectives.

V. The initial assessment form, upon completion, will be placed in the patient's permanent record.

VI. In the event there is no clear justification for the procedure, or there is a question of contraindication or a question regarding the appropriateness of the therapy, the following procedure will be enacted:
A. The therapist will include a SOAP note on the progress sheet indicating reason for the decision and that the physician will be consulted.

B. All such inclusions in the chart must be signed by the therapist, giving full name and title.

C. The therapist will follow-up by consulting with the requesting physician to determine if reassessment is necessary.

Note: At no time will oxygen therapy be indiscriminately discontinued prior to *final determination* of indication for therapy and its objectives.

Respiratory Therapy Department
Oxygen/Humidity Request Form

Room Number _____
Diagnosis _____   Date Ordered _____

Indication for Therapy: Please Check
- ☐ Shock
- ☐ M.I.
- ☐ Pulmonary edema
- ☐ Pulmonary embolism
- ☐ Sudden onset of dyspnea

- ☐ Hypoxemia of a cardiac or respiratory nature as evidenced by $P_aO_2 < 70$ mm Hg on room air
- ☐ Sleep hypoxemia
- ☐ Other: Specify

Therapy Desired:
Oxygen
- Nasal Cannula _____ liters/min
- Venturi mask _____ % O_2
- Oxygen tent _____ % O_2
- Partial rebreathing mask _____ % O_2
- Nasal catheter _____ liters/min

Humidity
- Venturi mask with high humidity _____ % O_2
- Aerosol tee _____ % O_2
- Tracheostomy collar _____ % O_2
- Continuous PEPB _____ % O_2 _____ cm of H_2O

_____
House Physician

Note: If, in an emergency situation, it is necessary for the nursing staff to initiate the therapy, this requisition must be forwarded to the respiratory therapy department immediately following such a procedure.

This order form must be filled out before any oxygen or humidity therapy is initiated by the respiratory therapy department. A new order is necessary when a change of equipment or percent is desired. *The responsible physician must document such therapies in the patient's chart by regularly recording the type, date, duration, indication, and effects of each respiratory care service provided to the patient, per the Joint Commission for Accreditation of Hospitals.*

D. If a mutually agreed upon decision cannot be reached, the matter will be referred to the medical director of the Respiratory Therapy Department for final determination.

VII. If the therapist determines that the patient is a candidate for oxygen therapy, he will so note on the assessment form and take necessary steps to continue the therapy.

VIII. Each day the complete setup will be changed by the Respiratory Therapy Department. At that time, the therapist will record on the Respiratory Therapy Flow Sheet in the patient's chart the following information: date, time, setup changed, FIO_2 ordered, FIO_2 analyzed, flow rates used, and temperature of gas as monitored weekly.

IX. If at any time during the course of the patient's therapy, there is a significant change in the patient's condition or an adverse reaction occurs, the therapist will so note on the patient flow sheet, SOAP a progress note, and notify the physician for advice.

X. At the time the therapy is discontinued, the therapist will include a final assessment of the effects of therapy in the progress notes. At that time, he will also place a sticker in the progress note requesting an evaluation by the physician.

USE OF THE PATIENT FLOW SHEET

1. This sheet is a *legal record*, and as such must be complete, accurate, neat, and written in *ink*.
2. When a patient is started on therapy, a flow sheet must be filled out with his/her name, respiratory diagnosis, objective of therapy, physician ordering, date ordered, and date of discontinue. The sheet is then placed in the patient's permanent record.
3. After each treatment administered, fill out the following information regarding the patient's therapy:
   a. Date
   b. Time administered
   c. Therapy
   d. Medication
   e. Assessment: patient's response to therapy, if adverse reaction occurs, indicate action taken.
   f. Technician's signature and title
   Use as many lines as necessary.
4. Do not use abbreviations or ditto marks on the patient flow sheets.

5. A patient flow sheet is to be filled out even if the patient receives only one treatment.
6. Flow sheets are to be kept on patients on oxygen–humidity therapy and should include:
   a. Type of therapy
   b. FIO_2 ordered
   c. FIO_2 analyzed (daily)
   d. Liter flows used
   e. Date setup changed (daily)
   f. Assessment of patient's response; indicate action taken if adverse reaction occurs

PATIENT FLOW SHEET

Diagnosis _____ Room Number _____

Objective of Therapy _____

Physician Ordering _____

Date Ordered _____ Date of Disc. _____

Initial Assessment Complete   Yes _____   No _____

Date	Time	Therapy	Medication	Assessment	Technician

PROTOCOL FOR INITIATION OF MECHANICAL VENTILATION

I. A written order, signed by the requesting physician, must be placed in the patient's chart before or soon after the application of the ventilator. The order must include the following information:
    A. Tidal volume
    B. Pressure limit
    C. Flow rate
    D. Respiratory rate
    E. FIO_2
    F. Sigh volume
    G. Sigh frequency
    H. Sigh pressure limit
    I. IMV
    J. Dead space
    K. PEEP

II. Immediately following application of the ventilator, the therapist will review the patient's chart and perform an initial assessment (see attached guide) of the patient to determine the indication for therapy and its objectives. The patient should meet at least one of the following criteria:
    A. Immediate postoperative period
    B. Comatose status, including drug overdose
    C. Postcardiopulmonary arrest
    D. Acute ventilatory failure as evidenced by increased P_aCO_2 with narcosis or respiratory acidosis
    E. Acute hypoxemic respiratory failure as evidenced by severe hypoxemia not corrected by simpler forms of oxygen therapy ($P_aO_2 < 60$ on 50% FIO_2)
    F. Thoracic trauma requiring stabilization
    G. Respiratory muscle paralysis

III. The initial assessment form, upon completion, will be placed in the patient's permanent record.

IV. In the event the patient does not meet at least one of the criteria, or the therapist feels that different settings may be indicated, the following procedure will be enacted:
    A. The therapist will include a SOAP note on the progress

sheet indicating reason for the decision and that the physician will be consulted.

B. All such inclusions in the chart must be signed by the therapist, giving full name and title.

C. The therapist will follow-up by consulting with the requesting physician to determine if reassessment is necessary.

D. If a mutually agreed upon decision cannot be reached, the matter will be referred to the medical director of the Respiratory Therapy Department for final determination.

V. The initial ventilator settings are to be recorded on the Ventilator Flow Sheet, as are any subsequent ventilator checks (at least twice a shift).

A. If the patient is being weaned at the time of the check, the length of the wean and the method are to be recorded on the flow sheets.

B. The Respiratory Therapy Department prefers to make any changes in settings that are necessary. However, if the physician deems it necessary to make such changes himself, he should so note on the flow sheet and on the order sheet in the chart. If there is no written order in the chart or no notation on the flow sheet of such changes, the therapist will make every effort to determine who made the change and to obtain a written order. If he is unable to determine this, he will return the settings to those in the last written order, as the possibility exists that the settings were changed accidentally.

C. Weaning orders should be ordered on a daily basis, indicating method, FIO_2, and length of time. No weaning will be carried out until such an order is received.

VI. If, at any time during the period of mechanical ventilation or its weaning period, the therapist notes a significant change in the patient's condition, particularly an adverse effect, he will so note on the flow sheet, SOAP a progress note, and contact the physician for advice.

VII. Upon completion of the weaning process, and subsequent discontinuation of the ventilator, the therapist will include a final assessment of the patient's condition in the progress notes. At that time he will also place a sticker in the progress note requesting an evaluation by the physician.

Respiratory Therapy Department
Ventilator Flow Sheet

Respiratory Diagnosis

			Arterial Blood Gas:			Arterial Blood Gas:			Arterial Blood Gas:
Date									
Time									
Ventilator			HCO_3^-			HCO_3^-			HCO_3^-
Assist/control									
Rate: SET/PT									
IMV Rate: SET/PT			P_aO_2:			P_aO_2:			P_aO_2:
Dilution/FIO_2									
Tidal volume ordered									
Tidal volume set			P_aCO_2:			P_aCO_2:			P_aCO_2:
Tidal volume—Wright									
Average Insp. pressure									
Pressure limit			pH:			pH:			pH:
PEEP (cm of H_2O)									
Peak insp. flow									
Sigh volume			FIO_2:			FIO_2:			FIO_2:
Sigh pressure limit									
Sighs/hr.									
Humidifier setting/temp.			Time:			Time:			Time:
Dead space added									
Alarm on									
Effective dynamic compliance									
Sensitivity									
Therapist									

Schedule of Respiratory Therapy Treatments

Number of Treatments per Day	7 am–3 pm	3 pm–11 pm	11pm –7 am
Daily or Qd	1 Rx		
Bid or 2x a day treatments given 8 hr apart	1 Rx	1 Rx	
Tid or 3x a day treatments given 4 hr apart	2 Rx	1 Rx	
Qid or 4x a day treatments given 4 hr apart	2 Rx	2 Rx	
Q1h or 24x a day treatments given 1 hr apart	8 Rx	8 Rx	8 Rx
Q2h or 12x a day treatments given 2 hr apart	4 Rx	4 Rx	4 Rx
Q3h or 8x a day treatments given 3 hr apart	3 Rx	3 Rx	2 Rx
Q4h or 6x a day treatments given 4 hours apart	2 Rx	2 Rx	2 Rx
Q6h or 4x a day treatments given 6 hr apart	2 Rx	1 Rx	1 Rx
Q8h or 3x a day treatments given 8 hr apart	1 Rx	1 Rx	1 Rx
H.S. or Hour of sleep		1 Rx 9 or 10 pm	
Q12h or 2x a day treatments given 12 hr apart	Depends on time started		
Stat	— IMMEDIATELY —		
PRN	— AS NECESSARY —		

Respiratory Therapy Department
Patient Assessment

I. Chart Review
   1. Respiratory diagnosis
   2. Chief complaint
   3. Objective of therapy
   4. Vital signs: Temperature
                   Pulse
                   Respiration
   5. X-ray reports ☐ Infiltrate (specify location)
                    ☐ Atelectasis (specify location)
                    ☐ Other significant abnormality
   6. Pulmonary function studies
                    ☐ Obstructive disease
                    ☐ Restrictive disease
                    ☐ Both obstructive and restrictive impairment
   7. Sputum reports (significant positive)
   8. Arterial blood gas reports — indicate FIO_2 (most recent sample)
   9. Cardiac status
      ☐ CHF   ☐ Cor pulmonale   ☐ Other — specify
      ☐ History of shock
  10. Past history of pulmonary problems (including side effects of pre-
      vious treatments, including pneumothorax)
  11. Occupation (exposure to pollutants)
  12. Medications (particularly bronchodilators)
  13. Other

II. Patient Interview and Examination
    1. Subjective respiratory symptomatology
       ☐ Dyspnea   ☐ Cough — describe
       ☐ Chest pain   ☐ Sputum — describe
       ☐ Hemoptysis   No Yes   No Yes
       ☐ Other   Smoking habits — Past ☐ ☐ Present ☐ ☐
                                        Months _____ Years _____
                                        Amount per day _____
    2. Objective respiratory signs (may be obtained from patient's chart)
       a. Pulse rate
       b. Respiratory rate
       c. Pattern of breathing   ☐ Labored
                                    ☐ Short of breath
                                    ☐ Shallow
                                    ☐ Rapid
                                    ☐ Use of accessory muscles
                                    ☐ Diaphragmatic breathing

☐ Stridor
☐ Wheezing
☐ Cheyne–Stokes

d. Hoarseness   ☐ Yes ☐ No

e. Inspection of chest
☐ Barrel chest
☐ Asymmetrical in shape
☐ Asymmetrical expansion
☐ Paradoxical movement
☐ Retraction
☐ Scars of prior surgery
☐ Scars of previous tracheotomy
☐ Kyphoscoliosis

f. Palpation
☐ Symmetrical expansion
☐ Asymmetrical expansion
☐ Diminished vocal fremitus
☐ Increased vocal fremitus

g. Percussion
☐ Dull — location
☐ Normally resonant

h. Auscultation   Sound   Location
☐ Rhonchi
☐ Rales
☐ Pleural rub

i. Volumes and capacities: Tidal   ml
Minute   liters/min
Vital capacity   liters/min

j. Color
☐ Cyanotic
☐ Ruddy

k. Level of consciousness
☐ Conscious and alert
☐ Lethargic
☐ Stuporous
☐ Semicomatose
☐ Comatose
☐ Confused, disoriented

l. Hydration of oral and nasal cavities
☐ Adequate
☐ Inadequate

m. Clubbing of fingers   ☐ Yes ☐ No

n. Sputum: Color
         Consistency
         Amount
         Odor
         Blood tinged

o. Mobility
☐ Active
☐ Difficult

p. Communication barriers ☐ Language
☐ Deaf
☐ Speech
☐ Other (specify)

q. Allergies — specify
r. Home respiratory therapy procedures
        ☐ O_2 — method
              FIO$_2$ or liters/min
        ☐ IPPB — Type of Unit
              Frequency
              Medications

3. Assessment
4. Plan

Signature _____
Title _____
Date _____

EXERCISES

1. Explain the importance of a *complete* physician's order.
2. Why should all ventilators have a controlled check sheet?
3. Develop a complete set of records for your Respiratory Therapy Department.
4. Why is documentation of all therapy so important?
5. What other records and statistics might your department want to keep?

UNIT 8

INFECTION CONTROL

INFECTION CONTROL IN THE RESPIRATORY THERAPY DEPARTMENT

I. *Introduction*

Because of the type of equipment used by the department, its widespread dissemination, and the destination (i.e., the respiratory tract) of the aerosol and gases used, the Respiratory Therapy Department must be alert to the possibility of the spread of microorganisms to those patients under their care. This may occur as a result of contaminated equipment taking an infection to a patient who has no previous infection or superimposing a new infection on one that is already present. Not only may the equipment be a source of contamination, but the personnel also may be responsible for the spread of infection through hands, clothes, and their own respiratory infections.

II. *Administrative Accountability*

Although each employee in the department is held accountable for maintaining good technique, the ultimate responsibilty is delegated as follows:

A. Medical director

B. Technical director

C. Chief respiratory therapist

The department must work closely with the microbiology laboratory, which processes the cultures. The nurse epidemi-

421

ologist aids in the formulation of policies. The infection control committee periodically reviews policies and procedures and makes recommendations as necessary, in areas that need improvement. The hospital epidemiologist is available for consultation should a problem arise.

III.   *Infection Control Policies*
  A. Patient–client population—The Respiratory Therapy Department is in the position to provide much health information to the patient, particularly as related to the spread of respiratory infections.
   1. All patients with whom the Respiratory Therapy Department personnel come in contact should be given instructions on covering their noses and mouths when coughing and sneezing, as droplet spread of infection is prevalent.
   2. All patients should be instructed to dispose of tissues and sputum in paper bags at the bedside.
   3. Patients, particularly those who have access to washing facilities, should be instructed in frequent handwashing practices.
  B. Personnel population
   1. All personnel in the Respiratory Therapy Department must be instructed in handwashing and gown technique. In addition, the department should hold infection control in-services four times a year under the direction of the nurse epidemiologist.
   2. All personnel must be instructed to wash hands between each patient cared for.
   3. Personnel must be instructed to follow the hospital dress code.
   4. All personnel should have chest x-rays once a year; personnel with negative PPD's should have them (PPD) repeated every 6 months.
  C. Equipment and materials
   1. All respiratory therapy equipment should be cleaned, processed and sterilized by the SPD Department.
   2. IPPB equipment
    a. If disposable mouthpieces and flex tubes are used, they should be disposed of after *each* treatment.
    b. Nondisposable parts are changed after *each* treatment.
    c. Each patient receiving IPPB treatments should have an IPPB machine for his individual use.

3. Oxygen–humidity and PEEP
   a. All equipment should be changed daily.
   b. When refilling humidifiers and the like, personnel should be instructed to dispose of any remaining solution and to refill with sterile water.
   c. Personnel should be instructed to drain condensation in tubing into another receptacle, not back into the nebulizer.

4. Ventilators
   a. Disposable ventilator tubing, if used, should be disposed of daily.
   b. Nondisposable ventilator parts should be changed daily.
   c. Terminal care of the ventilator
      (1) All parts are removed by the Respiratory Therapy Department prior to taking ventilator to SPD for cleaning.
      (2) Filters are wiped with 70% alcohol, packaged for steam autoclaving, and taken to SPD.
      (3) Thermometers, spirometer alarms, and black valves from spirometer are removed, wiped with 70% alcohol and taken to SPD for placement with the sterilized setup.
      (4) In the decontamination area of SPD, the ventilator itself is cleaned with 70% alcohol; nondisposable parts are washed and dried, and sent for packaging and gas sterilization.
      (5) No ventilator should be assembled for use until it is needed for patient care.
      (6) Each oxygen analyzer and Wright respirometer should be gas sterilized between patients.

5. Medications and solutions
   a. Only sterile solutions should be used in respiratory therapy equipment; if the entire amount of solution is not used, mark the container as to date and time opened; discard after 24 hr.
   b. Most medications are provided in single-unit dose containers.
   c. If a dosage of medication cannot be provided in a single-unit dose, the bottle must not be used, if opened, after 24 hr. Mark bottle as to date and time opened.

     d. The expiration date for each solution and medication must be strictly observed, and any expired solutions or medications discarded.

6. Miscellaneous equipment

     a. IPPB machines should be gassed between patients.

     b. Accessory and monitoring equipment (respirometers, oxygen analyzers, etc.) should be gas sterilized between patients according to manufacturer's recommendations.

     c. Equipment that is too large to place in a gas sterilizer should be cleaned with 70% alcohol. Wheels should be steam cleaned.

7. Supplies

     a. Disposable items are not reused.

     b. Sterile items received from SPD must be rotated; observe expiration date; if not used before expiration date, the item(s) must be resterilized.

     c. No used supplies or equipment should be in the work area of the Respiratory Therapy Department. Soiled equipment should be taken directly to the decontamination area of SPD.

8. Contaminated Equipment—Although all used equipment is essentially contaminated, this section refers to equipment used on patients who have a known infection that could be transmitted to other patients or personnel.

     a. Disposable supplies should be discarded in the patient's room.

     b. Equipment should be placed in a red plastic bag (*not* the water-soluble type), tied, and taken directly to the decontamination area of SPD.

     c. Handwashing before and after patient contact is essential.

     d. Gown technique must be followed, as indicated by the organism involved and type of isolation used.

     e. For equipment, such as a ventilator, that is too large to bag, after putting small parts in red plastic bag, place a red plastic bag over the arm of the machine. Also place a piece of red plastic tape on the cover to indicate that the machine must be aired. When the unit returns from SPD, place a sign on it: To be aired from *time and date* to *time and date* for 24 hours. At the end of that time, the Respiratory Therapy Department is responsible for removing all signs.

IV. Controls of the System
   A. Policies and procedures should be periodically reviewed and revised.
   B. Random cultures of respiratory therapy equipment should be done once a month.
      1. Ventilators, aerosol equipment, and IPPB units: cultures of the gas flow through the unit are done in three ways:
         a. Through a sterile funnel into BHI
         b. Onto a blood agar plate
         c. Sterile swab into thioglycollate
      2. Other equipment: a moist swab is taken and placed in thioglycollate.
   C. Once culture reports are received, they are reviewed with the medical director of the Respiratory Therapy Department. Any suspicious cultures are repeated and again reviewed. If a change in procedure is indicated, the necessary steps will be taken by the Respiratory Therapy Department.

STERILIZATION OF RESPIRATORY THERAPY EQUIPMENT

Whether or not the processing and sterilization of respiratory therapy equipment is done by a Central Supplies Processing and Distribution Department or by the Respiratory Therapy Department itself, the end result should guarantee that this equipment will not be a source of infection to the patient.

Discussed in this Unit will be the options available, their advantages and disadvantages, and quality control.

   I. Terminology
   A. *Antiseptic*—substance that can be applied to tissue and will either kill microorganisms or prevent their growth (bacteriostat).
   B. *Aseptic*—characterized by absence of pathogenic organisms.
   C. *Bactericidal*—causing death of bacteria; irreversible.
   D. *Bacteriostatic*—inhibition of bacterial multiplication; reversible (multiplication resumes when agent is removed).
   E. *Clean*—freedom of or removal of all matter in which microorganisms may find favorable conditions for continued life

and growth, such as by scrubbing with hot water and detergent.

F. *Disinfection*—chemical or physical process used to kill microorganisms on surfaces, but which is too toxic to be applied directly to tissues. Does not necessarily kill spores or tuberculin bacilli.

G. *Germicide*—anything that will kill microbes; does not necessarily kill resistant spores; may usually be applied to tissue as well as inanimate objects.

H. *Sterilization*—act or process of destroying completely *all* forms of microbial life (bacteria, spores, fungi, and viruses).

II. Cleaning of Equipment

No method of sterilization will be effective unless soil is first removed from the equipment. In this context, the word *soil* refers to blood, secretions, and the like, that may be on the outside or inside of any piece of equipment. The cleaning of such equipment may be accomplished in several ways:

A. *Manually*—after soaking in a solution of detergent and water, the equipment is scrubbed with a brush to remove visible soil, then rinsed.

　　1. Disadvantages

　　　　a. Inability to reach all surfaces (e.g., inside of long tubes).

　　　　b. Redeposition of soil on equipment unless water bath is changed frequently.

　　　　c. Cleaning of brushes is difficult.

　　　　d. Time consuming.

　　2. Advantages

　　　　a. Inexpensive equipment.

　　　　b. Allows for close inspection of individual equipment.

B. *Washer–Sterilizer*—machine automatically washes by means of a vigorously agitated detergent bath. This is followed by steam under pressure at a temperature of 270°F (132°C).

　　1. Disadvantages

　　　　a. Much respiratory therapy equipment will not tolerate temperature involved.

　　　　b. Sterilized equipment is not packaged and therefore must be handled.

2. Advantages

    a. Cleaning is usually quite thorough, unless soil is dried on. In that case, soaking in water prior to cleaning may be necessary.

C. *Ultrasonic Cleaner*—sound waves above 20,000 cycles/sec are used to generate minute bubbles. The bubbles expand until they burst inward, creating a vacuum. These minute vacuum areas are responsible for the cleaning process when coupled with detergent and heat [heat should not exceed 140°F (60°C), as protein tends to coagulate above this temperature and then is difficult to remove]. Ultrasonic cleaning must be followed by thorough rinsing, either by the unit itself or by hand.

1. Disadvantages

    a. The temperature of the rinse unit may deform some plastic items, necessitating individual rinsing.

    b. The drying cycle of the unit may also deform plastics.

    c. The rinse cycle does not always reach the inside of some equipment.

2. Advantages

    a. When properly operated and maintained, ultrasonic cleaning is much more thorough than manual scrubbing.

III. Methods of Sterilization

A. *Steam autoclave*—utilizes moist heat in the form of steam under pressure. It is probably the most reliable method of sterilization. The pressure is a means of attaining high temperatures and of itself does nothing to kill organisms. Temperatures between 250° to 270°F (121°C–132°C) are most frequently used. The higher the temperature, the shorter the period of time necessary for the load to be exposed.

1. *Disadvantages*

    a. Much respiratory therapy equipment cannot tolerate the high temperatures involved.

2. *Advantages*

    a. Destruction of most resistant bacterial spores in brief intervals of exposure.

    b. Economical.

    c. No toxic residue on equipment.

3. Procedure
   a. Before autoclaving any equipment, make certain that it is made of a material that can withstand the heat and pressure; many costly items have been destroyed because this was not done.
   b. Wash all equipment thoroughly.
   c. Drain and dry.
   d. Items may be packaged in paper or wrapped in linen, but, if possible, the two coverings should not be mixed in the same load, as the paper dries more quickly and becomes brittle.
   e. When packaging, arrange the items so that the steam can reach all areas of the equipment and air pockets do not form; covers should be at least partially removed from containers.
   f. Inside each pack, place a true sterilization indicator, which shows that saturated steam has been in contact for progressive periods of time.
   g. Seal the package.
   h. Label all packages as to date and contents; indicate "to be steam autoclaved."
   i. On the outside of the package place a strip of autoclave indicator tape that changes color when exposed to steam; however, it is important to note that such tapes do not mean that all requirements for sterilization have been met.
   j. Fortunately, most institutions have a central sterile supply department that is responsible for packaging and the operating of the autoclave and the drying of packs after sterilization; however, the respiratory therapist should still be responsible for checking the indicator in the pack when it is opened to see that at least the minimum requirements of sterilization have been met.

B. *Ethylene oxide gas sterilization*—ethylene oxide gas is microbicidal and sporicidal, provided that at least minimum standards of time, temperature, relative humidity, and gas concentration have been met. It is useful for sterilization of equipment that could not withstand the high pressures and temperatures of steam-autoclaving.

Heat of 120° to 140°F (49° to 60°C) is used. Vacuum

is drawn into the chamber for 5 to 45 min at 25 to 27 in. Relative humidity of 40% to 50% is injected following the vacuum period. Gas concentrations and exposure times depend on the size and type of sterilizer used, as well as temperature.

1. Procedure
    a. Wash equipment thoroughly.
    b. Drain and dry; a small amount of moisture left on the equipment is acceptable, as moisture is used in the sterilization process.
    c. Ethylene oxide gas easily permeates most packaging materials; however, moisture must also be able to enter the pack if the gas is to be effective; such materials as muslin, Kraft paper, and polyethylene film (up to 3 mils thick) may be used.
    d. Package equipment so that the gas and moisture are able to reach all areas of the item.
    e. In each pack place an ethylene oxide indicator, which assures the user that the proper sterilizing conditions have been met.
    f. Seal the package.
    g. On the outside of the package, place a strip of ethylene oxide indicator tape that changes color when exposed to ethylene oxide; however, as with autoclaving, such tape does not certify that sterilization requirements have been met.
    h. Label all packages as to date and content; indicate "to be gas sterilized."
    i. Once the equipment is sterilized, aeration is necessary to remove irritating residual gas from the materials; such time varies depending on the constituents: porous materials require longer periods of aeration than do nonporous materials. It is best to obtain the manufacturer's recommendations for such items; aeration cabinets are available that apparently reduce aeration time.

2. *Disadvantages*
    a. Ethylene oxide is flammable in both liquid and gaseous states and also has toxic properties. For this reason it is generally not used in its pure form but mixed with inert gases such as carbon dioxide or fluorinated hydrocarbons.

b. Certain acrylic plastic materials and polystyrene may be damaged if a mixture of ethylene oxide and hydrocarbon is used.

c. Equipment must be dry before gassing if packaged in plastic wrappers, as exposure to ethylene oxide may induce the formation of a film of ethylene glycol.

d. Many materials contain a residual of the gas at the end of the sterilization process, necessitating aeration. The time required for dissipation varies with the porous qualities of the material. This time can be accelerated by the use of an aeration cabinet. Whether such a cabinet is used or the equipment is aerated at room temperature in a well-ventilated area, the department will find it requires a greater inventory of equipment during this period.

3. *Advantages*

a. Equipment that is heat sensitive can generally be sterilized by this method without danger of melting or deformation.

b. Kills resistant spores.

C. *Pasteurization*—a means of disinfection by moist heat; equipment is immersed in a water bath of 170°F (77°C) for 30 min.

1. *Disadvantages*

a. When equipment emerges from the process, it is wet; commercial driers are available.

b. Equipment must be packaged *after* pasteurization, so that the danger of recontamination is always present. The individual department must establish its own standards; is it enough that the equipment be *clean* or must it be sterile?

c. Is not sporicidal.

2. *Advantages*

a. Is not harmful to heat-sensitive plastics and rubber.

b. The relatively short time from initial cleaning to drying cycle eliminates the need for a large inventory of equipment.

c. After the initial investment for the equipment (e.g., one system on the market consists of a washer, pasteurizer, and a drier), the cost of running the equipment is relatively low.

D. *Chemical Disinfection*—the use of chemicals in solution; many will kill vegetative (growing) bacteria, but not all will kill spores. There are several "cold sterilizing" agents on the market. However, to determine whether or not such an agent meets the standards of your particular department, it is necessary to work closely with the bacteriology department of your hospital to evaluate their effectiveness in relation to respiratory therapy equipment.

1. *Disadvantages*
   a. Many of the agents available are irritating to the skin, eyes, and respiratory tract. Care must be taken to avoid direct contact with the solution and to provide adequate ventilation.
   b. Those agents that are sporicidal often require soaking of equipment for extended periods of time and may eventually lead to some deterioration of equipment (particularly rubber.)
   c. If water from the cleaning process is left on equipment when it is immersed in solution, eventual deactivation of the disinfectant may occur.
   d. Most disinfectants require rinsing of equipment following the soaking period. Unless this can be accomplished as a sterile procedure, there is the danger of reintroducing pathogens.
   e. The final product must be dried and packaged; again, the result is a *clean* item, not a sterile one, if any handling of equipment is done. Air drying can also be a source of contamination.
   f. Some agents must be activated, requiring mixing of a powder with the solution; this is somewhat time consuming.

2. *Advantages*
   a. The entire disinfection process takes a relatively short period of time unless the department routinely is concerned about spores.
   b. Most agents may be used for a period of time, ranging from 14 days to 28 days.

IV. Special Considerations
   A. The area where soiled equipment is handled must be separate from the storage area for processed equipment.

B. Only personnel who have been thoroughly trained in decontamination and sterilization should be allowed to operate the equipment necessary for these vital processes.

C. Continuous monitoring of the efficiency of the sterilizer must be maintained, both by spore tests of the sterilizer itself, and by culturing of the finished product.

ISOLATION PROCEDURES

I. Transmission of infection
   A. Contact
      1. Direct contact—physically transferred from an infected individual to a susceptible person.
      2. Indirect contact—transferral of infection from articles belonging to infected individual to a susceptible person.
      3. Droplet—contact with infectious agents as a direct result of an infected individual's coughing, sneezing, or talking.
   B. Vehicle route—diseases transmitted via:
      1. Blood
      2. Water
      3. Drugs
      4. Contaminated food
   C. Vector route—diseases transmitted via insects.
   D. Airborne route—disease transmitted by droplet nuclei or dust, which contain infectious agents that may be inhaled by a susceptible individual.

II. Purpose of isolation—isolation is designed to:
   A. Prevent transmission of highly communicable diseases (strict isolation).
   B. Prevent infection of burn sites (sterile isolation).
   C. Protect those patients with impaired resistance from possible lethal infections acquired from other individuals (reverse isolation).

III. Handwashing—good handwashing is the basis for any isolation procedure.
   A. A sink with foot controls is preferable, but if not available, care should be taken not to touch the handles after washing.

B. A liquid washing agent, such as Betadine, which is dispensed from a foot-controlled unit, is preferred to bar soap, as the latter may harbor disease organisms.

C. Paper towel dispensers should be at sink level so that it is not necessary to reach the arms in such a manner as to allow water to run toward the elbows.

D. Procedure

1. Remove all jewelry.

2. Wet the hands and lower arms liberally with moderately hot water.

3. Apply a small amount of liquid washing agent; to make more suds, simply add more water.

4. If a scrub brush is used, it should be of the disposable variety; however, as these techniques are not for surgical purposes, a brush is not generally considered necessary.

5. Wash hands and lower arms for a minimum of 2 min.

6. Rinse well under running water, beginning at the elbow and rinsing downward over the hands.

7. Dry the hands thoroughly, using at least two paper towels.

8. If the sink does not have foot controls, turn off the handles with the paper towels used for drying the hands; do not touch the area of the towels which came in contact with the handles.

9. Dispose of the paper towels, being careful not to touch the waste container.

IV. Infections requiring isolation in a private room and the wearing of gowns, masks, and gloves:

A. *Staphylococcus aureus*

B. Group A *Streptococcus*

C. Diphtheria

D. Herpes simplex

E. Plague

F. Rubella, congenital syndrome

G. Smallpox

H. Varicella

I. Rubella

J. Herpes zoster, eruptive

K. Rubeola

L. Meningococcal meningitis

M. Mumps

N. Pertussis

O. Tuberculosis, pulmonary—sputum-positive (or suspect)

> *Note:* These patients must have respiratory therapy equipment for their individual use only.

V. Procedure for administering therapy to isolated patients:

A. Wash hands.

B. Assemble respiratory therapy equipment to be used.

C. Arrange a place for disposal of contaminated equipment, such as a paper bag placed on a cart outside the patient's room.

D. Use a clean gown each time you enter the patient's room; tie neck ties and waist ties, being sure that the back of your uniform is completely covered; individuals with unusually broad shoulders may find it necessary to wear two gowns: one tied in front, covered by one tied in the customary manner, in back; if the sleeves do not have knitted cuffs, pin the sleeves so that they fit closely to your wrists.

E. Put on mask, making sure that the nose and mouth are covered; the mask should be changed hourly.

F. Put on gloves, pulling cuffs up over cuffs on gown.

G. Upon completion of the therapy:

1. Place contaminated equipment in paper bag, outside patient's room.

2. Remove gloves and mask.

3. Remove gown, folding the inside to cover the outside, so that it is not necessary to handle the most contaminated areas of the gown; place in laundry.

4. Wash hands thoroughly.

5. Chart therapy.

VI. Sterile isolation for burn patients—as a form of protective isolation, a severely burned patient should be placed in a private room; as much as possible, all articles coming in contact with him should be sterile; persons entering the room should wear sterile gloves, masks, caps, and gowns.

A. Procedure
   1. Wash hands.
   2. Assemble all respiratory therapy equipment needed.
   3. Wash hands.
   4. Put on cap, being sure to cover all hair.
   5. Put on mask.
   6. Put on sterile gown in the following manner:
      a. Remove gown from its package by handling it by the neck ties only.
      b. Put on gown, being careful not to touch outside.
      c. Tie neck and waist ties; if necessary have someone do this for you; again, touch only the ties when you do this.
   7. Put on sterile gloves in the following manner:
      a. Reusable gloves are usually packaged in a folder that opens like a book.
      b. Open folder.
      c. With one hand lift the compartment holding one glove.
      d. With the other hand, remove the glove from the folder, being careful to touch only that part of the glove which is folded down into a cuff.
      e. Still holding the glove by its cuff, pull the glove over the other hand.
      f. Adjust the cuff of the glove over the cuff on the sleeve of the gown; if you are unable to do so without touching the outside (sterile area) of the glove, do not do so until after putting on other glove.
      g. Put on other glove in the same manner; however, pick the glove up by sliding the fingers of your gloved hand under the cuff on the other glove.
      h. Adjust both gloves, being sure to touch only the outside.
   8. Upon completion of the therapy, gloves, gown, mask, and cap should be discarded in containers set aside for that purpose.
   9. Wash hands.
  10. Chart therapy.

VII. Reverse isolation—reverse isolation to protect those patients with impaired resistance consists of a private room and the wearing of gown and mask by individuals entering the room; generally, sterile technique is not necessary but may be followed if the physician so desires.

VIII.   Other—because of the nature of the equipment used by the Respiratory Therapy Department, certain other infections require that equipment be isolated for individual patients; patients having these infections will not generally be isolated:

A.   Aspergillosis

B.   *Pseudomonas*

C.   Friedlander's bacillus

D.   Coccidioidomycosis (pneumonia)

CULTURING OF RESPIRATORY THERAPY EQUIPMENT

Respiratory therapy equipment has frequently been singled out as one of the leading sources of nosocomial infections. This can be related to the increasing use of these procedures, as well as the techniques of handling equipment by the personnel employing its use. The respiratory therapy field as a whole has become more cognizant of possible sources of patient and equipment contamination, and therefore has been vigilant regarding sterilization of equipment and establishment of infection control procedures.

It is imperative that sterilization procedures be monitored continuously to ensure that there is no breakdown in technique. Random cultures done at least monthly are necessary in order to provide meaningful information.

The culture samples may be taken either by personnel in the Respiratory Therapy Department or by the Bacteriology Laboratory. However, because Respiratory Therapy Department personnel are more familiar with the equipment, if they have been instructed in the technique of taking samples correctly, they are probably the logical ones to do so.

There is some controversy as to when culture samples should be taken. We prefer *sterilities*, cultures done on equipment after sterilization before use on a patient. These tell us that the equipment we apply to a patient at least initially will not be a source of infection.

Taking culture samples of equipment after it has been used by a patient for a period of time gives limited information, since the source of any contamination may be difficult to ascertain; it may be from the equipment, from the patient, airborne, or a result of poor technique by all personnel caring for the patient. However, such cultures are useful if they indicate that a change in procedure, such as more frequent equipment changing schedules, is necessary.

To be meaningful, culture samples must be done with the idea that, if contamination is there, you want to know about it—not just because a committee dictates that you do them. Therefore, the same technique to take culture samples cannot be used for all equipment. To take a swab of the outlet on a ventilator setup does not assure that there are no microorganisms farther back in the tubing. It is with this in mind that we have devised the following procedure. It may be modified to meet your particular needs. New products on the market, such as sterile disposable culture tubes and sampling chambers, if available to your department, will also be of assistance. Most of these products are reasonable enough in cost to warrant investigation of their use.

I. Culturing of Ventilators and Humidity Devices
  A. Equipment
    1. Sterile funnel—Pyrex funnels are convenient because they may be steam autoclaved and the stems may be cut to adapt to the length of the culture tube used. The stem should not touch the medium when inserted in the tube.
    2. Screw-top culture tube containing 5-ml trypticase soy broth or beef heart infusion.
    3. Alcohol lamp and matches.
    4. Culture tube containing thioglycollate
    5. Sterile cotton swabs with wooden sticks
    6. Blood agar plate
    7. Culture tube rack
    8. Sterile physiologic saline for moistening swab; may be poured into sterile medicine glass.
    9. Labels and cards as required by your laboratory.
  B. Procedure—we are modifying the procedure described by Sanford in the *American Review of Respiratory Disease*, vol. 94, 1966, p. 450.
    1. Collect culturing equipment and equipment to be sampled.
    2. Make out labels and laboratory cards for each piece of equipment. Include such information as serial numbers, expiration dates, and the like, to make identification as complete as possible.
    3. Wash hands thoroughly.
    4. Assemble equipment to be cultured, as you would when applying to a patient. Fill humidifying devices with the

sterile solution normally used and plug in any heating devices.

5. Wash hands thoroughly and between each culture.

6. Light alcohol lamp; however, be certain that no oxygen source is nearby.

7. Unscrew top of culture tube containing trypticase soy broth and *flame* tube by slowly rotating the top through the flame of the alcohol lamp. This is necessary to remove any organisms that might be on the outside top of the tube. Extinguish alcohol lamp. Do not lay screw top down while doing this, or at any other time, as organisms may be picked up that contaminate the inside of the screw top and therefore your culture sample.

8. Support culture tube in tube rack.

9. Open package containing sterile funnel. Funnel should be handled only on the outside of the very top.

10. Place funnel stem inside culture tube being careful not to touch stem of funnel to any part of tube.

11. With the unit in its operating mode, direct the flow of gas into the funnel for approximately 1 min.

12. Remove the funnel, flame the top of the tube and the screw top, and re-cover the tube immediately.

13. Label the tube immediately and set aside.

14. With the unit still in the operating mode, uncover the blood agar plate and expose the plate to the gas from the equipment for approximately 30 sec. Do not lay the cover down during this time for the same reason as described above. In addition, be careful not to touch the agar with the equipment.

15. Re-cover the plate and label immediately.

16. Pour sterile saline into a sterile medicine glass. Light alcohol lamp.

17. Open the package containing the sterile swab. Remove the swab by the extreme tip of the stick.

18. Moisten cotton swab in the sterile saline.

19. Wipe swab over surface of equipment to be sampled; generally, the best source is the *outlet* of the device.

20. Uncap the culture tube containing thioglycollate and flame.

21. Insert the swab into the culture tube, being careful not to touch the tube. The stick must be broken off below the area that you touch. Therefore, the farther down

you hold the stick, the more must be broken off to avoid contamination of the sample.

22. Flame the tube and cap. Replace cap. Extinguish lamp.

23. Label tube immediately.

24. Sterile, disposable culture tubes are available that greatly simplify this procedure.

II. Culturing of Other Respiratory Therapy Equipment

    A. Equipment with a *dry* surface may be cultured using thioglycollate and a sterile moist swab, such as parts of an IPPB setup. Try to obtain the sample from an area that would most likely be contaminated (e.g., the baffle and jet on a nebulizer or the ridges of a flex tube).

    B. Equipment with a *moist* surface may be cultured using thioglycollate and a dry swab (since moisture is provided by the surface itself). Moisture is necessary as any bacteria present are more easily sampled.

    C. Medications may be cultured by carefully dropping a small amount into the tube of thioglycollate.

III. Terminal Care

    A. Culture samples should be taken to the laboratory as soon as possible after completion. Then any additions to the medium may be made and the identification process started.

    B. Equipment from which samples were obtained should be reprocessed or disposed of.

IV. Interpretation of Results

    A. Most cultures are examined after 7 days of incubation and results are reported shortly thereafter. However the laboratory will generally notify the department if suspicious cultures appear prior to this time.

    B. Culture results that report the presence of pathogenic organisms are not necessarily the disaster they might appear to be.

        1. Examine the method in which the culture samples were obtained—could they have possibly been contaminated by the individual taking the sample? This is generally the problem. Could the culture tube and medium have been contaminated? Never use a tube in which the medium is cloudy and possibly contains bacterial growth.

        2. Repeat the culture on the same piece of equipment, if it is possible, or on similar equipment if it is not.

3. Quarantine the equipment until results are obtained.

4. If positive results are again reported, examine your sterilization procedure and the possibility that tubing or other parts may be contaminated when received from the manufacturer. A change in procedure may be indicated.

5. Positive results should be discussed with your medical director and your hospital infection control committee, both of whom may have further recommendations.

C. Culture results that report the presence of nonpathogenic organisms are of concern when they are present in large numbers. They indicate overhandling of equipment when assembling or prolonged exposure to airborne contaminants, two conditions that must be avoided.

D. A systematic method of filing culture reports should be devised so that they are readily available at all times. A large loose-leaf notebook is useful for this.

E. Do not become overly confident if a series of "negative" reports are obtained! This is no reason to discontinue taking cultures or to become less vigilant in sterilization procedures!

EXERCISES

1. When sterilizing with ethylene oxide, which organs in the body would be most affected if equipment were not properly aired?

2. How would you implement a program for culturing respiratory therapy equipment in your department?

3. Describe two methods of sterilization; include the advantages and disadvantages of each.

4. What are the most common methods of the transmission of infections in a hospital?

5. A patient has been isolated for a gas gangrene infection. He has been on an MA-1 with ultrasonic nebulization. Describe the terminal sterilization of this equipment.

TRACHEOSTOMY AND ENDOTRACHEAL TUBES AND SUCTIONING

TRACHEOSTOMY AND ENDOTRACHEAL TUBES

Mechanical ventilation requires the maintenance of a patent airway. This may be accomplished by the use of a variety of tubes (see Figures 9-1 through 9-4).

Endotracheal Tubes

These tubes are used primarily for short-term ventilation. They may usually be inserted rapidly and, since they do not require a surgical procedure for insertion, there is no scar and less danger of infection.

Endotracheal tubes are made of either rubber or a nonirritating plastic. Each tube is supplied with either a double- or single-wall inflatable cuff, which provides the airtight system necessary for mechanical ventilation. Each tube is also equipped with a 15-mm adapter for connection to the ventilator.

Tracheostomy Tubes

These tubes are usually inserted when it is determined that long-term ventilation will be required. For long-term ventilation, these tubes provide for more adequate removal of secretions. Their inser-

441

tion requires surgical intervention and thus constitutes a hazard in terms of infection.

Tracheostomy tubes are constructed of plastic, rubber, or metal. They are equipped with single- or double-wall inflatable cuffs, which may or may not be an integral part of the tube.

Comparison of Tube Sizes

Table 9-1 provides a comparison of various tube sizes.

TABLE 9-1

Endotracheal Tubes			
Diameter		English Size Magill Gauge	French Gauge
Internal	External		
2.5	4.0		12
3.0	4.5	00	12–14
3.5	5.0		14–16
4.0	5.5	0–1	16–18
4.5	6.0	1–2	18–20
5.0	6.5		20–22
5.5	7.0	3–4	22
6.0	8.0		24
6.5	8.5	4–5	26
7.0	9.0	5–6	28
7.5	9.5	6–7	30
8.0	10.0	7–8	32
8.5	11.5	8	34
9.0	12.0	9–10	36
9.5	12.5		38
10.0	13.0	10–11	40
10.5	13.5		42
11.0	14.5	11–12	42–44
11.5	15.0		44–46

Tracheostomy Tubes		
French Gauge	External MM	Jackson Trach Sizes
24	8	4
27	9	5
30	10	6
33	11	7
36	12	8
39	13	9
42	14	10

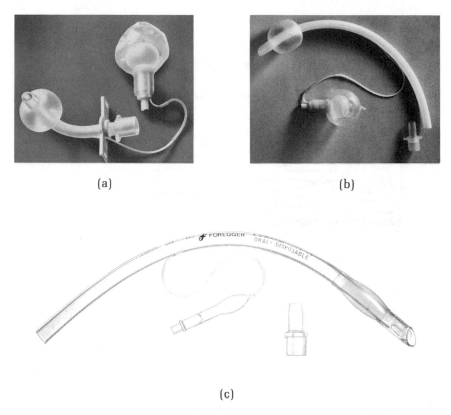

(a)

(b)

(c)

Figure 9-1. (a) Lanz Tracheostomy Tube. (b) Lanz Endotracheal Tube. (c) Forreger For-Clear Endotracheal Tube. (*Parts (a) and (b) courtesy of Extracorporal Medical Specialties, Inc., King of Prussia, Pa. Part (c) courtesy of Air Products and Chemicals Inc., Allentown, Pa.*)

SUCTIONING

I. Introduction

Nasopharyngeal and tracheobronchial suctioning are procedures that are frequently carried out on the respiratory patient, particularly one who has excessive or tenacious secretions that he is unable to clear.

It is important that the therapist and/or nurse understand the principles of the procedure as well as the problems that may arise. It is *not* a procedure that should be practiced without a great deal of initial supervision by someone proficient in the skill.

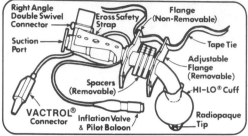

DIAGRAM OF ASSEMBLED pitt trach TUBE

Right Angle
Double Swivel
Connector

Eross Safety
Strap

Flange
(Non-Removable)

Suction
Port

Tape Tie

Adjustable
Flange
(Removable)

Spacers
(Removable)

HI-LO® Cuff

VACTROL®
Connector

Inflation Valve
& Pilot Baloon

Radiopaque
Tip

SUGGESTED PROCEDURE:

The tracheostomy tube is made adjustable by assembling the tube as
shown above.

To center tube within the trachea, remove the spacers and adjustable
flange as needed.

To secure spacers and flanges following adjustment, suture remaining
spacers and the two flanges together. Run the tape tie through both
flanges when tying around neck.

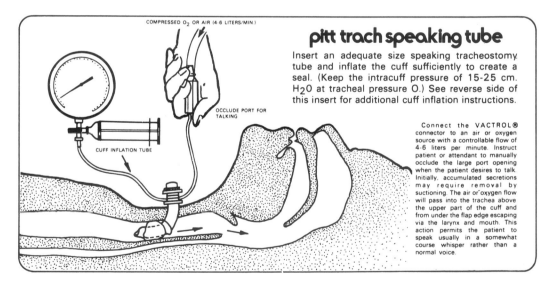

COMPRESSED O₂ OR AIR (4-6 LITERS/MIN.)

pitt trach speaking tube

Insert an adequate size speaking tracheostomy
tube and inflate the cuff sufficiently to create a
seal. (Keep the intracuff pressure of 15-25 cm.
H_2O at tracheal pressure O.) See reverse side of
this insert for additional cuff inflation instructions.

OCCLUDE PORT FOR
TALKING

CUFF INFLATION TUBE

Connect the VACTROL®
connector to an air or oxygen
source with a controllable flow of
4-6 liters per minute. Instruct
patient or attendant to manually
occlude the large port opening
when the patient desires to talk.
Initially, accumulated secretions
may require removal by
suctioning. The air or oxygen flow
will pass into the trachea above
the upper part of the cuff and
from under the flap edge escaping
via the larynx and mouth. This
action permits the patient to
speak usually in a somewhat
course whisper rather than a
normal voice.

Figure 9-2. Pitt Tracheal Speaking Tube. (*Courtesy of National Catheter Co., Argyle, N.Y.*)

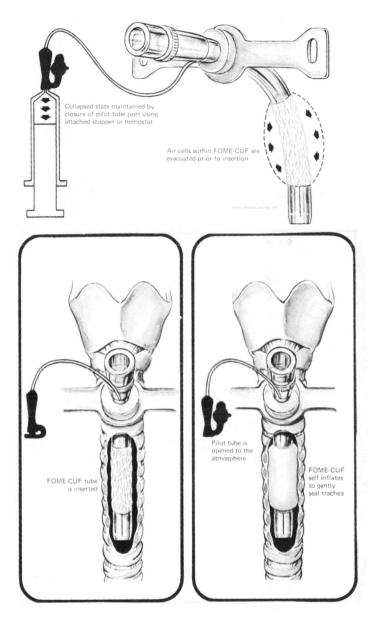

Collapsed state maintained by
closure of pilot tube port using
attached stopper or hemostat

Air cells within FOME-CUF are
evacuated prior to insertion

FOME-CUF tube
is inserted

Pilot tube is
opened to the
atmosphere

FOME-CUF
self inflates
to gently
seal trachea

Figure 9-3. Kamen-Wilkinson Fome-Cuf Tracheostomy Tube. (*Courtesy of Bivona Surgical Instruments, Inc., Hammond, Ind.*)

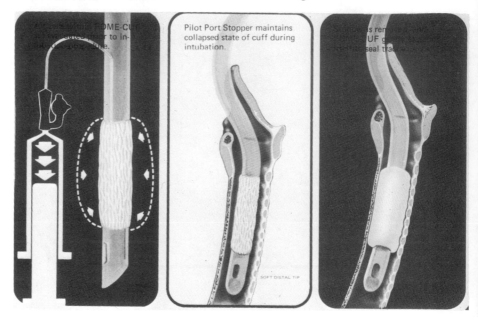

Figure 9-4.   Kamen-Wilkinson Fome-Cuf Endotracheal Tube. (*Courtesy of Bivona Surgical Instruments, Inc., Hammond, Ind.*)

II.   Definition—the act or process of sucking or of aspirating; to remove secretions from the nasopharynx and/or tracheobronchial tree by means of a suction catheter and negative pressure.

III.   Anatomical and Physiologic Considerations
  A.   The left and right main stem bronchi are asymmetrical, with the right bronchus larger and extending from the trachea at approximately a 25° angle compared to the more acute 45° angle of the left. For this reason, in some instances, the success rate for entering the left bronchus may be as low as 25%.
  B.   The respiratory tract functions to moisten the inspired air, filter it, and regulate its temperature. Heated nebulization may be needed to maintain the integrity of these regulatory mechanisms, especially if the patient has difficulty with tenacious secretions or if he has an endotracheal or tracheostomy tube in place that necessarily bypasses these functions.
  C.   Several reflexes may be stimulated in the respiratory tract. A reflex is an involuntary response to a stimulus. Because suctioning involves the introduction of a foreign

body (the catheter) into the respiratory tract, it is possible
to stimulate any or all of the following reflexes.

Reflex	Area Where Stimulated	Response
Cough	Pharynx Larynx Trachea Bronchi	Helps loosen secretions and perhaps raise them to a level where they can be reached by the catheter
Gag	Pharynx	Usually makes suctioning more traumatic for the patient; may induce vomiting, which could result in aspiration
Sneeze	Upper nasal passage	May aid in removal of secretions from upper passages
Spasm	Larynx Bronchi	Laryngospasm and/or bronchospasm could be fatal; resusitative measures may be necessary

D. Suctioning of the respiratory tract not only removes secretions, but also oxygen, and could lead to severe hypoxemia if prolonged. Therefore, it is necessary to provide the
patient with supplemental oxygen before, at intervals during, and following the procedure. If a patient is on a ventilator, this may be accomplished in two ways:

1. Set the ventilator to deliver 100% oxygen for several
minutes before the procedure. However, if the patient
has difficulty with retained CO_2, this must be monitored carefully. During the procedure, reattach the patient to the ventilator for 3 to 5 min. Once the suctioning is completed and the patient is again oxygenated
at 100% oxygen, *be sure to return the ventilator to its
previous oxygen setting.*

2. Use a manual resuscitator to ventilate the patient at
the necessary intervals. This accomplishes two
purposes:
   a. It provides additional deep breaths to the patient,
   usually at pressures greater than administered by
   the ventilator.
   b. It provides supplemental oxygen when the resuscitator is attached to an oxygen source. However,
   keep in mind that the design of most resuscitators
   is such that high percentages of oxygen cannot be

delivered without some modification of the bag–mask unit. Such a unit has the advantage that there is not the danger of forgetting to lower the oxygen percentage setting on the ventilator.

If the patient is not on a ventilator, it is still possible to provide supplemental oxygen. If a tracheostomy or endotracheal tube is in place, oxygen may be provided via the humidifying device. If such is not the case, oxygen may be provided by mask during this period. In some institutions this may be standard operating procedure; in others, a written order by the physician may be necessary.

IV. Indications for Suctioning
  A. Excessive secretions in the airways leading to dyspnea, fatigue, hypoxemia, hypercapnia, ciliary destruction, infection, and atelectasis. These secretions may be due to disease processes such as COPD or cystic fibrosis, and may have the additional feature of being tenacious.
  B. Inability to cough and/or swallow effectively due to a disease process that affects the respiratory musculature or nervous system—multiple sclerosis, myasthenia gravis, or Guillain–Barre syndrome, for example.
  C. Loss of cough reflex due to coma, drug overdose, head injury, or administration of neuromuscular blocking agents.
  D. Mechanical airway obstruction by tracheostomy or endotracheal tube.

V. Frequency of Suctioning
Frequency of suctioning is an individual need and should not be a standing order, such as "suction q1h." Assessment of the patient's condition and his need for suctioning must be made continually so that the health care professional involved in his care may intervene appropriately.
  A. Observe the patient's cough or inability to cough.
  B. Observe the secretions raised, if any.
  C. Listen for grossly audible signs that secretions are present. Although a pharyngeal gurgle may be present, such as when there is an air leak around a tube cuff, such a gurgle usually indicates the presence of a large amount of secretions. Although you want to avoid suctioning too frequently, this type of noise should generally be avoided.

D. Auscultate the patient's chest to ascertain the exact location(s) and type of secretions.

E. If the patient has a tracheotomy tube in place, secretions may be visible in the tube.

F. Monitor the patient's vital signs—changes in blood pressure, respiratory rate, pulse, and tidal volume may indicate a need for suctioning.

G. If the patient is on a ventilator, an increased system pressure, decreased tidal volume, or abnormal breath sounds can reflect the need for intervention.

VI. Procedure

A. Equipment—this procedure requires sterile technique in order to prevent introduction of microorganisms into the respiratory tract; therefore, the following equipment must be sterile and every effort must be made to maintain sterility.

1. Suction catheter—there are many manufacturers of sterile, disposable catheters. Most brands have a whistle-tip, built-in connector and vent. The term *whistle-tip* refers to a catheter with an open end and side holes. This allows for more complete removal of secretions with less damage to the delicate respiratory mucosa. The catheter should be packaged in a straight position, since coiling interferes with insertion, especially into the left main stem bronchus. In especially difficult cases, the use of a coudé catheter, one with an appropriate bend at the tip, is recommended. More than one catheter will be needed in most instances, one for the oral pharynx and one for the endotracheal or tracheostomy tube.

2. Sterile glove—although some people use two gloves, there is a greater chance of contaminating the glove that must remain sterile.

3. Sterile container for water.

4. Sterile water or saline.

Note: Several manufacturers now produce a *suction set* that includes all of these items—even bags of sterile water and the catheter.

5. Suction apparatus, which includes
   a. Collection bottle—should be changed daily and replaced by a sterile unit.

       b. Tubing system, which is connected to the suction catheter—replace with a sterile set at least daily.

       c. Gauge, either portable or wall mounted—registers the degree of vacuum (suction) from the suction pump.

     6. Sterile towel—needed to place ventilator connections on.

B. Positioning of the patient—a semi-Fowler's position produces the best results. Many practitioners recommend that you turn the patient's head to the opposite side to position the airways for easier insertion of the catheter. However, there seems to be little documentation that this is indeed effective.

C. Negative pressure settings (vacuum)—there is remarkably little written regarding which pressure settings to use for suctioning. Older references recommend pressures in the range of 115 to 150 mm Hg negative pressure. However, the current consensus is that settings above 100 mm Hg (one study used 200 mm Hg) are no more effective in removing secretions while greatly increasing tracheobronchial trauma, including denuded epithelium, loss of cilia, hemorrhage, inflammatory exudate, and edema. This is not to say that lower settings do not cause damage, just that it occurs to a lesser extent.

D. Technique of suctioning

    1. Wash hands.

    2. Collect equipment.

    3. Explain procedure to patient; this is at best a very uncomfortable procedure for the patient and at worst a traumatic one. Relief of his anxiety as much as possible is an important aid to its effectiveness. Suctioning a patient who has both feet braced against the foot of the bed, grasping both side rails for dear life, and who flings his head from side to side, makes for both physical and psychological trauma for the patient as well as the practitioner.

    4. Position the patient.

    5. Wash hands.

    6. Open the catheter package, but do not touch the catheter, in order to maintain its sterility.

    7. Pour sterile water or saline into sterile container.

    8. Put sterile glove on hand that will guide catheter.

9. Using ungloved hand to hold tubing from the suction unit, pick up catheter with the gloved hand and insert the catheter connector into the tubing; make sure that you do not touch the tubing itself with the gloved hand; it is usually helpful to hold the catheter in a coiled position, thus giving you more control.

10. Turn on the suction machine with your ungloved hand; check the pressure setting by placing the thumb of your gloved hand over the vent on the catheter and reading the gauge; adjust as necessary with your ungloved hand.

11. Lubricate the catheter by dipping it in the sterile water or saline.

12. If the patient is on a ventilator, remove the ventilator connection from the patient and lay on a sterile towel. Oxygenate the patient, using only your ungloved hand. As you gain experience, working one-handed will be much easier than it sounds.

13. Holding the catheter by the connecting tubing, turn the catheter until the natural curve points in the direction of the bronchus to be suctioned; use of this curve facilitates entry into the bronchus.

14. Hold the catheter itself 2 to 3 in. from the tip and *gently* insert the catheter into the nares, endotracheal tube, or tracheostomy tube, depending on the circumstances; as the catheter is inserted, gently rotate it between your thumb and forefinger. During insertion, *no vacuum* should be applied—in other words, *don't cover the vent*. If nasopharyngeal suctioning is being done, when the catheter reaches the larynx, have the patient inspire, if possible, to enable passage of the catheter past the vocal cords.

15. Only after inserting the catheter as far as you wish it to go should the vacuum be applied by closing the vent; at the same time, slowly withdraw the catheter with a rotating motion. This allows secretions on all sides of the airways to come in contact with the holes in the side of the catheter and thus allows for more complete removal of secretions.

16. Keep in mind that, as you remove secretions, you are also removing air, and thus oxygen; suction should not be applied for more than 5 to 10 sec at a time.

17. When the catheter has been fully withdrawn, rinse it

by flushing with water from the sterile container; observe the nature of the secretions removed—whether they are thin, tenacious, copious, bloody, foul-odored, and what color they are.

18. Unless the patient has such copious secretions that it would be dangerous to wait to continue with the suctioning procedure, allow the patient to rest for 3 to 5 min before suctioning again; if he is on a ventilator, replace the unit so that the patient is being oxygenated during this time.

Note: The order in which you suction the various cavities has been somewhat disputed. However, keep in mind that if you first suction the nasopharynx you must change the entire setup before suctioning an endotracheal tube or tracheostomy tube. If the patient has no tube, first suction the nasopharynx and then the oral cavity, as the oral cavity is more contaminated.

VII. Complications

In addition to the trauma and hypoxemia mentioned previously, the following complications could be encountered.

A. Laryngospasm—as evidenced by dyspnea, stridor, cyanosis, and increased, ineffective inspiratory effort with retraction of soft tissues around the thoracic cage. If this occurs, quickly remove the suction catheter; a physician should be notified immediately and measures taken by him to relieve the spasm. An emergency tracheostomy may be necessary, as well as cardiopulmonary resuscitation.

B. If during the suctioning procedure you feel the catheter "pull" as though it is holding onto tissue in the airways, take your finger off the vent and withdraw the catheter slightly before continuing; laryngospasm could occur if this is not done.

C. Coughing by the patient may occur during the suctioning process; this may be helpful in raising secretions to a point where they may be removed more easily by suctioning. If the coughing is not severe, simply remove your finger from the vent on the catheter and wait until it subsides. However, if the coughing is severe, remove the catheter, applying no suction, and wait until the patient relaxes.

D. No patient with a head injury or suspected head trauma should be suctioned through the nose, at least initially, because of the proximity of the cerebrum and nasopharynx. Nasal suctioning could cause additional severe brain damage or introduce infection.

VIII. Terminal Care of Equipment
   A. The catheter should be flushed with sterile water to remove secretions from the connecting tubing.
   B. Dispose of the catheter, glove, water, and container.
   C. Arrange the connecting tubing so that it will remain clean until the next time it is used.
   D. Replace used equipment so that it is available for the next suctioning procedure.

EXERCISES

1. Discuss the advantages and disadvantages of the use of low-pressure cuffs versus high-pressure cuffs on a tracheostomy tube.
2. Describe the complications of traumatic suctioning.
3. How does suctioning of a child differ from suctioning an adult?
4. Describe the difference between suctioning a patient with a tracheostomy tube and one with an endotracheal tube.
5. What are some of the complications of intubation?

PULMONARY FUNCTION TESTING

This unit is concerned with the general categories of pulmonary function tests and their clinical significance.

The major function of the lung is to maintain an adequate exchange of the respiratory gases, oxygen and carbon dioxide. To adequately perform this function a number of steps take place from the time air is breathed in to the time that oxygen is transferred to the blood and carbon dioxide to the alveolus. For the sake of clarification, pulmonary function testing has been divided into categories.

Before the categories of testing are enumerated, several salient features must be kept in mind. First, no pulmonary function test measures all facets of pulmonary function. Second, many tests measure the same thing, and hence, in many instances, there is some confusion as to the relative merits of each particular test. Third, it must be borne in mind with clarity that to adequately assess pulmonary function a battery of tests must be performed so that each step in the respiratory gas exchange pattern is carefully evaluated.

It has been conventional to divide pulmonary function tests into the following categories.

1. Volume evaluation
2. Ventilation evaluation
3. Distribution
4. Perfusion
5. Diffusion
6. Circulation
   a. The carrier for oxygen and carbon dioxide

b. The buffers of the blood for acid–base balance
c. The transport system, that is, heart and blood vessels

Volume (See Figure 10-1.)

The lung has been arbitrarily subdivided into four volumes:

1. *Tidal volume*—the volume of gas inspired and expired during each breathing effort.
2. *Inspiratory reserve volume*—the volume of air that can be inspired beyond the end of a normal inspiration.
3. *Expiratory reserve volume*—the volume of air that can be expired from the end of a normal expiration.
4. *Residual volume*—the volume of gas remaining in the lung at the end of a maximum expiratory effort.

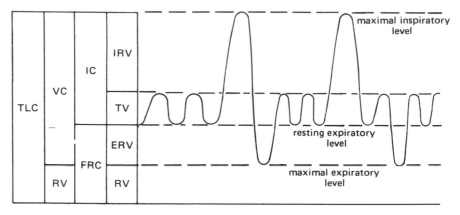

Figure 10-1.   Volumes and capacities of the lungs.

Capacities

A combination of two or more volumes can be referred to as a capacity.

1. *Inspiratory capacity*—the maximum amount of air that one can breathe in from a normal expiratory position.
2. *Vital capacity*—the maximum amount of air that can be breathed out after a maximum inspiration.
3. *Functional residual capacity*—the volume of gas remaining in the lungs at the end of a normal expiration.

4. *Total lung capacity*—the total amount of air in the lungs at the height of a maximum inspiration; this includes the forced vital capacity and residual volume.

By means of a number of devices, particularly a spirometer, the tidal volume, inspiratory and expiratory reserve volume, inspiratory capacity, and vital capacity can be measured directly. There are a number of indirect techniques for determining the remaining volumes and capacities. The most popular technique utilizes a trace gas such as helium and evaluates the degree of dilution of this helium from a known volume and concentration.

Abnormal changes in volumes and capacities are a very common manifestation of the majority of pulmonary diseases encountered clinically. For example, a low vital capacity is a common finding in diseases of the lung such as pneumonia, sarcoidosis, and fibrosis in which the air spaces of the lung have been decreased, thereby causing a decrease in the volume of air that the lung can hold. Likewise, in clinical conditions of incomplete airway obstruction there is a trapping of air in the lung; as a consequence, certain volumes may increase, particularly the residual volume. An increase in this volume is often seen in disease entities such as pulmonary emphysema and asthma.

Ventilation

The major function of the lung and breathing apparatus is to move air in and out of the alveolus so that there is an adequate exchange of oxygen and carbon dioxide. Hence, the process we call ventilation is referred to in terms of amount of air ventilated per unit of time (liters per minute). Unlike lung volumes, which are measured under static conditions, pulmonary ventilation implies a dynamic process going on minute to minute. Hence, when speaking of pulmonary ventilation we need to distinguish and to designate the particular circumstances. Usually testing situations are designated:

1. Resting
2. Standard exercise test
3. Maximum effort

Ventilation is concerned with the volume of air that is breathed in and out. We know that the functional unit of the lung is at the alveolar level, and, hence, air that remains in the air passageway itself does not actively enter into the gas exchange process. For this reason the volume of air moving in and out per breath, that is, the tidal volume, is subdivided into an alveolar portion and a dead-space portion. The alveolar portion is that volume of gas which enters into direct exchange at the alveolar capillary level, whereas the dead-space volume refers to that volume remaining either in the air passages themselves or in the alveoli that have been deprived of their blood supply. On this basis, dead space has been divided into anatomical dead space, which is the volume of air in the passageways, and physiological dead space, which is the volume of air in the passageways plus the volume of air in alveoli not adequately perfused.

To have an adequate exchange of air one has to look at the volume of air that is breathed in during each effort. The average size of airways in an adult is approximately 150 ml; a convenient rule of thumb to use is to estimate dead space at about 1 ml/lb of body weight. Hence, assuming a tidal volume of 500 ml in an average adult male weighing 150 lb, the dead space portion is 150/500 or 0.3 of total tidal volume, and the alveoli portion (which is 500 − 150) is 350/500 or 0.6 of the total tidal volume. In disease processes, these volumes change, and it is extremely important that the rate of breathing and, particularly, the depth of breathing and amount of tidal volume be carefully evaluated.

Techniques of Evaluating Alveolar and Dead-Space Ventilation

A meter such as a Drager Volumeter (Figure 10-2) or Wright Respirometer (Figure 10-3) can be used. In some instances a spirometer

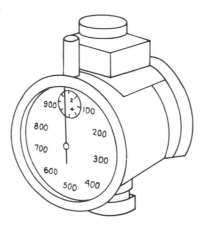

Figure 10-2. Drager Volumeter.

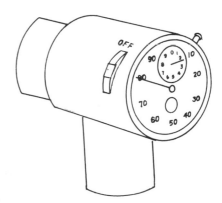

Figure 10-3. Wright Respirometer.

may be employed. An average tidal volume can be calculated by collecting the total volume for 1 min and dividing by the respiratory rate.

Clinical Significance

An individual in the process of breathing may ventilate normally and thereby maintain adequate exchange of the respiratory gases, oxygen and carbon dioxide. He can hypoventilate, in which instance the volume of air moving in and out of the lungs per minute is decreased, hence causing a decrease in gas exchange and resulting in a lowering of the oxygen tension and an increase in the carbon dioxide tension of the arterial blood. An individual may hyperventilate, in which instance the volume of air moving in and out of the lungs per minute is above normal. In this particular instance the major effect is seen on carbon dioxide; the carbon dioxide level is decreased. This may at times cause significant shifts in pH to the alkaline side. It also results in an increase in oxygen in the alveolus, but not to the same magnitude as the change in carbon dioxide.

In a number of disease entities, inadequate ventilation, particularly alveolar hypoventilation, is often seen. For example, this is true in the respiratory insufficiency seen in patients who have diffuse obstructive pulmonary emphysema. As a result of inadequate gas exchange, the oxygen level of the blood drops and the carbon dioxide level increases. As this increase continues, the carbon dioxide retention causes a drop in pH. With the pH change, respiratory acidosis develops.

The tidal volume dead-space ratio, V_D/V_T, has become a very useful indicator in making decisions regarding weaning of patients from ventilators in intensive care units. A V_D/V_T ratio of over 0.6 is usually indicative of continued need to support a patient's ventilations.

Spirometry

There are a number of techniques to perform spirometry. This evaluation continues to be the most commonly used technique in the appraisal of patients with pulmonary disease. There are essentially two broad categories of instrumentation. The first is mechanical; the Collins Respirometer and Vitalor (Figure 10-4) are examples of this category.

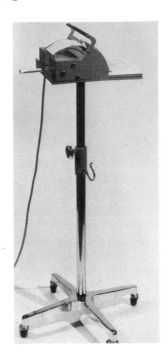

Figure 10-4. Vitalor. (*Courtesy of Air-Shields, Inc., Hatboro, Pa.*)

AIR-SHIELDS VITALOR

The Air–Shields Vitalor produces a permanent chart record of a patient's forced vital capacity, timed expiratory capacity (timed forced expiratory volume) and forced expiratory flow. This information is vital for comparison purposes or for evaluating the course of a disease and its response to therapy.

Operation

1. Place stylus in use position.
2. Release chart retainers and place Vitalor chart paper on chart carrier so that the two holes in the chart engage the two pins on the carrier. Refasten retainer to hold chart securely in place. *Note:* Be careful not to enlarge or tear pinholes on chart.
3. Gently lift the chart carrier (to avoid damaging gear) and slide

it to the starting position. Check to see that the thumb screw holding the stylus is tight, and that the stylus is on the base line.

4. Place a disposable cardboard mouthpiece over the chrome inlet to the bellows.

5. On the side of the Vitalor is a red pushbutton which controls the motor for driving the chart in conjunction with the automatic switch. The button must be pressed firmly and held during the entire test. The driver motor will start only when the patient exhales into the mouthpiece. The pushbutton may be pressed by the patient or by the operator or a remote starter switch (optional accessory) may be used by the operator. The unit can be changed to manual operation by adjusting the automatic switch so the motor will run continuously when using the pushbutton.

6. To make tracings, depress red start button. Instruct patient to take as deep a breath as possible, and hold it while placing mouth tightly around mouthpiece. Encourage the patient to blow as hard, fast and long as possible. Forceful, rapid exhalation is necessary to make the test meaningful. A nose clip may be used. *Note:* Red start button must be held down until maximum air is expired or until carrier stops automatically.

Calculation (Refer to Figure 10-5)

1. *FVC (Forced Vital Capacity)* This is calculated at the point where the curve reaches the highest level on the chart. In Figure 10-5 it would be 4.4 liters. Each heavy horizontal line represents one liter. Lines between are tenths of liters.

2. $FEV_{1.0}$ *(Forced Expiratory Volume)* This is the point where the curve intersects the one second line. In Figure 10-5 it would be 2.6 liters. Each heavy vertical line represents one second. Lines between are tenths of seconds.

3. *FEF (Forced Expiratory Flow)* This is found by placing a ruler so that it passes through the circled dot in the lower left hand corner of the chart, and extends to where the curve crosses the broken or dotted line at liters. A continuation of this line to the top of the chart will give FEF per minute. In Figure 10-5 it would be 360 liters.

The chart used with the Vitalor is pressure sensitive and does not require ink. A permanent record can be made by writing the pa-

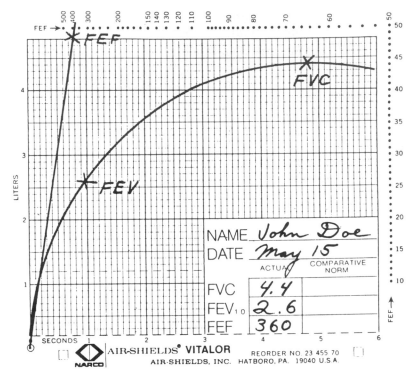

Figure 10-5. A typical Vitalor chart.

tient's name, date, and test results. Nomograms are provided with the Vitalor for comparison purposes.

COLLINS SPIROMETER

Equipment

A 13.5 liter Collins Chain Linked Water Sealed Spirometer with a 3-speed Kymograph (32, 160 and 1920 millimeters per minute) will be used in this procedure.

The patient should be connected to the spirometer by means of a disposable paper mouthpiece made from $1\frac{1}{4}''$ ID tubing or a large rubber mouthpiece connected to a free breathing bypass valve which is attached to the spirometer with two 34″ lengths of corrugated wire wound plastic tubing of $1\frac{1}{2}''$ ID with $1\frac{3}{8}''$ rubber ends. Lined chart paper is used for recording. *Important:* Be sure no unidirectional valves or CO_2 absorbers are present, as they will increase the resistance of the system.

Procedure: Before Testing Patient

1. Weekly calibration for FVC, should be done with a calibrated syringe with a volume of at least 3 liters.
2. Check spirometer bell for dents or any other observable problems.
3. Weight the spirometer to induce a positive pressure of several cms of water and monitor the bell position, looking for any leaks by recording the bell position with the pen for one minute.
4. Check speed of Kymograph drum, using a stopwatch.
5. Check to see that water is at proper level in the spirometer.
6. Inscribe first a vertical reference line on paper with Kymograph drum stationary. Second, inscribe horizontal lines by rotating the Kymograph drum, indicating the high and low points of the spirometer bell.
7. Record on paper:
   a. Date and time
   b. Patient's name, identification number and sex
   c. Patient's age in years
   d. Patient's height in cm
   e. Patient's weight in Kg
   f. Barometric pressure in mmHg
   g. Spirometer temperature in degrees Centigrade
   h. Patient's position during procedure (sitting, standing, etc.)

Procedure for Forced Expiratory Spirogram

1. Position the patient comfortably upright (except standing) for (MVV) Maximal Voluntary Ventilation.
2. Be sure all tight fitting clothing including undergarments are loosened.
3. Remove dentures if present.
4. Carefully explain the complete procedure before starting the test.
5. Place mouthpiece in the patient's mouth and check for possible leaks.
6. Place nose clips on the patient.
7. Vigorously encourage the patient to perform maximally.
8. Instruct the patient to breathe normally until a constant end-tidal point is reached for three consecutive breaths. (Kymograph speed at 32 mm/min.).

9. Instruct the patient to slowly but maximally exhale.
10. When the patient's expiration is maximal and RV (residual volume) has been reached, then instruct the patient to breath in as deeply as possible to TLC (total lung capacity.)
11. When the patient achieves full inspiration, change speed of drum to 32 mm/sec., when rapid rotation is observed.
    a. Order the patient to blow out all the air as fast as possible.
    b. Push the patient to keep exhaling, until the breath is completed as indicated by a constant level on the drum (Horizontal Line).
    c. In case the spirogram does not become horizontal, *do not terminate the study*, let the patient continue until he or she is able.
    d. At the point where expiration has been assessed to be complete, instruct the patient to maximally and rapidly inhale back to the point of maximal inspiration. Order the patient to breathe in.
12. When test is complete, have patient remove mouthpiece, remove nose clips, and have the patient relax; flush out the spirometer.
13. Repeat test until three good tracings are obtained.
14. Record assessment of patients' performances and cooperation.

Procedure for Maximum Voluntary Ventilation (MVV)

The Maximum Voluntary Ventilation procedure should be performed, when possible, with the patient in the standing position. Be sure to note the patient's respiratory rate on the recording. The procedure is performed by having the patient breathe the maximum amount of air for a time of at least 15 seconds. Ventilation in 12 seconds is calculated, corrected to body temperature and pressure saturated with water vapor, and multiplied by 5 to be expressed in liters BTPS per minute.

1. Instruct the patient to breathe normally until a constant end-tidal point is reached for three consecutive breaths.
2. Be sure to use both the intergrating pen and the direct recording pen.
3. Order the patient to breathe as deeply and rapidly as possible. Push the patient to maximal performance for 15 seconds.
4. Before repeating test, let the patient rest.

Calculations

FVC (Forced Vital Capacity)   Draw a tangent to the top of the expiratory curve, or the point where the full inhalation has stopped (A) and another tangent where the patient stopped exhaling and started to inhale more air (B). The difference between these two points is the FVC. The volume must be corrected by multiplying by 1.075 before reporting out. (See Figure 10-6.)

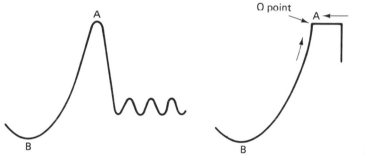

Figure 10-6.

FEV$_t$ (Forced Expiratory Volume)   Draw a line correlating with the steepest part of the FVC curve and intersect it with the tangent previously drawn for the top of the inhale. The point where this is made is the zero point. The exhale starts from point A; therefore, do the 1, 2, and 3 second time intervals. With the ruler, measure off one second from the zero point and mark it on the curve. Then, with the ruler at FEV$_1$, measure off another second (FEV$_2$) and finally another (FEV$_3$), in the same manner. Multiply all three by 1.075.

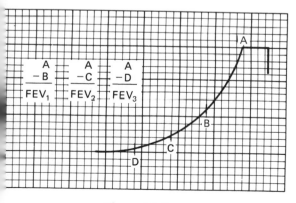

Figure 10-7.

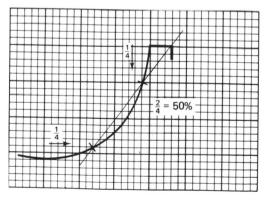

Figure 10-8.

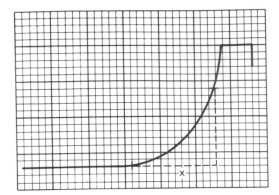

Figure 10-9.

MEFR 25-50% (Mid-Expiratory Flow Rate)   Divide the *uncorrected* FVC by four. Round off the answer to the nearest 25. (EX. 1263 to 1275). Subtract this number from the zero point and add it to the bottom of the curve. Draw a line through these two points and extend it to intersect a few time periods. Find where the extended line intersects the first time period after the FEV_1 marking. Subtract these two points and multiply the answer by 1.075.

MET (Mid-Expiratory Time)   Draw a vertical line down from the top quarter of the FEF and another horizontally from the bottom quarter (making a right triangle). Count the number of time divisions across the bottom. Correct the 12ths to 10ths of seconds by multiplying by .083.

MVV (Maximum Voluntary Ventilation)   Mark off where the tracing intersects a full-time period. Subtract the two points of intersection and multiply by 1.075. Then multiply by 5 (to correct 12 secs. to 1 min. 5 × 12 = 60 secs. = 1 min.) to bring the answer to liters/minute. Finally, multiply by 25, which is the pen factor. Count the

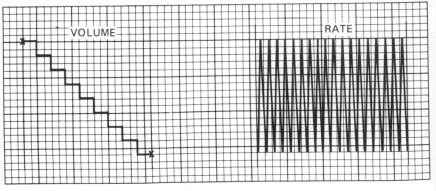

Figure 10-10.

number of respirations and multiply by 5. This will give you respirations per minute, or the rate.

Remember!

All volumes must be multiplied by the factor 1.075 before reporting out. The reason for this is that the patient is exhaling air at 37°C, while the volume is recorded on the spirometer at a usually lower temperature. The correction factor brings the volume back up to a 37°C reading.

LUNG VOLUMES USING THE SINGLE BREATH HELIUM DILUTION METHOD

Equipment

The Collins Helium Residual Volume and Single Breath Carbon Monoxide Diffusing Capacity Unit. (P-2100 W. E. Collins or equivalent apparatus)

Procedure for Patient Use

Calibration and procedure is identical to that described for carbon monoxide diffusing capacity single breath. It is important that you measure the vital capacity from the beginning of inspiration to the highest point of the spirometric tracing, and not the point at which the patient levels off, as some air may leak out of the patient's lungs.

Calculations

$$\text{TLCsb} = \text{FIVC ATPD} \times \frac{F_I He}{F_E He} \times (\text{ATPD to BTPS factor})$$

$$\text{TLCsb} = \text{Single Breath Helium Total Lung Capacity}$$

$$\text{FIVC} = \text{Forced Inspiratory Vital Capacity}$$

$$F_E He \text{ and } F_I He = \text{Expired and Inspired Helium Fractions}$$

Other Evaluation Methods

The second group has electronic components that are capable of translating the mechanical data into electronic signals to facilitate

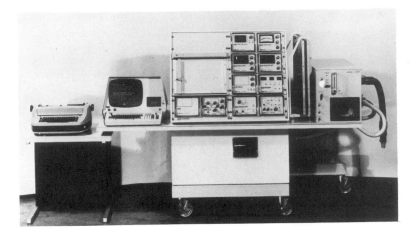

Figure 10-11. Med-Science Pulmonizer. (*Courtesy of Med-Science Electronics, Inc., Uxbridge, Mass.*)

recording and analysis. A number of instruments are available for this purpose.

In recent years instrumentation has been programmed that has greatly facilitated the technique of spirometry. It is possible to obtain an analysis of the patient's effort as related to the normal effort, including an interpretation of the study. Programmed spirometry with computer analysis opens up a number of possibilities for use, such as in screening programs and preoperative evaluation. With increased use of these tests, abnormalities of pulmonary function can be detected earlier and, in many instances, disease progression can be altered sooner. Increased alertness as to expectation of complications will improve our preoperative evaluation and postoperative care of surgical patients. (See Figure 10-11.) The utilization of computerized spirometry has made it possible for all hospitals, particularly smaller ones, to offer this service to the physicians and patients.

Mechanics

In the evaluation of the mechanics of lung function, the three variables considered are pressure, volume, and flow. The lungs are considered an elastic system, and the amount of pressure needed to change the volume of the lung by a certain amount can differ significantly in various disease states. This evaluation is referred to as compliance.

$$\text{Compliance} = \frac{\text{change in volume}}{\text{change in pressure}}$$

Compliance is usually expressed in volume per one centimeter of water of pressure change. The normal compliance of the lung is 200 ml or 0.2 liters.

When the texture of the lung changes, as in pulmonary fibrosis or edema, the lungs become stiffer and the pressure required to change the volume of the lung increases. In these situations the compliance is said to decrease.

In addition to pressure and volume, one has to consider airflow. The higher the airflow, the greater the pressure needed to create the flow. The airflow is also related to the diameter of the airway. The smaller the diameter, the greater the pressure needed to maintain the same flow. As a consequence, in many disease states such as asthma (bronchospasm), there is a decrease in flow of air in those airways with smaller diameters, while other airways with larger diameters are less affected. As a consequence, uneven distribution of ventilation is exaggerated. Likewise, as the resistance to airflow increases, the work of breathing increases in order to maintain adequate ventilation. In those disease states where this increase in work cannot be attained, respiratory insufficiency develops.

Spirometry is a very useful pulmonary function testing technique because it enables one to measure both volume and airflow. On the basis of spirometry, one can refer to pulmonary function as

1. Normal
2. Obstructive—there are normal volumes but a decreased airflow (e.g., bronchial asthma).
3. Restrictive—there are normal flows but decreased volumes (e.g., pulmonary fibrosis).
4. Combined—impairment of both volume and flow exists.

The utilization of spirometry in assessing lung function has become the standard yardstick for evaluation. One of the most common techniques employed is to record a spirogram on a patient, and then administer a bronchodilator aerosol and repeat the spirometry. In this way one can evaluate the degree of bronchospasm and its reversibility. An improvement in airflow of over 20% is considered significant.

More sophisticated assessment of mechanics has become part of evaluation in some laboratories. Pressure—volume curves, flow resistance, and frequency dependence compliance all add more understanding to assessing lung impairment; however, these are usually not employed routinely in day-to-day assessment. This technique assesses the volume level of thc lung at which the smaller airways close to airflow. It affords a technique of separating out and evaluating the smaller airways in the lung. Further clarification of this technique is needed, however, before it can become part of our standard or routine evaluation, since some controversy exists as to exactly what is being measured.

Flow-Volume Loops

In recent years the flow-volume curve has become a popular technique for assessment of volume and flow. Expired airflow is plotted against expired volume. Airflow on expiration increases rapidly to a peak and then decreases progressively as the lung volume decreases. A flow-volume loop is inscribed, which allows one to characterize the impairment to volume and/or flow. This maneuver allows one to obtain a clearer definition of smaller airway function, as well as assessment of the characteristics of the larger airways and volume. It is considered by most physiologists to be a more sensitive evaluation than standard spirometry.

Distribution

The next facet of pulmonary function centers around the evaluation of the distribution of air once it is inhaled. Ordinarily, in the normal individual, air is fairly evenly distributed to the millions of alveoli so that adequate gas exchange with the capillaries can take place. The imbalance between ventilation and perfusion at the capillary level is kept to a minimum. As a disease develops, this imbalance between ventilation and perfusion is exaggerated. In many clinical instances a serious decrease in oxygenation in the blood results.

The physician is clinically aware of this uneven distribution of ventilation when he listens to the chest with a stethoscope. Unfortunately, this is a very gross evaluation. By means of pulmonary function testing one can refine this to pick up manifestations of this abnormality earlier. Several tests are popular. The first is the nitrogen washout technique. In this test the rate of washout of nitrogen is measured as an individual is breathing 100% oxygen. The other popular technique is the utilization of a radioactive gas such as radioactive xenon. A study of the ventilatory pattern employing radioactive xenon can be compared with a technitium perfusion scan to help distinguish defects due to pulmonary emboli from defects caused by obstructive airway disease.

These tests to evaluate the imbalance between ventilation and blood flow are among the most significant measurements that one can make clinically to get a better understanding of the pathophysiology involved in any disease process. This imbalance between ventilation and blood flow is the most common cause of cyanosis in adults. As newer techniques are developed and simplified, this facet of pulmonary function testing will become more and more popular at the clinical level.

Diffusing Capacity

The next facet of pulmonary function is the evaluation of the rate of transfer of oxygen across the alveolar capillary membrane. Impairment of diffusion is present in a variety of disease entities. In the clinical pulmonary function laboratory, the usual test done is that of diffusing capacity. There are a number of variations on how the test is done, ranging from utilizing a single-breath technique to a rebreathing or steady-state technique. Each particular technique has its shortcomings; usually one particular technique is developed in a laboratory and refined to obtain reliable results.

The diffusing capacity utilizes a gas such as carbon monoxide, which has a high affinity for hemoglobin and lends itself very readily to evaluating the rate of exchange of oxygen. The concentration of carbon monoxide used is very low and is not toxic to the patient. It must be kept in mind that the evaluation of diffusing capacity is not a measurement of diffusion alone; it is also dependent on a number of other factors such as the pressure differences of the gas from the alveolus to the capillary and, particularly, the surface area for gas exchange. In the normal adult, the average surface area for gas exchange is about 70 m^2. In disease entities this surface area is significantly decreased. For example, in patients who have diffuse obstructive pulmonary emphysema, there is a tearing of interalveolar septae with a loss of surface area. As a consequence, patients with emphysema have an impaired diffusing capacity. Likewise, in other disease entities such as pulmonary fibrosis, there is a loss of surface area in addition to an interference with the integrity of the exchange membrane itself. Here, too, there is a drop in diffusing capacity. Hence, the measurement of diffusing capacity gives one an idea more of the pathophysiological process involved rather than differentiating a specific disease entity.

However, in certain specific circumstances the evaluation of diffusing capacity can be quite helpful in diagnosis. For example, we are able to separate reversible incomplete airway obstruction, such as bronchial asthma, from irreversible incomplete airway obstruction, such as pulmonary emphysema. In the former, the diffusing capacity would be within normal limits, whereas in the emphysematous patient the diffusing capacity would be impaired.

SINGLE BREATH CARBON MONOXIDE DIFFUSING CAPACITY

The most common gas utilized for determination of diffusing capacity is carbon monoxide, which is inhaled in very low concentration (0.3%). The ability for carbon monoxide to move from the alveolus to the capillary is diminished in patients with interstitial lung disease.

The patient inspires his vital capacity from a gas mixture containing CO, He, N_2 and O_2, holds his breath for 10 seconds and exhales into a collection bag. From the changes in gas concentrations between inspired and expired gas and the associated spirometric tracing, the D_{CO_2} and He dilution lung volumes may be calculated.

Equipment

1. Test gas containing approximately 0.3% CO, 10% He and O_2 in a concentration which will produce a PI_{O_2} of about 150 mmHg, with an average barometric pressure of 640 mmHg, 25% is required. The balance of the mixture is N_2.
2. A Box Balloon Respirometer (W. E. Collins, # P-2100)
3. Infrared CO Analyzer (0.3% CO Fullscale)
4. Linear He Analyzer (15% He Fullscale)
5. 5-Way Modular Valve (W. E. Collins, P-314)
6. T-shape Stopcock (W. E. Collins, P-321)
7. 1-Way Valve (W. E. Collins, P-315)
8. Rudolph Pulmonary Valve (non-rebreathing, Han Rudolph Model # 1400)
9. Stopwatch

Assembly

1. The spirometer should be connected to the air surrounding the latex bag in the Box Balloon with a flexible wire-wound plastic tube. The 5-way valve is connected to the latex balloon within a box. A 1-way valve permitting flow of gas out of the balloon should be inserted in the tubing as near as possible to its connection to the 5-way valve.

2. *Flush* port should be connected with a short piece of rubber tubing to a large T-shaped stopcock positioned in such a way that when the stopcock is turned to its right-angle connection, the *flush* opening of the 5-way valve is occluded.

3. Seal the gas sampling port of the stopcock to prevent a leak. The stopcock's straight-through fitting is linked by plastic tubing to the air within the box.

4. The *Room air* opening is connected by the shortest possible length of rubber tubing to the patient port of the Rudolph Valve.

5. The Flexible wire-wound plastic tubing joins the right-angle limb of the T-shape stopcock to the inlet of the Rudolph Valve.

6. The Rudolph Valve outlet is connected with plastic tubing to the spirometer.

7. A two-liter rubber bag which can be fully evacuated and sealed with a clamp is used to connect either to the mouth fitting of the 5-way valve or its *Alv-sample* port.

8. Test for leaks
   a. Lift the spirometer bell with the 5-way valve in the *Room air* position and the T-shape stopcock in right angle connection.
   b. Place a stopper at the mouth fitting of the 5-way valve.
   c. Weight the spirometer bell.
   d. Turn spirometer drum to low speed, monitor the volume of the system for five minutes.
   e. There should be no change in volume.

9. Gas measuring circuit
   a. A CO_2 absorber, H_2O absorber, CO analyzer and He meter.
   b. Place the water absorber between the CO_2 absorber and the CO analyzer.
   c. Gas to be analyzed should be pushed into the sample circuit and must not be aspirated through it by a pump or other means.

10. Test sample circuit for leaks
    a. Obstruct the outlet from the He meter sample cell.
    b. Attach a water manometer to the circuit inlet with a stopcock so that the system may be pressurized to about $5\,cmH_2O$ with a syringe of air.
    c. Observe pressure after 5 minutes.
    d. There should be no change in pressure.

Procedure For Patient Testing

1. Inspect CO_2 and H_2O absorbers to be sure they are no more than half exhausted. Change if needed.

2. Flush circuit with air and zero meter.

3. Test sample of pure gas and adjust the gain of the CO analyzer so that the CO concentration from the cylinder analysis corresponds to the appropriate meter reading taken from the calibration curve.

4. Flush analyzer with air and verify their zeroes.

5. Fill the reservoir balloon with test gas by turning the T-shape stopcock to its horizontal position.

6. Flush the air in the system's rebreathing circuit thoroughly by lifting and depressing the spirometer bell as far as it will travel several times.

7. Lift the spirometer bell, turn the stopcock to its vertical position and raise the pressure of the gas in the balloon above atmospheric by depressing the spirometer bell slightly.

8. Observe the spirometer pen, turn the 5-way valve to *Insp. hold*, and express about two liters of gas from the balloon, then quickly turn the 5-way valve back to the *Room air* position.

9. Connect the evacuated, clamped alveolar sample bag to the mouthpiece fitting of the 5-way valve. Depress the spirometer bell as before, turn the valve to *Insp. hold*. At the same time, open the clamp to the sample bag, and fill the bag with inspired gas mixture from the reservoir bag. Clamp the sample bag and return the 5-way valve to its *Room air* position. Analyze the contents of the sample bag and record data.

10. Attach rubber mouthpiece to the 5-way valve.

11. Inform the patient of the various maneuvers during the test.

12. With T-shape stopcock horizontal, position the recording pen about one-third from the bottom of the chart paper.

13. Attach nose clips to patient and have him breathe normally through mouthpiece. Set the spirometer at 32mm/minute, record enough normal breaths to obtain a stable level FRC.

14. Instruct the patient to exhale slowly and completely. When he reaches his residual volume, having smoothly expired until he can displace no more air, switch the Kymograph to 1920mm/min. (32mm/sec.), then turn the 5-way valve to *Insp. hold* and command the patient to inspire as rapidly as possible until his lungs are completely filled.

15. Start stopwatch at the beginning of the inspiration. When the subject reaches TLC, tell him to hold his breath, turn the 5-way valve to the *flush* position.

16. After eight seconds, remind the patient to hold his breath and turn stopcock to its vertical, straight-through position.

17. After nine seconds, instruct the patient to expire rapidly as much as he can. After 750 cc have been exhaled, turn the 5-way valve to the *Alv-sample* position, collect at least 500 cc of gas, then quickly turn the valve to the *Room air* position. Stop the drum and have the patient remove his mouth from the unit so that he may breathe normally.

18. Clamp and remove the alveolar sample balloon and analyzer and record its contents. Evacuate and replace the sample bag.

19. Flush the analyzer circuit with air and verify the meter zeroes. Flush the breathing circuit thoroughly. Wait at least three minutes from the start of the last test before beginning another, to ensure that all He and CO will be washed from the patient's lungs. Repeat the test three times.

Calculation

Example of a single breath D_{CO} and He dilution lung volumes with calculations.

1. Inspired He concentration from analysis of gas in Reservoir Balloon

$$HeI = 10.00\%$$

2. Expired He concentration from analysis of Alveolar Sample

$$HeE = 7.00\%$$

3. Ratio of expired to inspired He concentration $\dfrac{HeE}{HeI} = 0.70$

4. Inspired CO concentration from analysis of gas in Reservoir Balloon

$$CO_I = 0.300\%$$

5. Expired CO concentration from analysis of alveolar sample

$$CO_E = 0.097\%$$

6. Initial alveolar CO concentration $CO_{AO} = CO_I \times \dfrac{HeE}{HeI}$

$$= 0.300\% \times 0.70$$

$$CO_{AO} = 0.210\%$$

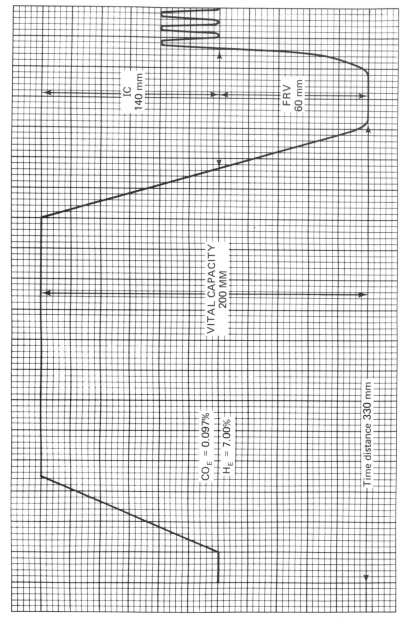

Figure 10-12. Tracing of D_{CO}.

476

7. Ratio of initial to final alveolar CO concentration

$$\frac{CO_{AO} = 0.210\%}{CO_E \ = 0.097\%} \qquad \frac{CO_{AO}}{CO_E} = 2.165$$

8. Natural logarithm of $\dfrac{CO_{AO}}{CO_E}$ $\qquad \ln\left(\dfrac{CO_{AO}}{CO_E}\right) = .7724$

9. Vital Capacity at ATPD

$$VC\ (ATPD) = 200mm\ \text{chart displacement} \times \frac{20.73\ ml}{mm}$$

$$VC\ (ATPD) = 4146\ ml$$

10. Vital Capacity at STPD

$$VC\ (STPD) = VC\ (ATPD) \times \frac{P_B\ mmHg}{760\ mmHg} \times \frac{273°C}{273°C + T°C}$$

$$= VC\ (ATPD) \times .0783$$
$$\text{(from above or ATPD-STPD Table)}$$
$$VC\ (STPD) = 3246\ ml$$

11. Alveolar volume (TLC at STPD)

$$V_A = \frac{VC\ (STPD)}{HeE/HeI} = \frac{3246\ ml}{0.70} \qquad VA\ (STPD) = 4637\ ml$$

12. Time from start to inspiration to beginning of alveolar sample collection

$$T = 330\ mm\ \text{chart displacement} \times \frac{1\ sec.}{32\ mm} = T = 10.31\ sec.$$

13. D_{CO}

$$D_{CO} = \frac{60\ sec./min. \times VA\ (ml)}{(P_B - 47)\ mmHg \times T\ (sec.)} \times \ln \frac{CO_{AO}}{CO_E}$$

$$\frac{60\ sec./min. \times 4637\ ml}{600\ mmHg \times 10.31\ sec.} \times .7724 = D_{CO} = 34.7\ ml/min/mmHg$$

14. D_L/V_A

$$V_A \ (L) = \frac{V_A \ (mlSTPD)}{1000 \ ml/L} = \frac{4635}{1000 \ ml/L} = 4.64 \ L \ (STPD)$$

$$\frac{D_L}{V_A} = \frac{34.7 \ ml/min/mmHg}{4.64 \ L(STPD)}$$

$D_L/V_A = 7.5 \ ml/min/mmHg/L(STPD)$

15. Corrected $D_{CO} \ \dfrac{measured \ D_{CO}}{0.06965 \times Hb}$

16. Helium dilution lung volumes multiplier for chart displacement in mm to L (BTPS)

$$\frac{20.73 \ ml}{mm} \times \frac{L}{1000 \ ml} \times \frac{P_B}{P_B - 47.0} \times \frac{310.0}{273.0 + T}$$

$$\frac{20.73 \ ml}{mm} \times \frac{L}{1000 \ ml} \times 1.126 = 0.02334 \ L \ (BTPS)/mm$$

(from above or ATPD—BTPS Table)

17.

VC

VC = 200 mm chart displacement
    × factor from P 0.02334 L (BTPS) mm   VC (BTPS) = 4.67L

18.

ERV

ERV = 60 mm chart displacement
    × factor from P 0.02334 L (BTPS)/mm   ERV (BTPS) = 1.40 L

19. TLC

$$TLC = \frac{VC \ (BTPS)}{HeE/HeI} = \frac{4.676}{0.70} \qquad TLC \ (BTPS) \quad 6.67 \ L$$

20. RV   RV (BTPS) = TLC (BTPS) − VC (BTPS)

    RV 6.67 L − 4.67 L   RV (BTPS) = 2.00 L

21. FRC

FRC (BTPS) = ERV (BTPS) + RV (BTPS)

$$= 1.40 \text{ L} - 2.00 \text{ L} \qquad \text{FRC (BTPS)} = 3.40 \text{ L}$$

22. IC

IC (BTPS) = VC (BTPS) − ERV (BTPS)

$$= 4.67 \text{ L} - 1.40 \text{ L} \qquad \text{IC (BTPS)} = 3.27 \text{ L}$$

Perfusion

The next facet of pulmonary function centers around the evaluation of perfusion of the lung. Perfusion of the lung can be estimated in a variety of ways. First, one can evaluate cardiac output. However, in this particular instance one has to assume that the shunting of blood through the lung is at a minimum. Perfusion of the lung can be evaluated by the use of radioactive material, such as in a lung scan. In this technique, macroaggregates of albumin tagged with radioactive technitium are employed to outline the flow characteristics through the lung; this material is injected intravenously and counts are taken usually with a gamma camera.

This technique has been of great practical value in diagnosing pulmonary emboli and has led to a better understanding of this disease process. One can also get an idea of the perfusion of the lung by an evaluation of some of the larger vessels with the use of contrast material by angiography.

Circulation

The evaluation of circulation centers around three facets. First is the carrier for oxygen and carbon dioxide. The major carrier of oxygen in the arterial blood is hemoglobin. Hence, the two most important measurements are the measurement of the amount of hemoglobin and the evaluation of the integrity of hemoglobin, in other words, making sure that the hemoglobin present has not been changed chemically to such a state that it is incapable of carrying oxygen. One gram of hemoglobin fully saturated is capable of carrying 1.34 ml of oxygen. If the normal hemoglobin concentration is 15 g%, this means that 15×1.34 ml or 20.1 ml of oxygen will be present in each 100 cm^3 of blood when fully saturated. In addition, a certain amount of oxygen is carried physically dissolved, and this is related to the pressure of oxygen in the blood. In the normal individual breathing room air, this amounts to about. 0.3 ml of oxygen/100 cm³ of blood (see Figure 10-13.) Clinically, the commonly used relationship is the expression of the saturation of hemoglobin with oxygen, as related to the pressure of oxygen in the blood, the *oxygen dissociation curve*.

A decrease in the oxygen of the arterial blood is referred to as hypoxemia. Essentially, four mechanisms cause hypoexmia:

1. Alveolar hypoventilaton—in this particular instance there is underventilation of the alveolus, with an increase in carbon dioxide level of blood and a decrease in the oxygen tension.
2. Uneven ventilation in relation to blood flow—this is the ventilation–perfusion ratio. In instances where this distribution of ventilation to perfusion is mismatched, there is a significant drop in oxygen tension.
3. Impairment of diffusion.
4. Venous to arterial shunts.

Normally, air contains 0.04% carbon dioxide. For practical purposes in the clinical laboratory, we can make the assumption

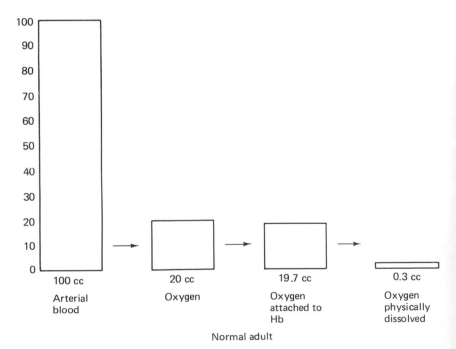

Figure 10-13.

that carbon dioxide is absent from inspired air. The loading, unloading, and transport of carbon dioxide by the blood is one of the most important functions in maintaining the pH, or hydrogen ion concentration, within normal limits. Carbon dioxide is carried in the blood in a variety of ways:

1. Physically dissolved in the plasma.
2. Chemically combined with an amine group of the hemoglobin.
3. A small amount of carbon dioxide dissolved in the red blood cell itself.
4. The carriage of carbon dioxide by means of bicarbonate.

The bicarbonate results from the combination of carbon dioxide and water to form carbonic acid with its subsequent dissociation into the hydrogen ion and bicarbonate ion. This particular reaction is enhanced by the presence of an enzyme, carbonic anhydrase, which is present in high concentration in the red blood cell. The amount of carbon dioxide carried in the blood is related to the partial pressure of carbon dioxide.

The only way carbon dioxide accumulates in the blood is when there is a decrease of air exchange or hypoventilation at the alveolar level. Ventilation is the only means that we have for ridding the body of carbon dioxide.

pH is an expression of the concentration of the hydrogen ion in the blood. This is a measure of the acidity or alkalinity of the blood. Normally, the pH of the blood is 7.40, and in most clinical laboratories the range for the normal is between 7.35 and 7.44. In instances of pulmonary disease due to hypoventilation, there is an accumulation of carbon dioxide in the blood. The overloading of the buffer system could eventually result in an excess of hydrogen-ion concentration and a drop in the pH to below the normal level. This retention of carbon dioxide accompanied by a drop in the pH below the normal level is referred to as respiratory acidosis. Some patients with pulmonary disease will hyperventilate and blow off too much carbon dioxide. This will result in a shift of the pH to above the normal level or into the alkaline range. This particular set of circumstances is referred to as respiratory alkalosis.

The evaluation of the oxygen tension, carbon dioxide tension, and pH of the blood has been facilitated greatly by the introduction of electrodes. By means of polarographic electrodes one can measure the oxygen tension, carbon dioxide tension, and pH of the blood very easily. These measurements have become extremely important in the evaluation and treatment of patients with respiratory problems, particularly in respiratory failure. Blood gas determinations are a necessity to adequate interpretation of acid–base balance. They are an integral part of the management of patients on ventilators.

Acid–Base Balance

A number of relationships exist among hydrogen-ion concentration, buffering ability, and oxygen-carrying capacity of the blood. A change in one variable is reflected in the other values. For example, an increase in pH (drop in H-ion concentration) will shift the O_2 dissociation curve to the left, thereby making it more difficult for hemoglobin to unload oxygen at the tissue level. (See Figures 10-14 and 10-15.)

Comprehension of acid–base balance demands an understanding of the electrolytes of the blood, particularly the common ones routinely measured in the clinical laboratory. Of the cations (positively charged ions), sodium and potassium are the most important. The anions (negatively charged ions) chloride and bicarbonate (Cl^- and HCO_3^-) are the most significant. Average cation values in the

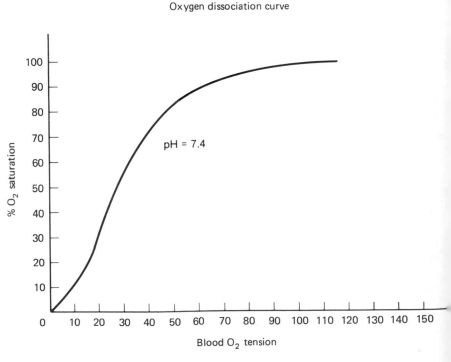

Oxygen dissociation curve

Figure 10-14.

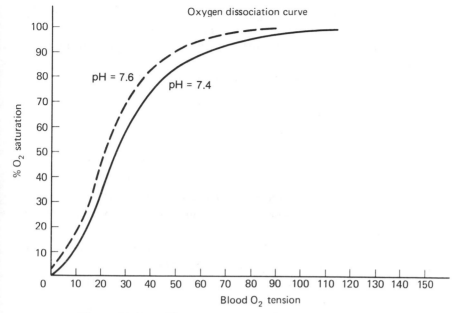

Figure 10-15.   Change in oxygen dissociation curve.

normal adult are Na^+, 140 meq/liter and K^+, 4.0 meq/liter. The relationship between the partial pressure of CO_2 and bicarbonate is the single most important determinant of the pH. The ratio of base to acid is important:

$$pH - pka + log \frac{base}{acid}$$

In pulmonary physiology, it is the ratio of bicarbonate to carbonic acid that is evaluated. In practical terms, in the approximation of these values assessed in the clinical laboratory, it is the bicarbonate to PCO_2 ratio that is evaluated.

A number of nomograms are available to plot the position or status of the patient. In the near future it is hoped that by repeated analyses and computer plottings, one can both follow the course of the patient and have the directions available to correct the acid–base imbalance in the patient being followed.

Summary

The clinical evaluation of pulmonary function by means of pulmonary function testing is an important aspect of care of patients. The sensitivity of pulmonary function tests available today enables one to assess degrees of impairment before they become manifest clinically. Pulmonary function assessment gives us a better understanding of how a disease affects the normal functioning of the cardiopulmonary system.

The relative merits of pulmonary function tests can be summarized as follows:

1. They can give us objective evidence on whether or not impairment itself exists.
2. This degree of impairment can be evaluated and quantitated.
3. By means of pulmonary function testing at intervals, the rate of progression of a disease process can be determined.
4. Likewise, the efficiency of treatment over a period of time can be evaluated.
5. The performance of pulmonary function tests can give us a better understanding of the pathophysiological mechanisms involved in the disease process, and can help us arrive at a specific diagnosis.

EXERCISES

1. What pulmonary function studies would be used to determine chronic obstructive lung disease? Restrictive disease?
2. What change in the residual volume is found in a patient with chronic obstructive lung disease, and why?'
3. Compare the information given by electronic spirometers, the Collins spirometer, and Vitalor.
4. What is meant by the term *compliance* of lung?
5. Do you feel that mass screening of all patients coming into the hospital is vital for early detection of respiratory disease? Explain.

UNIT 11

ARTERIAL PUNCTURES

Because the level of oxygen in venous blood varies so widely, arterial blood samples are felt by most practitioners to be the only accurate method of determining lung function. Although there are several problems associated with the obtaining of an arterial sample, these may be minimized by proper training of the individual therapist involved and by the use of techniques designed to minimize risk to the patient.

As with any procedure, the therapist must be supervised by someone proficient in the skill until such time as the instructor feels that the therapist is competent to perform.

I. Choice of Site: Adult
   A. The *radial artery* is the site most commonly used for an arterial puncture in the adult. Although the artery itself is small, it is easily accessible in most individuals, since there are relatively few anatomic structures to obscure the vessel. Hemostasis is facilitated because the artery may be compressed over the firm structures in the wrist. The ulnar artery generally provides collateral circulation to the hand so that, should thrombosis occur in the radial artery, the blood supply will be maintained. However, to ensure that the ulnar blood flow is adequate, an *Allen test* should always be performed prior to the puncture. This test will be described in detail later in this discussion.
   B. Until a few years ago, the *brachial artery* was the most widely used site for an arterial puncture. The fact that it is

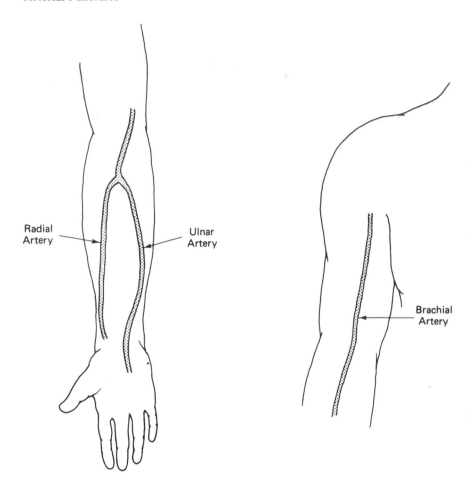

Figure 11-1.   *Left:* Location of Radial and Ulnar Arteries in Forearm.

Figure 11-2.   *Right:* Location of Brachial Artery in Upper Arm.

large in size is negated by its position deep between muscles and connective tissue, making it more difficult to palpate, particularly in the obese patient, and more prone to hematoma formation due to difficulty in compressing it adequately after the puncture. Collateral circulation is usually adequate when a single arterial puncture is performed. However, an arterial line (a cannula placed in the artery for obtaining multiple samples) may present a problem due to thromboembolism, as it does in any artery.

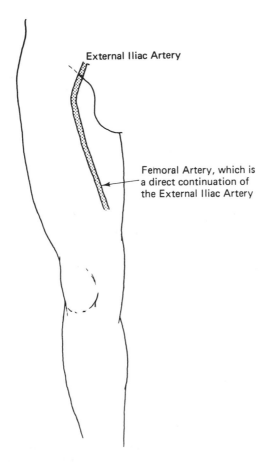

External Iliac Artery

Femoral Artery, which is
a direct continuation of
the External Iliac Artery

Figure 11-3. Location of Femoral Artery in Upper Thigh.

C. The *femoral artery*, because of its large size and easy access, would appear to some to be the site of choice for an
arterial puncture. However, most practitioners feel that the
disadvantages far outweigh these factors. Because it is
difficult to compress, significant hematomas can result.
Danger of infection at the site is more prevalent because
the area cannot be cleansed as effectively as the relatively
hairless arm. Particularly in the elderly, whose collateral
circulation to the lower extremities may already be impaired by atherosclerosis, this choice of site may lead to
further circulatory difficulties. Many feel that the femoral
artery should only be used when a sample cannot be obtained from the radial or brachial arteries.

II. Equipment
  A. Five-milliliter syringe—there is some controversy as to whether a glass syringe is preferable to a plastic syringe. Unless the PaO_2 is above 100 mm Hg, the fact that some plastics absorb oxygen is not significant, as in most instances the amount lost is so small that changes in PaO_2 are not vital. However, at PaO_2's above 100 mm Hg, this loss may be important.

  The fact that the plungers of some plastic syringes do not move freely enough to allow for filling of the syringe by arterial pressure has been the greatest reason expressed for not using them. If one must apply suction (by pulling back on the plunger), the incidence of air bubbles, and thus changes in PaO_2, is greatly increased. However, air bubbles introduced in this manner, if removed *immediately*, will not significantly change the PaO_2.

  Since there are many plastic syringes on the market, each institution must evaluate several to determine those that meet their individual requirements.
  B. Needle—no. 20 or no. 22 gauge, $\frac{5}{8}$ in.; usually a no. 25 needle is too small to allow blood to flow freely without use of suction; however, used skillfully, this small needle may prove less traumatic to the patient.
  C. Sodium heparin 1:1000, approximately 0.5 ml, to prevent coagulation of the blood and to fill the dead space of the needle and syringe. Most of the heparin will be expelled before the blood sample is drawn. Studies have shown that dilution of the blood sample by sodium heparin significantly reduces the measured $PaCO_2$ and the calculated bicarbonate and base excess in direct proportion to the amount of the dilution. This can lead to misinterpretation of the patient's acid—base status. For this reason, some practitioners recommend the use of a small-gauge needle (to reduce dead space) and filling of the syringe to its maximum (to reduce dilution).
  D. Antiseptic solution for skin cleansing.
  E. Cap to seal syringe after sample is drawn.
  F. Sterile gauze pads.
  G. Plastic syringe (1 to 2 ml) for local anesthetic if used; this may not be necessary if the person drawing the sample is skilled and the patient is psychologically prepared.
  H. Number 25 needle.
  I. One percent lidocaine or similar anesthetic.

J. Container for ice water, large enough to immerse the syringe; a zip-lock bag is very convenient for this.

K. Label and request slip.

III. Procedure

The following procedure relates to a single arterial puncture only, since the insertion of a cannula for multiple samples is usually the responsibility of a physician. The description includes the administration of a local anesthetic; however, in some institutions such a procedure may not be the responsibility of the therapist.

A. Preparation of the patient—a relaxed, comfortable patient is essential to the accomplishment of an arterial puncture. The procedure should be explained to him, and he must be allowed to ask questions and/or express anxieties. He must be reassured before, during, and after the procedure. This is especially important if he has endured previous traumatic punctures.

B. Allen test

If the radial artery is to be used as a puncture site, an *Allen test* should be administered before the infiltration of the area by local anesthesia. Then, if collateral circulation proves inadequate, you have not subjected the patient to unnecessary needle punctures.

1. Have the patient form his hand into a tight fist.

2. Apply pressure to the wrist, using two or three fingers; both the radial and ulnar blood flow should be obstructed.

3. Have the patient relax his hand slightly, so that the palm and fingers may be observed. Because of lack of blood flow, both will be blanched.

4. Remove the pressure that is compressing the ulnar artery (on the small-finger side of the wrist). Within 15 sec, the palm and the fingers should again become flushed as blood returns to the capillary bed via the ulnar artery.

5. Should the blood flow be inadequate to return the patient's color to its previous state, *do not* use the radial artery as a puncture site.

C. Administration of local anesthesia

1. Wash hands thoroughly.

2. Attach the no. 25 needle to the 1- or 2-ml syringe.

3. Swab the top of the lidocaine vial with antiseptic.

4. Draw up 1 ml of lidocaine.

5. Select the puncture site to be used. Swab the area well with antiseptic.

6. The skin overlying the puncture site and the tissue surrounding the artery should be infiltrated with a small amount of the anesthetic. Always pull back slightly on the plunger before inserting the anesthetic; a return of blood would indicate that the needle is in a blood vessel rather than tissue.

7. A period of only a few minutes is necessary for the anesthesia to take effect. During this period you may prick the area with a sterile needle to assure the patient that the anesthetic is working. This will help alleviate the common problems of hyperventilation, breath holding, and excessive movement, all of which will affect the blood gas results or ease of obtaining the sample.

D. Preparation of blood gas syringe

1. Wash hands thoroughly.

2. Swab the top of the heparin vial with antiseptic.

3. Withdraw 0.5 ml of heparin using the syringe intended for the blood sample. A different needle may be used for insertion into the vial if there is the possibility of the outside of the needle becoming contaminated with heparin or plugging of the needle with particles from the stopper.

4. Thoroughly wet the inside of the syringe with the heparin by moving the plunger slowly back and forth.

5. With the needle in an upright position, expel any air in the syringe.

6. Holding the syringe with the needle downward, expel some heparin, making certain that no air bubbles remain. Some heparin will remain in the needle and its hub, eliminating air in the dead space.

E. Preparation of label and laboratory slip

1. Stamp the label and laboratory slip with the patient's identification card so that all information is legible.

2. The following information should be monitored and recorded on the slip, so that accurate interpretation of the results is possible:

a. FIO_2 patient is breathing (not just what is ordered; this may vary!). If FIO_2 has been changed recently, a period of 20 min should elapse before the blood gas is drawn.

b. Method of oxygen administration—ventimask, cannula, or ventilator, and particulars as to liter flow where applicable (e.g., cannula, 2 liters/min).
c. Respiratory rate (if patient is on a ventilator on assist or IMV, record both patient's rate and ventilator rate).
d. Minute volume (if patient is on a ventilator).
e. Patient's temperature.
f. Procedure—radial site.
   (1) Support the wrist on a rolled towel; bend the wrist down and slightly back. However, do not bend the wrist to the extent that the pulse is obliterated.

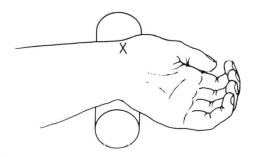

Figure 11-4. Position of arm and hand for radial puncture. "X" marks approximate site of puncture.

   (2) Palpate the location of the artery on the thumb side of the wrist.
   (3) Cleanse the area thoroughly with antiseptic; do not touch this area with the fingers after cleansing, as you will recontaminate it.
   (4) With the index finger of one hand, determine the exact point at which the needle should enter the artery.
   (5) Holding the syringe in the other hand at a 45° angle, with the bevel of the needle pointing upward, enter the skin about 5 to 10 mm distally to your index finger.
   (6) Advance the needle under the skin until the artery is entered; this is signaled by blood entering the syringe in a pulsating flow. (If the blood flow does

not pulsate, it is probably venous blood, in which case a new syringe must be prepared, and the procedure repeated.)

(7) Approximately 3 to 4 ml of blood should be obtained from an adult.

(8) When the blood needed is obtained, place a sterile gauze pad over the arterial puncture site, applying pressure as you withdraw the needle. Maintain pressure for a minimum of 5 *minutes*. However, this period of time may have to be extended if the patient is receiving anticoagulants or has a history of a bleeding disorder.

(9) A second person should handle the blood gas sample:

(a) Holding the syringe in a horizontal position (so that no air enters the sample), remove the needle.

(b) Cap the syringe to seal it.

(c) Rotate the tube gently to heparinize the sample.

(d) Label the sample.

(e) Immerse in ice water and transport to the laboratory immediately.

g. Procedure—brachial site

The procedure for obtaining an arterial sample from a brachial site is very similar to that using a radial site, with the following exceptions:

(1) The artery is palpated in the antecubital fossa.

(2) Because the artery is deeper and does not follow the bone, it is somewhat more difficult to enter.

(3) There is the possibility of hitting the median nerve with the needle, since it is located close to the artery.

(4) Hematoma formation is common, since there are no supporting structures to facilitate compression.

h. Procedure—femoral site

(1) Position the patient flat in bed with both legs extended.

(2) Using the index and middle fingers palpate the artery; the site of the puncture will be in the section of the artery supplying the upper third of the thigh, in the depression immediately below the fold of the groin. At this point, it is relatively superficial.

(3) Cleanse the puncture site thoroughly. It will be

necessary to use several applications of antiseptic to remove contamination.

(4) Because there are no firm supporting structures in the area, the artery must be stabilized by the middle and index fingers, spread 2 to 3 cm apart. (Palpating the artery before cleansing allows you to place the fingers without touching the point of insertion of the needle.)

(5) Hold the syringe perpendicular to the skin surface (90°) with the bevel of the needle facing away from you.

(6) Enter the skin between the fingers outlining the vessel.

(7) Compression of the femoral artery is especially difficult and must be maintained for a minimum of 5 minutes.

IV. Arterial Punctures: Infants and Children

Obtaining an arterial blood sample from an infant or child varies little from that of an adult, the difference being the concessions made to the size of the child.

A. Site of puncture

1. Radial artery—probably site of choice.

2. Brachial artery—frequently used.

3. Dorsalis pedis—passes forward from the bend of the ankle along the tibial side (inside) of the foot to the first intermetatarsal space, where it divides into two branches.

4. Posterior tibial—extends downward along the tibial side of the leg to the fossa between the inner ankle and the heel.

5. Temporal—located just above the ear; usually requires that the hair be shaved from the head. Arterial line best.

6. Femoral—least favorable, since penetrating through the artery can lead to aseptic necrosis of the hip.

7. "Arterialized" capillary sample—the heel is heated for a period of 10 min; after cleansing, the heel is stabbed with a sharp blade, and the free-flowing blood collected anaerobically in a capillary tube. The PCO_2 and pH obtained by this method are reasonably accurate; however PO_2's above 45 mm Hg are not interpretable. Sometimes, however, this is the most accessible site and may therefore be used initially in the child's course of therapy as a "starting point." As one physician stated, "You some-

times have no choice; for instance, if you are treating a chubby, 4-month-old asthmatic, who is alert and crying, it's by far the easiest and least traumatic."

B. Equipment
   1. For the premature infant, a no. 25 gauge tuberculin syringe and needle are adequate and easier to handle.
   2. For the older infant, a no. 23 gauge butterfly may be used. This needle is attached to a capillary tubing and enables you to determine that you truly are in the artery. (Use of a syringe usually requires suction, since arterial pressure in a child is not great enough to fill the syringe spontaneously. Therefore, a venous sample could be obtained erroneously.)
   3. For repeated samples, an arterial line may be used.

C. Procedure
   1. The procedure for obtaining an arterial sample is basically the same as for an adult. Local anesthesia with lidocaine should be used, since the procedure is probably even more traumatic for a child; he just can't tell you so!
   2. Compression of the artery should be maintained for 5 minutes.

EXERCISES

1. Explain why the patient's temperature is important to the interpretation of an arterial blood gas.
2. Describe what you feel would be the problems associated with an "arterial line."
3. At what specific stages in a patient's care would arterial blood gases be necessary?
4. Explain the procedure of an arterial puncture to a classmate, as you would to an anxious, acutely ill patient.

CHEST PHYSIOTHERAPY

In the last few years, chest physiotherapy has developed into one of the most important areas of care for the patient with respiratory problems. In both the acute and chronic stages of his disease, the removal of secretions from the airways of such a patient is essential.

An effective program of chest physiotheraphy should be instituted as soon after admission to the hospital as possible. The program should utilize the efforts of the nursing staff, the physical therapist, and the respiratory therapist.

For the patient with chronic obstructive lung disease, such a program should be based on the premise that it will become an integral part of a continuing rehabilitation regimen and will be used even after discharge.

COUGHING TECHNIQUES

One aspect of patient care that has been frequently overlooked in literary material is the actual process of teaching a patient effective (productive) coughing techniques. Nurses and therapists are admonished to "encourage the patient to cough." However, without proper instruction, the patient will soon become fatigued and depressed over his inability to raise secretions.

The patient who suffers from postoperative pain will also present a challenge; the pain will be greatly increased by a forceful paroxysmal cough. He will soon refuse to carry out the procedure and most likely will be labeled as "a baby" or "uncooperative" by the staff. Ideally, the surgical patient's teaching should begin pre-operatively when he will most likely be alert and more receptive. This, coupled with the judicious use of his "pain medication" given approximately 30 min before his coughing sessions, should prove more beneficial.

To avoid the fatigue of lengthy practice sessions, the staff involved in patient teaching of coughing techniques should initially *explain* and then *demonstrate* what the patient must do. This will help the patient conserve his strength for the actual procedure.

I. Position
   A. In bed:
      1. Elevate head of bed.
      2. Have patient flex knees toward chin.
      3. Support feet on mattress.
                        OR
      1. Have patient turn on side with upper body flexed forward.
      2. Knees should be flexed toward chin.
   B. Sitting position:
      1. Feet should be supported on floor or on chair.
      2. Have patient sit with shoulders rotated inward, with head and spine slightly flexed.
      3. Forearms should be relaxed or supported.

II. Procedure
   A. Instruct the patient to inhale slowly and deeply through his mouth, using the diaphragm and lower intercostal muscles.
   B. Exhale slowly and fully, with slightly pursed lips.
   C. Repeat several times; on the last expiration, cough out two to three times in stages.

III. Special Notes
   A. The patient with chronic obstructive lung disease may find that bending forward slowly on each expiration, using slightly pursed lip breathing, will further aid his coughing and expectoration.
   B. Postoperative patients may be taught to support their incision when coughing to ease the pain. This may be accomplished by the use of their hands, a pillow, a towel, or even their gown pulled tightly over an abdominal incision.

POSTURAL DRAINAGE AND PERCUSSION

Postural drainage is a form of therapy that utilizes the force of gravity to advance secretions from the smaller airways to the main bronchi, from which they can be removed by coughing or suctioning.

Postural drainage requires that the patient be placed in a variety of positions related to the bronchopulmonary segments of the lungs and the airways that drain them. Although some positions require more effort by the patient, many are such that even a cardiac patient, with assistance, may assume the positions without strain or probability of further damage.

The length of time a session of postural drainage should last will depend on the areas of the lungs to be drained and the patient's tolerance. The length of time and the positions may be modified to meet individual patient needs.

I. Indications for Postural Drainage
   A. Any time excessive secretions are present, or whenever they are extremely thick and tenacious.
   B. Any time a patient is *unable* to cough voluntarily or *will not* cough due to pain.
   C. Any time coughing proves ineffective and leads to exhaustion.
   D. As a prophylactic measure when a patient is very obese or inactive.

II. Contraindications
   A. Any time the changes in position adversely affect the patient's vital signs.
   B. Usually, postural drainage is avoided directly after meals as some positions may induce vomiting and aspiration.
   C. If a patient is to receive IPPB treatments, the IPPB should precede the postural drainage, as an aid to mobilization of secretions.

III. Equipment
   A. Bed—preferably adjustable; if not, a jack is also required. However, close observance of the jack is necessary as such equipment has a tendency to slip.
   B. Tissues for sputum.

IV. Clapping or Percussion

This maneuver is used at intervals during postural drainage.

A. Should be performed only over the thoracic cage. This is especially important when the patient has a chest deformity, such as a barrel chest; care must be taken not to percuss below the level of the ribs as organs other than the lungs would be exposed.

B. Is accomplished by cupping your hands and rhythmically clapping the patient's back or chest wall, using your wrists to perform most of the work. The resulting noise will resemble the "clip-clop" of a horse's hooves.

C. Be sure to keep the hands cupped, as this provides an air cushion and prevents discomfort to the patient.

D. It is not necessary to apply percussion for the entire period of time the patient is in a position. Three to four minutes is adequate per side of the chest. Do not percuss on bare skin or in the same spot continuously; move the hands around on the chest.

V. Postural Drainage Positions

A. Upper lobes

1. *Apical segment*—bed flat; have patient lean back at a 30° angle onto a pillow. Percuss over the area between the clavicle and top of scapula on each side (see Figure 12-1).

2. *Anterior segment*—bed flat; have patient lie flat on back; support knees with a pillow. Percuss between the clavicle and nipple on each side of the chest (see Figure 12-2).

3. *Posterior segment*—bed flat; have patient lean forward at a 30° angle. He may support himself on an over-the-bed table; however, be certain that the wheels are locked.

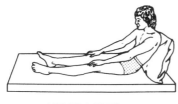

UPPER LOBES
Apical Segment

Figure 12-1.

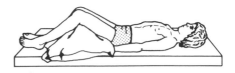

UPPER LOBES
Anterior Segment

Figure 12-2.

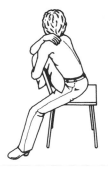

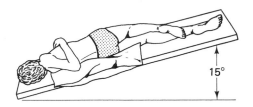

15°

UPPER LOBES
Posterior Segment

RIGHT MIDDLE LOBE
Lateral Segment
Medial Segment

Figure 12-3.   **Figure 12-4.**

Percuss over the upper back on each side of the chest (see Figure 12-3).

B. *Right middle lobe*—foot of bed elevated 15°; have patient lie with his head in a downward position on his left side; rotate chest one quarter-turn backward, flex knees; support back with pillows. Percuss over the right nipple area. However, on a female patient, it may be necessary to position breast tissue so that you do not percuss directly on the breast, causing the patient a great deal of discomfort (see Figure 12-4).

C. *Left upper lobe* (lingular segment)—foot of bed elevated 15°; have patient lie on right side with his head in a downward position; rotate chest one quarter-turn backward; flex knees; support back with pillows. Percuss over left nipple area, but again, not directly on breast tissue of a female patient (see Figure 12-5).

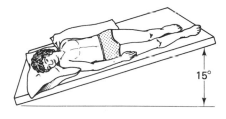

15°

LEFT UPPER LOBE
Lingular Segment
Superior   Inferior

Figure 12-5.

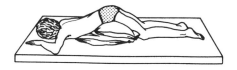

LOWER LOBES
Superior Segment

Figure 12-6.

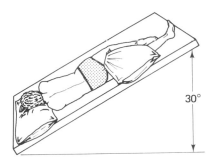

LOWER LOBES
Lateral Basal Segment

Figure 12-7.

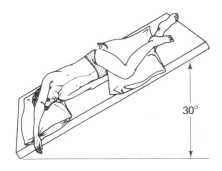

LOWER LOBES
Anterior Basal Segment

Figure 12-8.

D. Lower lobes

1. *Superior segment*—bed flat; have patient lie on his abdomen with pillows under his hips; this position may be difficult for a COLD patient to assume. If so, modify the position somewhat by removing some of the pillows. Percuss over the middle of the back below the tip of the scapula on either side of the spine (see Figure 12-6).

2. *Anterior basal segment*—elevate foot of bed 30°; have the patient lie on his side with his head in a downward position; place a pillow between his knees. Percuss over lower ribs just beneath the axilla (the patient must lie on the opposite side also, if both lungs are to be drained). See Figure 12-7.

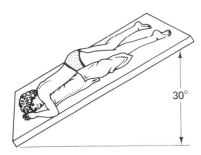

LOWER LOBES
Posterior Basal Segment

Figure 12-9.

3. *Lateral basal segment*—elevate foot of bed 30°; have the patient lie on his abdomen and then rotate his chest one quarter-turn upward. Place a pillow between his knees for support. Percuss over the uppermost portion of the lower ribs (position the patient on his opposite side if both lungs are to be drained). See Figure 12-8.

4. *Posterior basal segment*—elevate foot of bed 30°; have the patient lie on his abdomen with his head in a downward position; place a pillow under his hips. Position his legs for comfort. Percuss over the lower ribs close to the spine on each side of the chest (see Figure 12-9).

EXERCISES

1. Discuss the role of chest physiotherapy in the treatment of chronic obstructive lung disease.

2. Discuss the effectiveness of (1) chest physiotherapy without IPPB and (2) IPPB without chest physiotherapy for a patient with chronic obstructive lung disease.

3. How could the procedures described be adapted for home care use?

APPENDIX

THE HOLISTIC APPROACH TO PATIENT CARE

The holistic approach to patient care is a very controversial subject. Today, many physicians, as well as others in the health field, are specializing in a different part or section of the human body. Pulmonary specialists, kidney specialists, ear, nose, and throat physicians, and cardiologists, for example, can be found listed in the telephone directories of any large city. Nurse clinicians, those nurses specializing in cardiology, respiratory therapy, and other fields, are becoming more numerous in our society. You, as respiratory therapists, have also joined the ranks of the paramedical specialists participating in the care of patients. This is not to say that these individuals do not provide adequate and good care; however, it has been established that man usually responds as a unified whole, and not in a series of unintegrated parts. Ask yourself the question, "How do I see the chronic asthmatic being admitted to the hospital for a hernia repair?" You may discover that every illness is an illness of the entire person. Patients are usually treated out of context of family, home, and work; however, an individual does not leave his problems at home or at work when he walks into the admission area of a hospital. Consider yourself; during your last bout with the flu or a cold, how did you react when your children asked you for help with their homework, or how well did you balance your check book with an elevated temperature and a severe headache? Mind and body are not separate, man is a single entity; when something happens to a part, it happens to the whole. Therefore, we shall try to examine the holistic approach: "looking at man as a whole, from every view, and in the circumstances of his total environment, considering every part as related to every other part." As respiratory therapists we are concerned with caring for our patients. Our patients are people; the same as you and I. Although we may have individual differences, we have very comparable biologic characteristics, we all experience certain universal problems, and we share universal needs. We gain this type of knowledge through courses in sociology, psychology, and the other behavioral sciences in our respiratory therapy schools, giving us insight into our own behavior. The care of our patients depends on the respiratory therapist's ability to perceive and understand the behavioral cues that tell us the patient's state of comfort and his ability to cope with problems brought about by illness.

Let's take a look at a portion of your assignment today. You have the following patients to care for:

In room 505, Mr. Geldar, a 57-year-old male, who has recently had a lobectomy due to a malignancy of the right lung. Until his surgery he worked every day to support his wife and two sons. He had "passed out" while at work three weeks ago and was admitted to the hospital for a work up. He had been a smoker for many years; however, he had no major complaints except for a "smoker's cough" and slight shortness of breath. He nods a "Hello" to you as you approach his bed. He looks somewhat tired, but is very willing to work with you as you prepare for his chest physiotherapy. You think about Mr. Geldar and the many problems he will face. Will he be able to work again and provide for his wife and family? How much pain is he having, and how difficult is it for him to respond to your therapy to his one good lung? You have been in his room when his wife and family visit him. He appears to be cheerful, but how does he really feel about his condition? Does he fear the "spread of cancer," and what are his personal feelings about death? What about smoking? You chat with Mr. Geldar a few minutes and discover he loves to hunt and fish. He fears he will be unable to participate in these activities when he recuperates. He also tells you he doesn't care to eat, "food doesn't taste good anymore." You leave Mr. Geldar, still wondering about all his problems.

Mr. Abell, the patient in room 506, greets you with a "breathless" good morning as you enter his room. He has been in the hospital many times before; however, this is the first time you have been assigned to his care. He is 69 years of age, retired, and has severe emphysema. His wife passed away a few years ago, and he lives with his daughter and her family. His color is somewhat cyanotic this morning and his breathing difficult. He receives IPPB treatments four times a day to assist him in bringing up secretions. A very recent pulmonary infection made this hospitalization necessary. He rarely has visitors; his daughter has four young children and they keep her busy at home. You think a minute about how Mr. Abell feels about his home situation; is this busy environment proving to be more than he can cope with? Is he cleaning his IPPB equipment thoroughly at home? Do the children play with his equipment? Does he miss his wife, and the "tender loving care" she no doubt gave him? He had mentioned "what a wonderful wife" she had been. You are only 22 years of age, healthy and active, and yet you must be able to communicate with this older gentleman who can no longer work or play. You also know that the chronic chest patient needs a somewhat set or scheduled routine to his everyday living to help him adjust to his environment. Does he feel he is contributing to life in his daughter's home? What can you do about these problems?

Now to report to the trauma intensive care unit. John Blanchard, the patient in room 3, is your responsibility. "Gee! He's the same age I am!" He's so still and pale and is being maintained on a ventilator. He was working yesterday in a machine shop, and on his way home another automobile struck him head on. Crushed chest, broken pelvis, he doesn't move his legs either—spinal cord injury? Hard to tell, as his lower extremities were injured when it took the rescue team over an hour to cut the car from around him in order to free him. His family sits quietly as you check out the ventilator, change the setup, and make any necessary adjustments. Should I speak to John, and/or to his family, and just what should I say? Will he live long enough to come off from the ventilator? Wonder if he ever thought about dying; have I? What are his parents thinking; wonder what the doctors have told them about John's condition? He has a brother and sister; how do they feel about John and the accident? Can John hear me adjusting the ventilator? Does he have pain? What are my responsibilities toward this young man—a peer of mine?

There are a few different approaches you, as a respiratory therapist, can take regarding the care of these patients. Your care can be purely technical, mechanical, and very impersonal. You can do just those things absolutely necessary, such as "just administering Mr. Geldar's physiotherapy" in an abrupt, businesslike manner. You can ignore all the personal problems Mr. Geldar has and treat him with "robot-type" care. You can treat Mr. Abell in a similar manner, "just giving him his morning treatment." You can close your "eyes and ears" to "why" he contracted an upper respiratory infection and hospitalization again became necessary. You can readily avoid any conversation with these two patients, who might want to enjoy a little "TLC"—a very basic need of all of us. You do not have to talk to Mr. Geldar about perhaps encouraging his sons to become interested in his hobbies, hunting and fishing. You are well trained in ventilator care, so just "changing the tubing" can become almost automatic. You don't have to converse with John, "he may not hear you anyway." John's parents may be very interested in what you are doing, but you think "it doesn't matter anyway." In other words, you can totally ignore very personal relationships and still think you have given thorough care to your patients. Unfortunately, this ignoring of "patients are people" just like you and I continues everyday in many hospitals.

On the other hand, you can realize that your patients do have problems and needs, but you approach them in a very disorganized manner. You are unable to sort out the "signs and symptoms" and relate to them. You do not see or comprehend any threads that might link these patients together. You fail to see any connections between the problems of your patients, yourself, and your own problems. Your plan of care becomes disjointed, and you become quite frustrated. It's like preparing a load of people for a picnic in the country, but, then ask, "who will drive the bus?"

You now really begin to think about your patients as real people. Think of yourself the last time you were a patient in the doctor's office or in the hospital. Which people who attended you gave you the most help and care? Patients are not really so much different than we are ourselves. All of us have basic needs; some of these are fulfilled and some may never be. Our environments have great effects on each of us. We use different methods of adaptations in our lives and environments, but nevertheless we all "adapt" in some way. It is really "people" we care for in our professions—not all the facts and theories. If people were not involved, we, as respiratory therapists, or any other paramedical specialties would not even exist. As a result, let's turn our attention to the holistic approach; the aims and goals of good respiratory therapy center around looking at the *total* man—the *total* patient. He is a complex, thinking, and feeling person living in our social environment side by side with us.

Let's take a look at man from a biological standpoint. We are not really that different or distinguishable from some of the lower forms of life that exist around us. We have a very similar chemical background, and we all evolve from a cell which can be called "the unit of life." Respiration is essential to all life, and a state of internal homeostasis is necessary. The need to grow, develop, and reproduce also are biologic processes we all share. If man and the lower forms of life are to survive, we must also be able to adapt to changes in our environment. If we examine the preceding facts regarding man, we begin to wonder just what makes man different and sets him apart from other organisms. What characteristics does man share with his fellowman?

During your course of work you have certainly heard the remark, "people as patients are all alike." We, however, like to think of our own individuality and uniqueness, yet we all tend to "group" our patients, and particularly those with a chronic illness. Nothing, however, is further from the truth. Each patient we care for is an individual and feels there is no other patient as important, and no one else exactly like him. What makes these differences? Each of us comes from different backgrounds. We have each experienced different stress, trauma, and success in our lives. It is these experiences that play an important role in facing and adjusting to illness. Mr. Geldar, with his diagnosis of cancer, may respond very differently than another patient with a similar diagnosis. Therefore, we must use a wide variety of approaches to patients, even those with the same diagnosis. Mr. Geldar may be a devoutly religious individual, he may have witnessed another family member face the same situation and still not "fall apart," so he does not view his diagnosis as fatal. The care of Mr. Abell, the older patient, should indicate to us that we certainly need to be familiar with the general characteristics of the older patient. John, our younger patient, has needs that are different from the characteristics of the mature adult. Various ethnic groups share different characteristics; however, there are cultural differences that must be considered when planning their care. Therefore, as a participant in total health care, the more knowledgeable you are and become regarding age, racial, economical, and occupational differences, the more intelligently you can care for patients. It can be said then that, while we are biologically similar, and all have our individual and group differences, we still all continue to share universal problems and needs. It is these universal experiences and needs that give us the opportunity to understand and interact with our patients as human beings.

Man has many basic needs, some more vital than others. Instead of going into detail about survivial needs, stimulation needs, and those involving safety and security, I would simply like to offer you some suggestions. You certainly will not ignore Mr. Abell's color, and when his cyanotic status becomes worse, you know he needs oxygen. In addition, you know the need of John to have side rails on his bed due to his unconscious state. We have to remember that it is a part of our job to help our patients meet needs within the hospital setting and within the limitations of his illness. The needs for love and respect, though sometimes much less obvious, are equally important to our patients. Our chronic chest patients confined to limited areas in the hospital, as well as at home, need great mental stimulation as well as physical mobility. Patients do not want to simply have their survival needs attended to; they want to live as completely as possible and be as independent as they can. Think a few minutes. What needs do you have and want satisfied? Then perhaps you will understand your patient better!

We have briefly discussed basic needs; however, we have not discussed universal problems or experiences that we all have in common. The one word that comes to mind first in our century is *stress*. Stress can be defined as force, strain, a pressure that tends to distort a body, and that may induce both body and mental tension. Stress, however, may occur in normal living, for example, just getting back and forth to work; this act does not involve any bodily injury or disease. Stress can also occur and yet individuals can benefit from it; for example, competitive sports help us vent our emotions. Patients, however, are very susceptible to stress, and we as health workers must be knowledgeable as well as patient about how our clients "adapt" to stress. Adaptation, meaning to adjust or accommodate at the human level, is very complicated. Man attempts to face the challenges of life today with his body, intellect, and emotions. An example of man's ability to adapt from a physiological point of view can be demonstrated and experienced by all of us when we are exposed to extreme cold: we begin to shiver, rub our hands together, and move our feet; these activities will aid our bodies in producing and conserving heat. If we are attacked by a virus or a bacteria, our white cells will increase, thereby attempting to fight off the infection. Adaptation on a psychological level can be experienced by everyone who has ever attended school. School teachers and professors are all different types of people, some very strict and some more lenient and understanding; when we go to different classrooms for various subjects, we are constantly changing our attitudes and our behavior, as well as our methods of approach. As a result of these adjustments, we are able to remain in school and gradually reach our own goals. However, adjustment and adaptation do not always result in what is best for an individual.

Our patient, Mr. Abell, whom we discussed previously, may be the type of individual who does not adjust or adapt in a healthy manner. He may wish to be dependent on his daughter and her family, and as a result does not help himself to carry out his daily routine to the best of his ability. He may feel "sick people can be dependent," and therefore he experiences no guilt feelings when not performing some of the everyday activities he could do for himself. This type of adaptation, although not considered to be successful adjustment, may be the very best a patient can make to protect himself in order to continue to live out his life span.

Everyone has to adjust to his present society and to his particular culture. Consider yourself when you first entered the respiratory therapy course at school. You were exposed to many new circumstances and experiences very rapidly: a new vocabulary, establishment of ethics particular to respiratory therapy, exposure to patients, and standards you had to meet. Gradually you learned medical terminology, developed confidence in taking care of your-patients, and learned how to use various types of respiratory therapy equipment, and thereby managed a healthy adjustment. There are a few facts to remember whenever adaptation takes place. None of us really loses our identity when using adaptive procedures. These adaptive procedures are all attempts to maintain a homeostatic state of being, a condition that may vary, but which is fairly constant. Each individual may alter his adaptive responses; for example, the rigid and strict individuals may be less likely to cope easily with stress and change. In addition, however, a physical illness does not always result in failure to adapt. Patients such as Mr. Geldar, whose diagnosis is a malignancy of the right lung followed by lobectomy, may suddenly have to change their occupation and entire life style.

To look further at the holistic approach to patient care, we need to discuss briefly the concepts of health and disease. Disease is quite predictable; it usually reaches all of us in one way or another and affects us personally, as well as professionally. Today, both health and disease are not static conditions; both appear to be in a continuous state of change and growth. It is therefore critical to all of us to learn and continue to learn as much as possible about diseases and their current treatment. However, we must also continue to be open-minded when looking at the causes of disease, treatment, and the like, because what was true yesterday may prove to be untrue tomorrow.

We are only really beginning to become involved with man as a total being, and just beginning to study the states of health and disease from a broad view, looking at the physical, emotional, social, and adaptive measures of man—the holistic approach! In addition, today we understand that each individual has his own definitions of health and disease. Today patients have and are familiar with the "Patient's Bill of Rights." One's own life experiences and social and cultural backgrounds will affect one's outlook on health and disease. Today, we realize more and more that when an individual is physically ill, his mental status and outlook are affected also. Despite all the technological advances made by modern medicine, one questions if man is really suffering less, or perhaps his suffering has merely changed in nature. Modern medicine is just now beginning to consider a multicausal theory of disease taking into account all the factors that can, and do, affect health and disease. Instead of just examining man's bodily processes, medicine is looking at and examining the total person, the relationships of the various organs, and the relationship of mind and body, as well as man's total environment.

This being the case, it only makes sense that treatment of diseases, as well as patient care, must also take place on a multidimensional level. Let's take a patient and explore the importance of total care. A member of your family, your favorite uncle, has experienced shortness of breath for the past several years. Yes, this shortness of breath has been increasing, becoming more frequent, and for longer periods of time. However, because he has been a smoker for a number of years, he attributed his morning cough and sputum production to his cigarette smoking. He is a little heavier in weight than he should be and is just 52 years of age. He has worked in the steel plant in maintenance for a number of years. Recently, the plant offered a special 12-week course that he took to be able to upgrade himself to work in the mill as a foreman. He was successful in obtaining this upgrading, and his wife and three teen-age children were as thrilled as he regarding this accomplishment. This particular job involved much more physical exertion and exposure to pollutants; therefore, his shortness of breath increased. He was seen by the plant physician, and after a thorough physical examination and testing, he was diagnosed as severe emphysema and early retirement was advised. A decision had to be made that would involve the entire family. The chief "breadwinner" and "provider" of this family for many years had been struck with a disabling illness.

What advice would you be able to give him? After all, you are a "professional." You are well acquainted with emphysema, its progressive symptoms, and its treatment. Yes, he should and can quit smoking. How will you advise him in order to accomplish this? No doubt he will need advisement, regarding his condition, and further treatment, and you as a respiratory therapist can help him with this aspect of his illness. He will need good emotional help and support in making his adjustment from employment to retirement. How will you be able to help him meet and cope with his new life style? Who will provide financially for his family now; will his social security benefits get them through, or will his wife have to seek employment to assist this family? How will all these changes in his own life and the lives of his family affect all of them? Will all these changes affect his status as the "father figure" and his male role? Will his children view him as an unsuccessful father and provider? It will be necessary to evaluate and treat his social and psychological problems, as well as treating his physical problems to help him from deteriorating further. Special care as well as treatment need to be included in all phases of his problems.

There is one additional human need that has not been discussed in this chapter. Nevertheless, it must be considered, as it may affect our patient's general well-being, as well as his mental and emotional health. This is the spiritual need, a need that relates to sacred or spiritual matters. Each of us may have to search our own mind and soul first to discover how we ourselves feel about this need in order to be of help to our patient and his family. We must be prepared, if this need arises during patient contact, to know the patient's religion and religious background. At the very least, we should be able to tell our patient or his family who to contact within the hospital setting, the individual to get in touch with if he requires the services of a pastor, priest, or rabbi. In addition, it might be helpful to patients if we can tell them the time and day of the various religious services that might be held at the hospital. If the hospital has a chapel, we should be able to direct the patient or his family to it.

Just helping the patient cope with his disease alone is not enough. We have to consider his total life situation, his adjustment to his environment and to society. The aims and goals of the respiratory therapist must involve the total man—the total patient and the *holistic approach* regarding the care of our patients.

It is not only necessary, but most important that the entire health team maintain an attitude of accountability to all patients. The respiratory therapist must not only be skilled in the technical aspect of his work, he must be able to assess patients needs and help the patient achieve optimum health.

EXERCISES

1. Spend some time thinking about your own experiences with illness. From these experiences, determine ways in which you can better understand how your patient feels, and record specific ways in which you can help him.
2. Discuss in writing the pro's and con's of the holistic approach to patient care.
3. Attempt to determine how you feel about death and dying. Then write down important factors in giving care to the dying patient.
4. List two basic needs of the patients for which you have provided respiratory therapy this morning.
5. Define stress, and discuss some of the adaptive mechanisms patients may utilize during their hospital stay.

OTHER COMMON PROCEDURES

There are a variety of procedures with which the respiratory therapist will come in contact. Some will be his responsibility and others will not. We feel that a brief discussion of several of these will enable the therapist to administer better overall patient care.

I. CVP Readings

The central venous pressure (CVP) gives an indication of the pressure under which blood is pumped to the superior vena cava or the right atrium. The normal pressure within the superior vena cava, and thus the CVP reading, is 5 to 10 cm of water. Variations below this are indicative of a decreasing circulating blood volume (such as due to hemorrhage), while readings above 10 cm of water are indicative of overloading of the right heart and impaired venous return.

A. Indications for measurement of the CVP

1. To guide the physician in the treatment of congestive heart failure.

2. To guide the physician during replacement of massive fluid or blood volume, as in the treatment of hypovolemic shock and severe burns. Therefore, CVP monitoring can also assist the physician in reducing the patient's period of hypotension to a minimum by indicating how quickly the blood volume can be restored without danger of circulatory overload.

3. Guides the physician in differentiation between hypovolemic (low volume) and nonhypovolemic shock (shock due to other causes).

4. Guides the physician in determining whether true renal shutdown exists or dehydration and/or hypovolemia is the cause of a decreased urine output.

5. May be used postoperatively:
   a. To prevent or correct inadequate blood volume and thereby improving cardiac output.
   b. To prevent hypervolemia (overloading the circulatory system), which increases work of the heart.
   c. To aid in early detection of signs of complications.
   d. To aid in maintenance of normal circulation.

B. Procedure

Under aseptic conditions, a special catheter is inserted into the superior vena cava or right atrium using the median basilic, cephalic, jugular, or subclavian vein as a pathway. The catheter is attached to a manometer, four-way stopcock, and an intravenous infusion setup.

1. Baseline—the manometer is positioned at the level of the right chest (midchest). This presents somewhat of a difficulty in patients with a barrel chest, making it necessary to use the lower third of the lateral chest as a guide-

line. All readings, to be accurate, must be taken at this point, preferably with the patient in a flat, supine position.

2. Fluid from the intravenous setup is allowed to run into the catheter until approximately the 25 cm of water level.

3. The stopcock is then repositioned for the actual pressure reading, which is read at the maximum level the meniscus of the fluid reaches after it stabilizes. This indicates an equilibration of pressure between the vena cava and the manometer.

4. The system is kept functioning by returning the stopcock to its original position and controlling the flow of intravenous solution by a microdrip method.

C. Special considerations

1. After the insertion of the catheter, an x-ray film should be taken to be certain that the catheter placement is correct.

2. If all connections are not tight, air embolism could occur.

3. Pneumothorax could occur during insertion of the catheter if force is used.

4. For accurate readings, if a patient is on mechanical ventilation, the ventilator should be disconnected. However, in some institutions this is not the practice, since some physicians feel that the trend of changes is more important than the actual readings. Whichever method is used, therefore, it must be consistently practiced in order to give usable data.

5. If venous spasm occurs due to irritation by the needle, wait for a few minutes before taking the reading.

D. Causes of an elevated CVP

1. Improper placement of the catheter

2. Vasoconstrictor drugs

3. Myocardial failure

4. Obstruction to venous return by an embolus

5. Increases in intrathoracic pressure, as due to pneumo- or hemothorax or mechanical ventilation.

E. Causes of a lowered CVP

1. Hypovolemia due to hemorrhage, severe burns, or dehydration

2. Vasodilator drugs

II. Dialysis
There are two basic forms of dialysis, peritoneal and hemodialysis, and either may be used to temporarily relieve symptoms of renal failure. Dialysis may also be used to sustain life
(the well-known "artificial kidney") in those patients having
irreversible renal disease. It is also helpful in preparing a patient physically for a renal transplant.
Dialysis is a diffusion process as discussed in Unit One.
In this instance, however, the procedure substitutes for renal
function utilizing the peritoneal membrane (for peritoneal dialysis) or an artificial membrane (for hemodialysis). These
membranes have pores that are large enough to allow electrolytes, urea, and creatinine to pass through, but which are too
small to allow blood cells and other proteins to move across.
A special electrolyte solution is infused on one side of the membrane, while the patient's blood occupies the area on the other
side.
A. Goals of dialysis therapy
1. Remove urea and creatine from the blood (end products
of protein metabolism).
2. Maintain serum electrolytes at a stable, safe level.
3. Replenishment of the blood's bicarbonate buffer system
and correction of metabolic acidosis.
4. Removal of excess water from the blood.
B. *Peritoneal dialysis*—a catheter is inserted into the peri-
toneum under strict aseptic conditions (peritonitis can result if any contamination is permitted). Approximately 2000
ml of a specially prepared electrolyte–dextrose solution
(dialysate) is inserted through the catheter, from where it
enters the peritoneal space. There it comes in contact with
the peritoneal membrane and is allowed to remain for 20
min. The amount of dextrose determines how much water
leaves the blood, depending on the patient's particular
needs. At the end of the 20 min, the solution is allowed to
drain by gravity, carrying with it the toxic substances that
have been removed from the blood. Accurate records of fluid
intake and output are extremely important.
C. *Hemodialysis*—requires the performance of a surgical shunt
between a vein and artery, utilizing a cannula in each which
is then connected externally. This shunt remains in place
for an indefinite period of time. When the patient is to be
dialyzed, the arterial cannula is connected to the membrane
of the dialysis machine by means of tubing. Blood thus fills

the membrane compartment, returning to the patient through tubing connected to the venous cannula.

Fresh dialysate solution is continuously pumped around the outside of the membrane compartment. As the dialysate is used, it is allowed to flow out and down a drain.

Hemodialysis lasts for a period of 6 to 10 hours at a time, and is usually performed three times a week, for patients having irreversible renal failure.

Upon completion of each treatment, the arterial cannula is clamped and any blood remaining in the membrane compartment is returned to the patient via the venous cannula. The venous cannula is then clamped. The shunt is then reestablished by connecting a U-shaped piece between the artery and vein.

III. Electrocardiograms (ECG)

In many institutions, the respiratory therapist is responsible for obtaining electrocardiograms. The function of the ECG machine is beyond the scope of this discussion. However, the resultant graphic information obtained is of use not only to the medical staff, but to the therapist who is administering drugs that have cardiac effects. The tracing is also similar to that seen on cardiac monitors, to which many of the acutely ill patients we care for will be attached.

An ECG is a graphic tracing of the electrical impulses generated by depolarization and repolarization of the heart muscle (myocardium). The impulses are detected by electrodes placed at various points on the body and measured by a galvanometer.

It is important to keep in mind that an ECG is not foolproof. Unless there is a disturbance in the electrical discharges of the heart, an ECG will not depict heart disease as such.

A brief review of the functioning of the heart is necessary to understand how the pattern of an ECG is made.

A. The S–A node, the "cardiac pacemaker," is located at the point where the superior vena cava joins the right atrium. It is in the S–A node that each heart beat originates. This node is under the control of the sympathetic nervous system, which increases the rate of electrical discharge, and the parasympathetic nervous system, which decreases the rate. Normally, electrical discharges occur 60 to 100 times/min, resulting in atrial contraction, followed by ventricular contraction. This contraction is termed depolarization because it causes an electrical imbalance in the cells of the myocardium. This depolarization is represented on the graphic strip as the P wave (the initial upward wave) which is the electrical discharge of the atrium, and the QRS complex, or depolarization of the ventricle.

B. Repolarization occurs during the relaxation of the atria and ventricles. During this period of time, the cells are recharged. This repolarization of the ventricles is represented on the graphic chart by the T wave.

C. ECG paper consists of a graph comprised of small and large squares. Each small square represents 0.04 sec. Five small squares, linearly, represent 0.2 sec. These five small squares make up one large square. Five large squares represent 1.0 sec. (The vertical squares represent voltage.)

Figure A-1 is an example of a normal ECG strip. This is known as *sinus rhythm.*

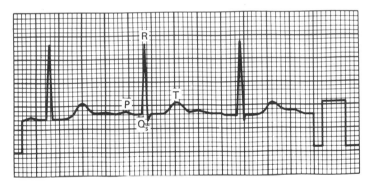

Normal sinus rythm, rate
within normal limits

Figure A-1.   Normal ECG strip.

D. Impulses formed in the atrium have to pass through the A–V node; this delays passage of the impulse. This delay is represented on the graph by the PR interval. To find this, you measure from the beginning of the P wave to the beginning of the QRS complex. Normal is 0.1 to 0.2 sec.

1. *First-degree heart block*—the PR interval is greater than 0.2 sec, but the QRS follows

2. *Second-degree heart block*—not all P waves are followed by a QRS complex. If there is a QRS complex, the PR interval may or may not be normal.

3. *Third-degree (complete) heart block*—no impulse passes through the A–V node. There is no relationship between

the P wave and the QRS complex. The ventricles beat independently.

E. Other arrhythmias

1. *Atrial fibrillation*—P wave is replaced by a series of vibrations; impairs life, but can sustain life.

2. *Ventricular fibrillation*—no QRS complex; no cardiac output; arrest.

3. *Asystole*—straight line on graph; arrest.

4. *Agonal rhythm*—dying heart.

IV. Vital Signs

Every respiratory therapist should be familiar with the vital signs—how to measure them and what relationship they have to the patient and his respiratory problems.

A. Temperature

1. May be taken orally or rectally.

2. An increased temperature increases metabolism and, therefore, increases oxygen consumption.

3. An increased temperature often indicates the presence of an infectious process.

4. A decreased temperature slows all body functions.

B. Pulse

1. Each time the heart beats it forces a spurt of blood into the blood vessels, causing an alternate contraction and expansion of the arterial wall. Therefore, the pulse rate is normally the same as the heart rate.

2. Factors that increase the pulse rate.
   a. Exercise
   b. Emotion
   c. Disease processes—disease produces *stress;* infection increases pulse; electrolyte imbalances may increase pulse as may cardiac dysfunction.
   d. Medications—bronchodilators, particularly vasodilators, increase pulse rate.

3. Where to measure pulse rate.
   a. Most convenient place to feel pulse is usually over the *radial artery* on the thumb side of the wrist. This is because the radial artery is situated over bone and is close to the surface at this point. Place the first two fingers gently over the wrist; do not press too firmly as this obliterates the pulse. Never use your thumb to take a pulse, as it has a pulse of its own, which could easily be mistaken for that of the patient.

       b. Other sites to use.
         (1) Temporal artery
         (2) Carotid artery
         (3) Femoral artery
    4. Rate of pulse
       a. Usually 60 to 100/min
       b. Bradycardia—below 60 beats/min
       c. Tachycardia—over 100 beats/min
    5. Rhythm of pulse
       a. No regular rhythm—arrhythmia
       b. Double beat (soft pulse)—dicrotic: counted as one beat
    6. Volume of pulse
       a. Normal—strong and full
       b. Thready—weak and thin (volume suddenly diminished)
    7. Apical–radial pulse—normally should be almost the same; one person takes radial pulse while another takes apical pulse with a stethescope placed over the apex of the heart. If the radial pulse is less than the apical pulse, the difference is termed *pulse deficit*. This indicates impaired cardiotonic efficiency.

C. Respiration

Respiration is usually an unconscious process, but may be under some voluntary control. Therefore, when counting respiration, you should do so without the patient being aware; otherwise, he may not breathe normally. This may be accomplished by counting respirations while still holding the patient's wrist; he will think you're still taking his pulse.

Because you are treating primarily patients with respiratory problems, it is important to count respiration for *one full minute*, since the pattern can change significantly in that period of time.

    1. Types of respiration
       a. Periods of difficult respiration followed by periods of no respirations—Cheyne–Stokes respirations.
       b. Painful or difficult respirations—dyspnea.
       c. Inability to breathe while lying flat—orthopnea.
       d. Lack of respiration—apnea.
       e. Noisy respiration—stertorous.
       f. Deep, rapid respiration—hyperpnea.
    2. Rate of respiration—usually 14 to 18/min; regular rhythmic, effortless, and quiet.

3. Factors increasing rate of respiration:
   a. Exercise
   b. Eating
   c. Posture
   d. Extremes of environmental and body temperature
   e. Emotions
   f. Drugs
   g. Increased metabolic rate

Note: Except when brain pathology is involved, most disease processes tend to increase the respiratory rate. However, factors such as increased intracranial pressure and some drugs (especially morphine) will decrease the rate.

D. Blood Pressure

As the heart contracts it sends spurts of blood through the blood vessels. This contraction is heard as the systolic portion (the first sound) of a blood pressure reading. When the heart relaxes, this is termed diastole, and is heard as the last sound in a blood pressure reading. Some clinicians consider the diastolic pressure to be that point at which there is a definite change in the sound.

1. Factors influencing blood pressure
   a. Activity
   b. Emotion
   c. Disease
   d. Force of heartbeat
   e. Elasticity of arteries
2. Blood pressure readings
   a. Normal is 120/80 mm Hg.
   b. Hypertension—high-pressure readings; may be due to decreased elasticity of blood vessels.
   c. Hypotension—low-pressure readings; may be normal for some people; may indicate hemorrhage and/or shock.
3. Measurement of blood pressure—taken by use of a sphygmomanometer; a cuff containing a bladder is placed securely around the arm at the brachial artery. The cuff is inflated by squeezing a rubber bulb; this pressure compresses the artery. Upon the slow release of air from the cuff, the pressures may be read on a manometer containing mercury or a spring-type gauge, while simultaneously listening with a stethescope held against the brachial artery.

4. Pulse pressure—the numerical difference between the systolic and diastolic pressures. A marked increase or decrease in pulse pressure is indicative of the heart's inability to pump effectively.

Note: Blood pressure readings require some experience by the practitioner before they may be made accurately. There are double stethescopes available that allow both the student and instructor to listen simultaneously, which are therefore a useful tool for teaching.

V. Chest Tubes and Water-Seal Drainage
A chest tube (catheter) may be inserted into a patient's chest to:

1. Remove air (pneumothorax)
2. Remove blood (hemothorax)
3. Remove air and blood (hemopneumothorax)
4. Remove purulent material (empyema)

The insertion of such a tube may be an emergency procedure following trauma or a spontaneous pneumothorax, or may be done as part of the surgical closing procedure following thoracic surgery. The latter is required to reexpand a collapsed lung caused by the entry of air at atmospheric pressure into the pleural space when the chest is opened.

The insertion of a chest tube is considered a surgical procedure since an incision must be made. Frequently, more than one such tube may be inserted, one in the anterior aspect of the chest through the second intercostal space to permit the escape of air rising in the pleural space, and one posteriorly through the eighth or ninth intercostal space in the midaxillary line to drain off fluid accumulating in the lower portion of the pleural space. This lower tube is generally larger in diameter to aid in free drainage. Although the two tubes may be connected by a wye junction, it is generally best to attach them separately to two different water-seal drainage systems. This allows you to monitor air and fluid drainage from each tube and to remove a nondraining tube without disrupting the other. Flexible drainage tubing connects the chest tube with the drainage apparatus.

A. One-bottle water-seal apparatus—consists of a sterile bottle containing 100 ml of sterile normal saline or sterile water; a tight-fitting stopper containing two holes is placed in the opening of the bottle and is taped securely in place. Two hollow tubes are placed in the holes in the stopper; one tube is short and acts as an air vent, and the other tube is longer and acts as a water seal when it is placed so that it extends into the bottle about 3 to 5 cm below the fluid level. The other end of this tube is attached to the patient's chest tube. Water-seal drainage acts as a one-way valve, permitting one directional flow of air and fluid out of the pleural space, but allowing none to enter from the drainage system. Although suction may be used with some water-seal systems, it is not used with the one-bottle system, as this is simply drainage by gravity.

B. Two-bottle water-seal apparatus—consists of an empty drainage bottle placed between the patient and the water-seal bottle. Fluid collects in the empty bottle, allowing you to accurately measure the amount. If gravity drainage is insufficient for lung reexpansion, suction may be applied by an electrical pump or from a wall suction outlet. If suction is applied, the water in the water-seal tube will fluctuate, thus giving you an indication of proper functioning; on inspiration, the fluid level will rise, while on expiration it will drop.

C. Factors affecting chest drainage
   1. The apparatus for closed chest drainage must always be located at a level lower than the patient's chest in order to maintain drainage by gravity.
   2. Always be careful not to accidentally knock over the bottles or to break them when using a high–low bed or the side rails.
   3. If for some reason the chest tube is clamped, never unclamp the tube if the apparatus is above the patient's chest or the fluid in the drainage bottle will run down or be siphoned into the patient's pleural cavity.
   4. Avoid kinking or compressing the tubing.
   5. Closed chest drainage systems must be kept airtight.
   6. Aseptic technique must be used when caring for the chest tube and drainage system.

D. Clamping chest tubes
   Do not clamp chest drainage tubes without an order to do so (this is usually a nursing function) except in an emergency. If the tube is clamped, only rubber-shod Kelly clamps should be used.
   1. When to clamp the chest tube
      a. To locate a malfunction in the system.

    b. If the water-seal bottle breaks, and you know that no bubbling of the water has been taking place prior to the breakage (the lung is almost completely reexpanded), clamp the chest tube and then wipe the exposed end of the tube with an antiseptic solution and reconnect to another water-seal bottle. If the tube is clamped and the patient is in respiratory distress, *unclamp the tube and notify the physician immediately.*

    c. Ordinarily, if the chest bottle breaks and you know that bubbling of the water has been taking place prior to the breakage, indicating incomplete expansion of the lung, you *do not* clamp the tube before reconnecting to another water-seal bottle.

DISCHARGE PLANNING AND HOME CARE FOR THE RESPIRATORY PATIENT

The care of a patient with chronic obstructive lung disease does not end with his discharge from the hospital. Indeed, careful discharge planning and a well-defined home care program are essential if the patient is to spend an extended period of time at home. Such planning should be initiated as soon after admission as one can reasonably predict the type of long-term therapy he will require.

Many different members of the health team should be involved in helping the patient and his family adjust to the limitations of his disease. They include members of social services, vocational rehabilitation counseling, the public health nurse, the pharmacist, the physical therapist, the dietician and the respiratory therapist.

Many institutions have established a routine referral procedure, which is modified as necessary, to meet the needs of each individual patient and his family. It is important, however, that the referring physician allow sufficient time before discharge for each department to visit the patient. Nothing is more frustrating than to receive a call in the morning that "Mr. Smith is being discharged this afternoon. Could someone please teach him how to use his IPPB machine!"

Departments that will be giving the patient detailed instructions for use of equipment and procedures, such as respiratory therapy and physical therapy, will find it helpful to provide the patient with *simple* written instructions to take home with him. Diagrams should be included if possible. Even the most competent patient will feel more secure if he has something to refer to should he forget how to assemble his equipment or how to clean it. You will find, also, that the patient will usually be more conscientious about following his therapy regimen.

Let us examine how such a program could be used effectively for one patient.

Mr. George Robinson is a 45-year-old steel worker who was admitted to the intensive care unit in respiratory failure. He was diagnosed as having moderate to severe emphysema of several years duration. Initially he required a tracheostomy and assisted ventilation.

While still on the ventilator, Mr. Robinson was visited regularly by the physical therapist, who initiated a program of percussion, coughing, and postural drainage to mobilize secretions. Mrs. Robinson was frequently present for these sessions so that she could become accustomed to the procedures used. Later the therapist worked with both Mr. and Mrs. Robinson to instruct them in the correct manner to carry out the procedures at home. Before discharge, the therapist supervised them as they performed the entire regimen and offered suggestions for improvement, as necessary. He also supplied written instructions and diagrams for reference.

Because Mr. Robinson was initially on a ventilator, the respiratory therapist was in constant attendance. Frequent monitoring of blood gases and ventilator setting was required and changes were made as necessary. The ventilator tubing was frequently drained to prevent buildup of condensation and the tubing system was changed every 24 hours to prevent contamination of Mr. Robinson's respiratory tract by organisms found in such tubing.

The respiratory therapist was also present during the critical weaning process. He monitored Mr. Robinson's vital signs, tidal volume, minute volume, and so on and provided much needed psychological support.

As Mr. Robinson's condition improved, it was decided that he would require supplemental oxygen and IPPB therapy even after discharge. The physician consulted the respiratory therapist as to the best type of unit to purchase. Arrangements were made through social services for the acquisition of the equipment. Using similar equipment in the hospital, the respiratory therapist began teaching Mr. Robinson the mechanics of a good IPPB treatment. He supervised Mr. Robinson as he assembled the unit, measured out the prescribed medication, positioned himself, and took the treatment. The therapist reviewed the instruction manual, which is provided with the IPPB unit, with both Mr. and Mrs. Robinson, so they would be familiar with it should questions arise at home. He also gave them written instructions regarding the frequency and method to be used for cleaning the equipment.

As Mr. Robinson would require continuous low-flow oxygen via nasal cannula, the physician decided that a portable oxygen unit that could be refilled from a reservoir would best meet his needs.

The therapist then instructed Mr. and Mrs. Robinson in the use of the unit, refilling of the portable unit, and discussed placement of the reservoir in their home for greatest safety. Arrangements were made for the reservoir to be delivered the day before Mr. Robinson's planned discharge so that it would be available upon his arrival home.

Other areas that the respiratory therapist might discuss with the patient and/or his family would include:

1. Side effects of medications used for IPPB.
2. The importance of taking IPPB treatments—when and how they are prescribed.
3. The importance of reporting changes in amount, color, and quality of sputum to the physician.
4. The importance of using only the liter flow of oxygen prescribed by the physician and why.
5. The importance of reporting colds or other infections to the physician so that therapy can be initiated.
6. The importance of avoiding crowds and particularly those individuals with colds or the "flu."
7. The importance of observing safety precautions associated with the use of oxygen.

As is frequently the case with a patient with a chronic disease, Mr. Robinson's appetite was poor. This was partially due to the fact that the eating process caused great fatigue and dyspnea.

The dietician visited Mr. Robinson to determine the types of foods he most enjoyed. These were then incorporated into six small nutritious feedings. The food was mostly of a soft nature at first so that less body energy was used for the chewing process. Eventually more solid foods were introduced; however, Mr. Robinson preferred to continue on six feedings per day, as he became less tired.

The dietician explained to Mrs. Robinson the importance of nutritious meals and advised her of low-cost methods of preparing foods.

The physician determined that Mr. Robinson would not be able to return to his job at the steel plant. The vocational rehabilitation counselor was consulted regarding other opportunities of employment that would be within the limits of the patient's disability, but that would also help him maintain his role of provider and "head of the house." A desk job that did not call for much physical work and for which he could be easily trained was eventually found once his convalescence was over.

It is important to note that many areas have rehabilitation programs that, by various means, fund educational programs for individuals with disabilities such as Mr. Robinson. Age, motivation and the extent of disability are necessary determining factors.

The physician determined that Mr. Robinson would be on several medications at home. The hospital pharmacist was contacted to explain the goals of Mr. Robinson's drug therapy to him in relation to his disease. He then supervised Mr. Robinson for several days before discharge, while he self-administered his medications. The importance of taking his medications at the prescribed times was emphasized. Side effects of the various drugs were discussed, as well as care of the drugs, as some required refrigeration.

It was suggested that the Robinsons find a pharmacy in their neighborhood where they could obtain all their drugs. There would then be a complete record of all medications that Mr. Robinson takes, and any problems that might arise would be more easily solved. The hospital pharmacist helped them choose such a pharmacy, which could provide them with several medications that are not normally stocked in the form required.

It is no surprise to anyone that hospitalization is an expensive process. Even those with insurance may find themselves in need of financial assistance and advice. Such was the case with the Robinsons. The Social Service Department was therefore consulted to help them. Community resources and assistance were enlisted and therapy equipment purchased. The family was also given listings of other sources available, such as groups in the community who provide transportation and information.

The physician requested that the public health nurse initially supervise Mr. Robinson's home care. The hospital-based public health consultant visited Mr. Robinson in the hospital, and later the public health nurse visited the home. Frequent follow-up visits were made by the nurse to determine Mr. Robinson's progress. She observed the procedures he and his family used regarding chest physiotherapy, respiratory therapy, and taking of medications. She also encouraged him to keep his doctor's appointments and discussed with him any changes in his therapy. Although the nurse advised and assisted the family with problems, she always referred them to their physician when major problems or questions arose.

Little has been said about the hospital nurse's role in Mr. Robinson's care. This is not an oversight. Because of the multitude of services performed by the nurse, it is not within the scope of this study. However, it is important to note that, since the nurse spends more time with the patient than possibly any other member of the health team, she will frequently be the individual to recognize and identify patient needs. The nurse then communicates these to the individual most able to provide assistance.

Mr. Robinson has been discharged from the hospital for 9 months. He visits his physician regularly, follows his treatment regimen, gets sufficient rest, and eats nutritious food. Although he will never be cured of his disease, its progress will probably be significantly slowed by the program that was instituted soon after his admission to the hospital.

EXERCISES

1. Why should the therapist be familiar with procedures such as CVP readings, dialysis and others, if they are not his responsibility?
2. Choose a patient you have cared for, and explain what part the holistic approach has played in his care.
3. How can the holistic approach be applied to home care?

BIBLIOGRAPHY

BOOKS

Bendixen, H. H. *Respiratory Care.* St. Louis: C. V. Mosby Co., 1965.

Bland, John H. *Clinical Metabolism of Body Water and Electrolytes.* Philadelphia: W. B. Saunders Co., 1963.

Brainerd, H., S. Morgen, and M. Chatton. *Current Diagnosis and Treatment.* Los Altos, Calif.: Lange Medical Publications, 1968.

Bryan, A. H., C. A. Bryan, and C. G. Bryan. *Bacteriology; Principles and Practice,* 6th ed. New York: Barnes & Noble, 1962.

Burton, G., et al. *Respiratory Care—A Guide to Clinical Practice.* Philadelphia: J. B. Lippincott Co., 1977.

Cherniack, R. M., and L. Cherniack. *Respiration in Health and Disease.* Philadelphia: W. B. Saunders Co., 1961.

Comroe, H., Jr., et al. *The Lung: Clinical Physiology and Pulmonary Function Tests.* Chicago: Year Book Medical Publishers, 1962.

Comroe, H., Jr. *Physiology of Respiration.* Chicago: Year Book Medical Publishers, 1965.

Davenport, H. *The ABC of Acid–Base Chemistry,* 4th ed. Chicago: University of Chicago Press, 1958.

Dejours, P. *Respiration.* Trans. by Leon Farhi. New York: Oxford University Press, 1966.

Dutcher, I. E., and S. B. Fielo. *Water and Electrolytes: Implication for Nursing Practice.* New York: Macmillan Publishing Co., Inc., 1967.

Egan, Donald F. *Fundamentals of Respiratory Therapy,* 2nd ed. St. Louis: C. V. Mosby Co., 1973.

Fluid and Electrolytes. North Chicago, Ill.: Abbott Laboratories, 1970.

Frobisher, M., L. Sommermeyer, and R. Fuerst. *Microbiology in Health and Disease,* 12th ed. Philadelphia: W. B. Saunders Co., 1969.

Gaskell, D. V., and B. A. Webber. *The Brompton Hospital Guide to Chest Physiotherapy.* Philadelphia: J. B. Lippincott Co., 1973.

Gebhardt, I. P., and D. Anderson. *Microbiology,* 3rd ed. St. Louis: C. V. Mosby Co., 1965.

Gray, Henry. *Anatomy, Descriptive and Surgical.* Edited by T. Pickering Picte and Robert Howden. New York: Bounty Books, 1977.

Greenwood, M. E. *An Illustrated Approach to Medical Physics.* Philadelphia: F. A. Davis Co., 1966.

Grenard, Steve. *The Hazards of Respiratory Therapy.* Monsey, N. Y.: Glenn Educational Medical Services, 1973.

Grenard, S., G. Beck, and G. Rich. *Introduction to Respiratory Therapy.* Monsey, N.Y.: Glenn Educational Medical Services, 1970.

Grenard, S., et al. *Advanced Study in Respiratory Therapy.* Monsey, N.Y.: Glenn Educational Medical Services, 1971.

Guyton, A. C. *Function of the Human Body,* 2nd ed. Philadelphia: W. B. Saunders Co., 1964.

Kempe, C. Henry, et al. *Current Pediatric Diagnosis and Treatment.* Los Altos, Calif.: Lange Medical Publications, 1978.

Kimber, D. C., C. E. Gray, and C. E. Stackpole, *Anatomy and Physiology,* 14th ed. Edited by Lutie C. Leavell. New York: Macmillan Publishing Co., 1961.

Levine, Myra. *Introduction to Clinical Nursing.* Philadelphia: F. A. Davis Co., 1973.

Lough, M., C. Doershuk, and R. Stern. *Pediatric Respiratory Therapy.* Chicago: Year Book Medical Publishers, Inc., 1974.

Luckmann, J., and K. Sorensen. *Medical–Surgical Nursing.* Philadelphia: W. B. Saunders Co., 1974.

Massachusetts General Hospital Manual of Nursing Procedures. The Department of Nursing. Boston: Little, Brown and Co., 1975.

Metheny, N., and W. D. Snively. *Nurses Handbook of Fluid Balance,* 2nd ed. Philadelphia: J. B. Lippincott, 1974.

Petty, Thomas. *Intensive and Rehabilitative Respiratory Care,* 2nd ed. Philadelphia: Lea & Febiger, 1974.

Roe, J., II. *Principles of Chemistry,* 10th ed. St. Louis: C. V. Mosby Co., 1967.

Sackheim, G. I. *Practical Physics for Nurses,* 2d. ed. Philadelphia: W. B. Saunders, Co., 1962.

Safar, P. (ed.). *Respiratory Therapy.* Philadelphia: Davis, 1965.

Schaffer, Alexander J., and Mary E. Avery. *Diseases of the Newborn,* 3rd ed. Philadelphia: W. B. Saunders Co., 1971.

Shapiro, Barry A. *Clinical Application of Blood Gases.* Chicago: Year Book Medical Publications, 1973.

Secor, J. *Patient Care in Respiratory Problems* (Saunders Monographs in Clinical Nursing 1). Philadelphia: W. B. Saunders Co., 1969.

Vaughan, Victor C., III, et al. *Nelson Textbook of Pediatrics.* Philadelphia: W. B. Saunders Co., 1979.

Wade, Jacqueline F. *Respiratory Nursing Care—Physiology and Technique.* Saint Louis: C. V. Mosby Co., 1973.

Weisberg, H. *A Better Understanding of Anion–Cation (Acid–Base) Balance*

(The Surg. Clinics of N. Am., 39:1). Philadelphia: W. B. Saunders Co., 1959.

INSTRUCTION MANUALS

Air-Shields, Inc., A. Narco Medical Company, Hatboro, Pa. Ambu Resuscitator. Air-Shields Croupette. Air Shields Vitalor Operating and Maintenance Instructions.

American Review of Respiratory Diseases (July 1978), Recommended Standardized Procedures for Pulmonary Function Testing.

Beckman Instruments Inc., Electronic Instruments Division, Schiller Park, Ill. Beckman Model D2 and Model OM 15 Oxygen Analyzers.

Bendix Health Care Products, Davenport, Iowa. Respiratory Support System.

Bio-Marine Industries, Inc., Devon, Pa. Bio-Marine Oxygen Analyzer and Digital Display, Model OA288.

Bio-Med Devices Inc., Stamford, Conn. Instruction Manual IC-2 Ventilator.

Bird Corporation, Palm Springs, Calif. Instruction Manuals: Bird Mark 1, Bird Mark 7, Bird Mark 8, Bird Mark 10, Bird Mark 14, Neonatal CPAP Generator Form L924, IMV Bird Form L 925, Baby Bird Ventilator Form 795.

Bivona Surgical Instruments Inc., Hammond, Ind. Kamen-Wilkinson Fome-Cuf Endotracheal and Tracheotomy Tubes.

Bourns, Inc., Life Systems Division, Riverside, Calif. Bourns Infant Ventilator, Bourns Ventilation Monitor Model LS 75, Ventilator Monitor Model LS 160, Bear I Adult Volume Ventilator PN 50000-10500, Bourns Infant Pressure Ventilator Model BP 200.

John Bunn Company, A Division of Greene & Kellogg, Inc., 11035 Walden Avenue, Alden, N.Y. Bunn Universal Oxygen Tent, Bunn LT 60 Alarm System.

Chemetron Medical Products, St. Louis, Mo. Gill I Volume Controlled Respirator.

Clinical Pulmonary Function Testing: A Manual of Uniform Laboratory Procedures for the Intermountain Area, Intermountain Thoracic Society, Salt Lake City, Utah.

Clinical Spirometry Instructions for use of Collins Respirometer, Warren E. Collins, Inc., Braintree, Mass.

DeVilbiss Company, Somerset, Pa. Service Manual DeVO$_2$ Oxygen Concentrator, 35B Ultrasonic Nebulizer.

J. H. Emerson Company, 22 Cottage Park Avenue, Cambridge, Mass. Emerson Postoperative Ventilator Instruction Manual.

The Harris-Lake, Inc., 10910 Briggs Road, Cleveland, Ohio. The Wright Respirometer Instruction and Maintenance Manual, Teledyne Percent Oxygen Detector Model 330A.

Healthdyne, Inc., Smyrna, Ga. Healthdyne IMV Controller, Healthdyne Micromonitors.

Hudson Oxygen Therapy Sales Co., Temecula, Calif. Operating Manual Model 3000 Cloud Chamber, Ventronics Polarographic Oxygen Monitor Model 5570, Oxygen Analyzer Model 5575.

IMI Division of Becton, Dickinson and Company, 4321 Birch Street, Newport Beach, Calif. IMI Portable Oxygen Analyzer Instruction Manual.

LKB Medical Incorporated, Rockville, Md. Engstrom Respirator ER 300.

Micro-Mist Corporation, P. O. Box 569, Hudson, Ohio, Micro-Sonic Nebulizer Instruction Manual.

Monaghan: A Division of Sandoz-Wonder, Inc. Littleton, Colo. Monaghan 670 Ultrasonic Humidifier, Monaghan 225 Volume Ventilator.

National Catheter Co., Argyle, N.Y. Form 13215 9/76, Pitt Trach Speaking Tube.

OEM Medical, Inc., Edison, N. J. OEM Mix-O-Mask, OEM Tracheotomy Mix-O-Mask.

Ohio Medical Products, Division of Airco, Inc., Madison, Wis. hand-E-vent II, Form 9879 (rev. 1970), Hope Resuscitator, Form 9760 (rev. 1968), Model 560 Respirator, Form 1887, Ohio-Armstrong Care-ETTE Isolation Type Incubator.

Olympic Surgical Company, Inc., 1117 Second Avenue, Seattle, Wash. Olympic Oxyhood.

Owens—Illinois Health Care Products, Toledo, Ohio. Hydro-Sphere Nebulizer.

Puritan-Bennett Corporation, Kansas City, Mo. Operating Instructions.
    All-Purpose Nebulizer, Form 433044, (rev. 1-67).
    Bennett Model TA-1, Form 8046 B.
    Bennett Temperature Alarm, Form 7722 B (rev. 6-1-74).
    Bubble Humidifier, Form 433040 (3-64).
    Cascade Humidifier, Form 2271 (rev. 1-66).
    IPPB Therapy Units, Models TV-2P, PV-3P, Form 1008B, 1969.
    MA-2 Volume Ventilator Form AA-450 (2/79).
    MA-2 Ventilator Operating Instruction Form 11407 (5/78).
    Monitoring Spirometer and Alarm, Form 2582C, 1969.
    Pressure Breathing Therapy Unit, Model AP-4, Form 2768 (rev. 11-68).
    Puritan Flowmeters, Form AA244 (rev. 10-69).
    Puritan Manual Resuscitator, PMR, Form 433031 (rev. 5-67).
    Respiration Units:
        Bennett Model PR-1, Form 1693B, 1969.
        Bennett Model PR-2, Form 2131B, 1969.
        Bennett Model MA-1, Form 5030J, 1969.

Respiratory Care Inc., Arlington Heights, Ill. Concha Pak System, Form LL-0012-1 4/78.

Retec Developmental Laboratory, 9730 S. W. Schools Ferry Road, Portland, Ore. Instruction Sheets, Retec NC-30.

Searle Cardio-Pulmonary Systems, Inc. Emeryville, Calif. Searle Adult Volume Ventilator.

Siemens-Elema AB, Solna, Sweden, Siemens Corporation, Union, N.J. Operating Manual Servo Ventilator 900/900B.

Timeter Instrument Corporation, Lancaster, Pa. Operation and Service Manual, Low/High Pressure Alert Model C 1070.

Union Carbide Corporation, Linde Division, 270 Park Avenue, N.Y. Linde Walker Instruction Manual, Linde Oxygen Walker System Mark II.

Veriflo Corporation, Medical Products Division, 250 Canal Boulevard, Richmond, Calif. Instruction Manual Ventilator Oxygen Controller Model MR-1.

JOURNALS

Amborn, Sylvia A. "Clinical signs associated with the amount of tracheo-bronchial secretions." *Nursing Res.* 25, no. 2: 121–126, 1976.

Anthony, J. S., and D. J. Sieniewicz. "Suctioning of the left bronchial tree in critically ill patients." *Critical Care Med.* 5, no. 3, p. 161 ff., 1977.

Cournand, A., et al. "Studies on intrapulmonary mixture of gases: IV. Significance of pulmonary emptying rate." *J. Clin. Invest.* 20, 1941.

Filley, G. F., D. J. MacIntosh, and G. W. Wright. "Carbon monoxide uptake and pulmonary diffusing capacity in normal subjects at rest and during exercise." *J. Clin. Invest.* 30, 1954.

Hansen, James E., and Daniel H. Simmons. "A systematic error in the determination of blood PCO_2." *Amer. Rev. Resp. Dis.* 115: p. 1061 ff, 1977.

Ishikawa, Sadamu, et al. "The effects of air bubbles and time delay on blood gas analysis." *Ann. Allergy* 33, p. 72, Aug. 1974.

Journal of the American Medical Association, [Supplement] February 18, 1974, Vol. 227, No. 7 "Standards for Cardiopulmonary Resuscitation (CPR) and Emergency Cardiac Care (ECC)."

Kory, R. C., R. Callahan, H. G. Boren, and J. C. Snyder. "Clinical spirometry in normal men." *Am. J. Med.* 30, 1961.

Kuzenski, Barbara M. "Effect of negative pressure on tracheobronchial trauma." *Nursing Res.* 27, no. 4, 260–263, 1978.

Sandham, Gayle, and Barbara Reid. "Some Q's and A's about suctioning." *Nursing* 7, no. 10. 60–65, 1977.

Segal, M. S., M. M. Goldstein, and E. O. Attinger. "Some recent advances in physiologic management of chronic dyspneic diseases." *Tex. J. Med.* 53: 137–146, 1957.

Segal, M. S., A. Salomon, M. J. Dulfano, and J. A. Herschfus. "Intermittent positive pressure breathing: its use in the inspiratory phase of respiration." *New. Engl. J. Med.* 250 (6): 225–232, 1954.

Severinghaus, J. W., and A. F. Bradley. "Electrodes for blood pO_2 and pCO_2 determination." *J. Appl. Physiol.* 13, 1958.

PUBLICATIONS

"Nonflammable Medical Gas Systems," NFPA No. 56F, 1974 Edition. National Fire Protection Association, 470 Atlantic Avenue, Boston, Mass.

U.S. Department of Health, Education, and Welfare, Public Health Service, "Isolation Techniques for Use in Hospitals," Publication No. 2054. Washington, D.C.: 1970.

INDEX